PRINCIPLES *of*
ICD-10-CM
CODING

Deborah J. Grider, CPC, CPC-H, CPC-I, CPC-P, CPMA, CEMC, CPCD, COBGC, CCS-P

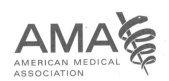

AMERICAN MEDICAL
ASSOCIATION

Executive Vice President, Chief Executive Officer: James L. Madara, MD

Chief Operating Officer: Bernard L. Hengesbaugh

Senior Vice President, Publishing and Business Services: Robert A. Musacchio, PhD

Vice President, Business Operations: Vanessa Hayden

Vice President, AMA Publications and Clinical Solutions: Mary Lou White

Senior Acquisitions Editor: Elise Schumacher

Manager, Book and Product Development and Production: Nancy Baker

Senior Developmental Editor: Michael Ryder

Production Specialist: Mary Ann Albanese

Director, Sales, Marketing and Strategic Relationships: Joann Skiba

Director, Sales and Business Products: Mark Daniels

Manager, Marketing and Strategic Planning: Erin Kalitowski

Marketing Manager: Lori Hollacher

Content Reviewers: Grace Kotowicz, Nancy Spector

Internet address: www.ama-assn.org

The American Medical Association ("AMA") and its authors and editors have consulted sources believed to be knowledgeable in their fields. However, neither the AMA nor its authors or editors warrant that the information is in every respect accurate and/or complete. The AMA, its authors, and editors assume no responsibility for use of the information contained in this publication. Neither the AMA, its authors or editors shall be responsible for, and expressly disclaims liability for, damages of any kind arising out of the use of, reference to, or reliance on, the content of this publication. This publication is for informational purposes only. The AMA does not provide medical, legal, financial, or other professional advice, and readers are encouraged to consult a professional advisor for such advice.

The contents of this publication represent the views of the author[s] and should not be construed to be the views or policy of the AMA, or of the institution with which the author[s] may be affiliated, unless this is clearly specified.

Please visit www.ama-assn.org/go/ICD10principles for potential updates.

Additional copies of this book may be ordered by calling 800 621-8335 or from the secure AMA Web site at www.amabookstore.com. Refer to product number OP 103511.

ISBN 978-1-60359-532-2

BQ41: 11-P-096:11/11

Contents

Acknowledgments

During my 32 years in the health care field, I have educated numerous physicians, students, colleagues, and instructors who have directly and indirectly contributed to my career success. A book is never the product of one individual: Many colleagues have shared their knowledge and experiences and took the time to answer my questions along the way. I wish to express my thanks to all of them. They have truly been instrumental in the writing of this book, and they have enriched my life.

In particular I wish to thank Elise Schumacher, Senior Acquisitions Editor, AMA Press, for her ideas, confidence in my abilities, and continued encouragement, which has helped with each writing project I have undertaken. Also, Michael Ryder, Senior Developmental Editor, AMA Press, who offered support, suggestions, and encouragement to complete this project. He has been instrumental in helping me meet my deadlines on the project and in helping through the rough spots. Others at AMA Press who participated in making this first edition a reality are Mary Ann Albanese and Nancy Baker.

I thank the many physicians I have worked with who, with their questions, helped me understand their confusion with complex coding issues and helped me to develop tools to overcome it.

Thank you to my family and friends, who have helped me turn this project into a reality. Without their day-to-day support in keeping me focused, this project would not have been a reality. Special thanks to Michelle Yaden, CPC, CPC-I, CEMC, my colleague and an avid health care consultant. My family has also encouraged me and made sacrifices to see that I accomplished the things in my life that were important to me, including my career, even when it meant sacrificing our personal life.

Lastly, thank you to all the coders, educators, and colleagues I have met and worked with throughout my career. Their knowledge and wisdom have truly made this an adventure of a lifetime.

Deborah J. Grider, CPC, CPC-H, CPC-I, CPC-P, CPMA, CEMC, CPCD, COBGC, CCS-P

Reviewer

Judy B Breuker, CPC, CPMA, CCS-P, CHCA,
PCS, CEMC, CHC, CHAP
Medical Education Services, LLC

About the Author

Deborah J. Grider is a Certified Professional Coder (CPC), a Certified Professional Coder—Hospital (CPC-H), a Certified Professional Coder—Payer (CPC-P), a Certified Professional Medical Auditor (CPMA), an E/M Specialist (CEMS), a Certified OB/GYN Coding Specialist (COBGC), a Certified Dermatology Coding Specialist (CPCD) with the American Academy of Professional Coders, and a Certified Coding Specialist—Physicians (CCS-P) with the American Health Information Management Association. Her background includes many years of practical experience in reimbursement issues, procedural and diagnostic coding, and medical practice management.

Ms Grider teaches and consults with private practices, physician networks, and hospital-based educational programs. Under a federal retraining grant, she helped develop and implement a Medical Assisting Program for Methodist Hospital of Indiana. She conducts many seminars throughout the year on coding and reimbursement issues and teaches several insurance courses and coding courses for various organizations.

Ms Grider is a well-known national speaker on coding and revenue cycle issues for physicians and hospitals. Deborah was a national advisory board member for the American Academy of Professional Coders and past president of the National Advisory Board. Prior to becoming a consultant, Ms Grider worked as a billing manager for 6 years, and a practice manager in a specialty practice for 12 years.

Deborah previously owned her own consulting firm and currently works with Blue and Company, LLC, as a Senior Manager in the Revenue Cycle Advisory Division. Ms Grider continues to provide consulting and educational services to medical groups, physician practices, and hospital organizations and provides coding training education to various organizations and medical societies.

Her professional affiliations include the American Academy of Professional Coders (AAPC), AAPC National Advisory Board member 2002–2005;

President-Elect of the American Academy of
Professional Coders National Advisory Board
2005–2007; President of the American Academy
of Professional Coders National Advisory Board
2007–2009; member of the American Health
Information Management Association (AHIMA);
and member of the Indiana Medical Group
Management Association (IMGMA) and the

Healthcare Financial Management Association
(HFMA).

Deborah has authored, among other titles, *Coding with
Modifiers*, Fourth Edition (to be released in 2011 by
AMA), *Medical Record Auditor*, Third Edition (AMA,
2011), and *Preparing for ICD-10-CM* (AMA, 2010).

Preface

Diagnostic coding began in Great Britain in 1839 as part of the London Bills of Mortality, an ongoing statistical study of disease that evolved into the International List of Causes of Death in 1937. Over the years, revisions were made and the title was changed to the International Classification of Causes of Death.

In 1948, the classification came under the direction of the World Health Organization (WHO), which used this information to track morbidity and mortality in order to make statistical assessments of international health and disease trends. The classification name was changed to the International Classification of Diseases. By 1950, hospitals in the United States used the listing to classify and index diseases.

The International Classification of Diseases has been revised periodically to incorporate changes in the medical field. ICD-9-CM is based on the official version of the WHO's ninth revision of the International Classification of Diseases. In February 1977, the National Center for Health Statistics convened a committee to provide advice and counsel in the development of a clinical modification of the ICD-9. The term *clinical* was used to emphasize the intent to use the modification as a tool when classifying morbidity data for indexing of medical records, medical care review, ambulatory care, other medical care programs, and basic health statistics. This resulted in the International Classification of Diseases, 9th Revision, Clinical Modification (ICD-9-CM).

Introduction

The Health Insurance Portability and Accountability Act (HIPAA) of 1996 includes provisions for the standardization of health care information. These administrative simplification provisions include standards for electronic transmission of claims, provider identifiers, privacy, and code sets. A national committee of the Department of Health and Human Services has worked extensively over the past several years to develop recommendations that meet the HIPAA requirements. Committee discussion of code sets has been lengthy and controversial due to potential costs of the transition to new and revised code sets in terms of infrastructure (computer software), anticipated delays in billing at startup, and costs associated with training and education.

The National Center for Health Statistics (NCHS) developed ICD-10-CM (*International Classification of Diseases, 10th Revision, Clinical Modification*) in consultation with a technical advisory panel, physician groups, and clinical coders to ensure clinical accuracy and utility. There are no codes for procedures in the ICD-10-CM; procedures are coded using the procedure classification appropriate for the encounter setting (eg, Physicians' Current Procedural Terminology [CPT®] and ICD-10-PCS).

The NCHS notes that this 10th revision, Clinical Modifications, represents a significant improvement over ICD-9-CM and ICD-10 mortality (cause of death) codes in terms of the increased number of codes. Improvements were also made to content and formatting and include the addition of information relevant to ambulatory and managed care encounters; expanded injury codes; the creation of combination diagnosis/symptom codes to reduce the number of codes needed to fully describe a condition; and the addition of alphanumeric subclassifications with up to 7 digits, which will increase the level of specificity with the addition of laterality in code assignment.

The term *clinical* is used to emphasize the intent to use the modification as a useful tool when classifying morbidity data for indexing of medical records, medical care review, ambulatory and other medical care programs, as well as for basic health statistics. To describe the clinical picture of the patient, the codes must be more precise than those needed for statistical groupings and trend analysis.

Origins of the International Classification of Diseases

This 10th edition of the International Classification of Disease is the latest in a series that originated in the 1850s. The first edition, known as the International List of Causes of Death, was adopted

by the International Statistical Institute in 1893. At its inception in 1948, the World Health Organization (WHO) took over the responsibility for the ICD when the sixth revision, which included causes of morbidity for the first time, was published. In 1967, the World Health Assembly adopted the WHO Nomenclature Regulations, which stipulate use of ICD in its most current revision for mortality and morbidity statistics by all Member States. ICD-10 was endorsed by the 43rd World Health Assembly in May 1990 and came into use by WHO Member States in 1994.

The ICD is the international standard diagnostic classification for all general epidemiological issues, many health management purposes, and clinical use. Included are analysis of the general health situation of population groups and monitoring of the incidence and prevalence of diseases and other health problems in relation to other variables such as the characteristics and circumstances of the individuals affected, reimbursement, resource allocation, quality, and guidelines.

ICD is used to classify diseases and other health problems recorded on many types of health and vital records, including death certificates and health records. In addition to enabling the storage and retrieval of diagnostic information for clinical, epidemiological, and quality purposes, these records also provide the basis for the compilation of national mortality and morbidity statistics by WHO Member States.

FINAL RULE FOR THE ADOPTION OF ICD-10-CM AND ICD-10-PCS

On January 15, 2009, the Department of Health and Human Services released the final regulation that supported the move from the current ICD-9-CM coding system to the ICD-10 coding system beginning October 1, 2013. This time line allows for planning for and implementing this regulatory change. The final rule to update the current 4010 electronic transaction standard to the new 5010 electronic transaction format for electronic health care transactions was also published, with an implementation date of January 1, 2012. Version 5010 provides the framework needed to support ICD-10 diagnosis and procedure codes and is the prerequisite to implementing ICD-10. The current 4010 format will not allow for the 7 digits of specificity necessary for ICD-10. Information systems for submitting electronic claims must be converted to the 5010 format by the implementation date in 2012.

ICD-10-CM includes some terminology, conventions, classifications, and other features that are similar to those in ICD-9-CM. This publication will cover the basic information that every user will need in order to successfully use ICD-10-CM. Coders can expect to see numerous changes in ICD-10-CM, including:

- The addition of information relevant to ambulatory and managed care encounters

- Expanded injury codes in which ICD-10-CM groups injuries by site of the injury, as opposed to grouping by type of injury or type of wound, as was done in ICD-9-CM

- Creation of combination diagnosis/symptom codes, which reduces the number of codes needed to fully describe a condition

- The length of codes being a maximum of 7 characters, as opposed to 5 characters in ICD-9-CM

- Greater specificity in code assignment with the use of up to 7 characters

- V and E codes being incorporated into the main classification in ICD-10-CM

- ICD-10-CM codes being alphanumeric and including all letters except U

The systematic arrangement of ICD-10-CM makes it possible to encode, computerize, store, and retrieve large volumes of information from the patient's medical record. Hospitals, physicians' offices, and other health care providers can use ICD-10-CM to code and report clinical information required for participation in various government programs, such as Medicare, Medicaid, and professional standards review organizations. Even though diagnostic coding is important to the reimbursement process, it is equally important for tracking disease and compiling statistical data.

The US National Center for Health Statistics and the Centers for Medicare and Medicaid are responsible for the annual update of ICD-10-CM, which occurs every year on October 1. The changes are published in 3 publications—*Coding Clinic*, published by the American Hospital Association; the *American Health Information Management Association Journal*, published by the American Health Information Management Association; and the *Federal Register*, published by the US Government Printing Office.

The Official Coding and Reporting Guidelines were developed and approved by the following Cooperating Parties for ICD-10-CM: American Hospital Association; American Health Information Management Association; Centers for Medicare and Medicaid, formerly the Health Care Financing Administration; and the National Center for Health Statistics, to assist the user when coding and reporting situations where the ICD-10-CM manual does not

provide direction. Coding and sequencing instructions in ICD-10-CM take precedence over any other guidelines. When these guidelines appear within the text of the book, they are identified as the Official ICD-10-CM Guidelines with the appropriate section number for reference. A copy of the Official ICD-10-CM Guidelines for Coding and Reporting is included in Appendix C for your convenience.

PURPOSE OF ICD-10-CM

Physicians' offices, hospitals, clinics, home health care agencies, and other health care providers use ICD-10-CM coding to substantiate the need for patient care or treatment and to provide statistics for morbidity and mortality rates. ICD-10-CM coding serves the following purposes:

- Establishes medical necessity

- Translates written terminology or descriptions into a universal, common language

- Provides data for statistical analysis

Establishes Medical Necessity

The first step in the reimbursement process is to establish medical necessity. Each service or procedure performed for a patient must be reported with a diagnosis that justifies the care provided by presenting the appropriate diagnostic facts. An insurance company will "link," or match, the diagnosis submitted with the procedure or service performed. If the diagnostic code submitted does not establish medical necessity, the insurance carrier may deny the service or procedure. An example of this would be a provider who submits an insurance claim for a chest X-ray with a diagnosis of foot pain. The insurance carrier would not be able to associate the need for the chest X-ray with the diagnosis reported (foot pain) and would deny the service.

Translates Written Terminology or Descriptions into a Universal, Common Language

When health care professionals submit claims for procedures or services performed or supplies issued, they must establish medical necessity through specific diagnoses, signs, symptoms, and/or complaints reported on the claim form. Prior to the Medicare Catastrophic Coverage Act of 1988, most health care professionals included a simple written description of the injury, illness, sign, or symptom that was the reason for the encounter on the insurance claim. This meant that insurance carriers who used ICD-10-CM coding had to code the diagnostic descriptions before entering them into the computer system. Today, most third-party payers, Medicare included, require the use of ICD-10-CM codes to report diagnoses on insurance claim forms. Health care professionals who accept assignment on a Medicare claim and fail to include ICD-10-CM codes will have their claims returned for proper coding, may be subject to postpayment review by the Medicare contractor, and may be subject to payment denials.

Provides Data for Statistical Analysis

Diagnostic coding has evolved from the initial efforts to classify causes of death to more sophisticated statistical data sets and analyses. ICD-10-CM is used as a statistical reporting medium and allows researchers to calculate everything from the leading causes of death, to the number of cases of certain infectious diseases, to the number and percent distribution of physician office visits by principal diagnosis. This same data can be used to study health care costs associated with a diagnosis or group of diagnoses to research the quality of health care and even to predict and plan for health care trends and needs.

Coding involves far more than assigning numbers to services and diagnoses. It involves abstracting information from patient records and/or other source documents and combining that information with reimbursement and coding guidelines to optimize payment for services and/or procedures provided to the patient. The consequences of inaccurate ICD-10-CM codes are numerous. For example, it can affect a physician's level of reimbursement as well as cause claims to be denied, fines or penalties to be levied, and sanctions to be imposed.

How to Use This Book

This book introduces the reader to the principles of ICD-10-CM coding for outpatient and physician services. The information provided herein will prepare the reader to accomplish the following objectives:

- Understand the purpose of ICD-10-CM and its relationship to the reimbursement process

- Understand and apply coding conventions when assigning codes

- Interpret basic coding guidelines for outpatient care

- Assign ICD-10-CM codes to the highest level of specificity

- Properly sequence ICD-10-CM codes

Principles of ICD-10-CM Coding contains 12 chapters. The first 4 chapters provide an overview of the material contained in ICD-10-CM, including the following: content, format, general coding guidelines, the coding process, and supplementary classifications. Chapters 5 through 11 present the basic guidelines for the coding in each chapter of ICD-10-CM. These chapters provide concrete instructions on how to code the diseases and injuries categorized in ICD-10-CM. Chapter 12 covers conventions and terminology.

Also included is a CD-ROM with checkpoint exercise answers, along with PowerPoint slides for each chapter that instructors or readers can use as an overview of each chapter. An exam testing module is included with a midterm examination, final examination, and answer keys for both exams.

The text is designed for use by community colleges, career colleges, and vocational school programs for training medical assistants, medical insurance specialists, and other health care providers. It can also be used as an independent study tool for new medical office personnel, physicians, independent billing services personnel, and any others in the health care field who want to obtain additional skills.

Resources

National Center for Health Statistics, International Classification of Diseases, 10th Revision, Clinical Modification (ICD-10-CM); About the International Classification of Diseases, 10th Revision, Clinical Modification ICD-10-CM, http://www.cdc.gov/nchs/about/otheract/icd9/icd10cm.htm.

Centers for Medicare and Medicaid Services, 2008; ICD-10-CM July 2007 release; http://www.cms.hhs.gov/ICD10.

American Hospital Association; NCVHS Committee recommendation for I-10; http://www.ahacentraloffice.org/ahacentraloffice/html/icd10resources.html.

September 2005 joint AdvaMed, AHA and Federation of American Hospitals letter in support of ICD-10 implementation; http://www.ahacentraloffice.org/ahacentraloffice/images/ICD-10McClellanJGLogo.pdf.

Library of Congress, Senate bill 628; http://thomas.loc.gov/cgi-bin/query/D?c110:3:./temp/~c110LF7pnB.

Lumpkin, John. Letter to Tommy Thompson on ICD-10, November 5, 2003. Available online at http://ncvhs.hhs.gov/031105lt.htm.

Introduction

Before focusing on the diseases and injuries covered in the *International Classification of Diseases, 10th Revision, Clinical Modification* (ICD-10-CM), it is important to understand how the code book is organized and how the coding process is designed. The first part of this book introduces the history, content, format, and structure of ICD-10-CM. Chapter 1 provides the history of the *International Classification of Diseases* and presents the rationale for the migration to ICD-10-CM. Chapter 2 covers the structure and function of ICD-10-CM and examines how the content is formatted for coding purposes. Chapter 3 focuses on the symbols, notes, acronyms, and conventions used in ICD-10-CM. Chapter 4 focuses on the coding.

Chapters 5 through 11 use a step-by-step presentation to give the reader easy access to correct coding and provide examples and exercises to amplify learning.

A review of medical terminology is provided in Chapter 12.

CHAPTER 1

History and Background

LEARNING OBJECTIVES

- Understand the history and background of the *International Classification of Diseases*

- Understand the purpose of moving to ICD-10-CM

- Review the Final Rule for an understanding of the industry impact

ICD History and Background

BACKGROUND

The *International Classification of Diseases* (ICD) "is the international standard diagnostic classification for all general epidemiological [uses], many health management purposes and clinical use."[1] Published by the World Health Organization (WHO), ICD "is used to classify diseases and other health problems recorded on many types of health and vital records including death certificates and health records. In addition to enabling the storage and retrieval of diagnostic information for clinical, epidemiological and quality purposes, these records also provide the basis for the compilation of national mortality and morbidity statistics by the World Health Organization Member States."[1] Uses of ICD-based statistics include "the analysis of the general health situation of population groups and monitoring of the incidence and prevalence of diseases and other health problems in relation to other variables such as the characteristics and circumstances of the individuals affected, reimbursement, resource allocation, quality and guidelines."[1]

The ICD is used today not only for disease classification but as the standard for payment justification and supporting medical necessity for a procedure or service provided to a patient in a health care setting. It has become the core classification system used to code claims for commercial and government health insurance reimbursement.

HISTORY OF THE ICD

The ICD has its roots in the 1600s when the study of disease statistics began with the work of John Graunt on the London Bills of Mortality. "The classification is the latest in a series which has its origins in the 1850s. The first edition, known as the International List of Causes of Death, was adopted by the International Statistical Institute in 1893. WHO took over the responsibility for the ICD at its creation in 1948 when the Sixth Revision, which included causes of morbidity for the first time, was published. The World Health Assembly adopted in 1967 the WHO Nomenclature

Regulations that stipulate use of ICD in its most current revision for mortality and morbidity statistics by all Member States."[1]

The WHO convened the international conference for the ninth revision of the *International Classification of Diseases* in Geneva in 1975. The governing bodies at this conference were interested in using the ICD for their own statistics. Some subject areas in this classification were inappropriately arranged, and the classification needed to include more detail to make it more relevant for:

- Evaluating medical care
- Classifying conditions into chapters according to affected body parts
- Producing statistics and indexes oriented toward medical care

The resulting *International Classification of Diseases, Ninth Revision* (ICD-9) provided additional detail in the 4-digit subcategories and optional 5-digit subdivisions. ICD-9 also included alternative methods of classifying diagnostic statements to capture information about the organ or site of manifestation as well as the underlying disease. This system, known as the dagger and asterisk system, is retained in the *International Classification of Diseases, 10th Revision* (ICD-10). Technical innovations were included in ICD-9 to increase its flexibility for worldwide use.

In 1977, the National Center for Health Statistics (NCHS) formed a committee to help develop a clinical modification of ICD-9 for use in coding and reporting. The *International Classification of Diseases, Ninth Revision, Clinical Modification* (ICD-9-CM) was implemented by the United States in 1979 to classify patient morbidity (illness) and mortality (death) for statistical purposes and for indexing health records by disease and operation for data storage and retrieval. In addition to its use to identify mortality and morbidity, ICD-9-CM was adopted to classify diseases and health conditions for health care claims for hospitals, physicians, and other health care providers. ICD-9-CM has been used in the United States since 1979 not only to report diagnoses to facilitate payment for health services but also to evaluate utilization patterns, predict health care trends, analyze health care costs, research the quality of health care, and plan for future health care requirements.

The clinical modification added additional detail at the fourth- and fifth-digit subdivisions of the codes. Also, alternative methods of classifying diagnostic statements were added, which included information regarding underlying conditions and manifestations in a particular organ or site. This modification was designed to provide greater flexibility in many situations. "The term *clinical* is used to emphasize the modification's intent: to serve as a useful tool in the area of classification of morbidity data for indexing of medical records, medical care review, and ambulatory and other medical care programs, as well as for basic health statistics. To describe the clinical picture of the patient the codes must be more precise than those needed only for statistical groupings and trend analysis."[2]

In the late 1970s, the United States developed Volume 3 of ICD-9-CM to report inpatient hospital procedures to use along with Volumes 1 and 2 of ICD-9-CM, which are used to classify morbidity and mortality data. Volume 3 has been used since 1979 to report procedures performed in the hospital for hospital claims and statistics.

Beginning in 1983, when the inpatient prospective payment system was adopted, Volumes 1, 2, and 3 of ICD-9-CM were used for assigning cases to diagnosis related groups (DRGs). Because of advances in medicine, the system must be updated and revised periodically. The need for providing greater clinical detail was evident. The ICD-9-CM Coordination and Maintenance Committee established a process to update ICD-9-CM on an annual basis.

In 1988, Congress passed the Medicare Catastrophic Coverage Act (MCCA), which required the use of ICD-9-CM codes for processing Medicare claims. Many commercial and other third-party payers followed Medicare's lead and adopted ICD-9-CM as the standard for reporting diagnoses to support medical necessity for procedures performed.

DEVELOPMENT OF ICD-10 AND ICD-10-CM

"ICD-10 was endorsed by the Forty-third World Health Assembly in May 1990 and came into use in WHO Member States as in 1994."[1] ICD-10 is the current international standard diagnostic classification for all general epidemiological and many health management purposes. ICD-10 is used throughout the world for reporting causes of mortality and for reporting data nationally to the WHO. ICD-10 has been used in the United States for coding of death certificates since 1999.

The development of ICD-10 by the WHO was based on the reality that greater expansion of the system would be needed. The need for expansion required a rethinking of the structure to achieve a stable and flexible classification that would not require revision for many years. ICD-10 was developed to replace ICD-9 and is already being used in Canada, Australia, and many European countries with clinical modifications for the specific needs of each country.

In 1992, ICD-10 was first released by the WHO. With the release of the ICD-10 Tabular List in 1992 by the World Health Organization, the United States was granted permission to develop an adaptation of ICD-10, which is referred to as ICD-10-CM (Clinical Modification), for use in the United States for government purposes. ICD-10-CM contains significantly more codes than the current system. ICD-10-CM codes are alphanumeric and have up to 7 digits of specificity.

The National Center for Health Statistics (NCHS) first awarded a contract to the Center for Health Policy Studies (CHPS) to evaluate ICD-10 for use for morbidity statistics in the United States. A technical advisory panel developed a prototype of ICD-10-CM in 1994. Based on the panel's findings, it was recommended that the NCHS proceed with implementation of ICD-10-CM with revisions. Further work on ICD-10-CM was performed by the NCHS, along with the review of proposals from the ICD-9-CM Coordination and Maintenance Committee and input from medical and surgical specialty groups.

The draft of ICD-10-CM along with a preliminary crosswalk between ICD-9-CM and ICD-10-CM was developed in December 1997 and was available for comment for 3 months. More than 1200 comments were received, analyzed, and categorized into draft categories from which some comments were rejected, some were incorporated into ICD-10-CM, and some required further analysis for possible inclusion in ICD-10-CM. The preliminary data compiled in 2001 were published in March 2003. These comments and preliminary data were posted on the NCHS Web site. ICD-10-CM development has continued with changes made in response to comments obtained during the open comment period as well as from physician specialty groups.

A prerelease draft published on the NCHS Web site in June 2003 included the Tabular List, Alphabetic Index, Table of Neoplasms, External Cause of Injury index, and Table of Drugs and Chemicals. The Rand Science and Technology Policy Institute was awarded a contract to conduct an impact analysis study of moving to ICD-10-CM and ICD-10-PCS (discussed below). The purpose of the analysis was to identify costs associated with the transition, including information system changes, rate negotiation, changes to reimbursement methodologies, training, and revisions to forms; the impact of costs and benefits; and the potential return on the investment of implementation.

Also, the American Health Information Management Association (AHIMA) and the American Hospital Association (AHA) conducted a pilot study of ICD-10-CM. The study involved coding records using ICD-9-CM and ICD-10-CM concurrently. More than 180 participants were drawn from a cross section of health care entities. This study indicated general support for adoption of ICD-10-CM as an improvement over ICD-9-CM. The study also showed that ICD-10 could be implemented without excessive staff training costs or changes in documentation practices. Training ICD-9 users to use ICD-10 has been shown to be relatively straightforward. In-depth knowledge of anatomy, physiology, and pharmacology, however, will be necessary for ICD-10-CM coders.

The NCHS, which maintains the ICD-10-CM code set, has continued to update the draft version of ICD-10-CM, with the latest update published in July 2007. (The ICD CM code set has been updated every year since 2007.) ICD-10-CM is located on the Web site of the Centers for Medicare and Medicaid Services (CMS) and can be downloaded at www.cms.hhs.gov/ICD10.

ICD-10-PCS

CMS, the agency responsible for maintaining the inpatient procedure code set in the United States, contracted with 3M Health Information Systems in 1993 to design and develop a procedural classification system that would replace Volume 3 of ICD-9-CM. The *International Classification of Diseases, 10th Revision, Procedure Coding System* (ICD-10-PCS) was developed for CMS and the Department of Health and Human Services (HHS) to replace ICD-9-CM Volume 3 as the new standard for coding of inpatient hospital procedures. Current Procedural Terminology (CPT®) will remain the coding standard for procedures and services in office and outpatient settings.

ICD-10-PCS was initially released in 1998. Although not in use until 10/01/2013, it has been updated annually since that time. ICD-10-PCS, which is maintained by CMS, is located on the CMS Web site and can be downloaded at www.cms.hhs.gov/ICD10.

Supporting ICD-10-PCS is a logical, consistent structure that informs the system as a whole, down to the level of a single code. This means that the process of constructing codes in ICD-10-PCS is also logical and consistent: individual letters and numbers, called "values," are selected in sequence to occupy the 7 spaces of the code, called "characters." Once the coding system is learned, the process of coding is simple.

All codes in ICD-10-PCS are 7 characters long. Each character in the 7-character code represents an aspect

CHARACTER 1	CHARACTER 2	CHARACTER 3	CHARACTER 4	CHARACTER 5	CHARACTER 6	CHARACTER 7
Section	Body System	Root Operation	Body Part	Approach	Device	Qualifer
Medical and Surgical	Upper bones	Repair	Radius, Right	External	No Device	No Qualifer
0	P	Q	H	X	Z	Z

The code selection is: 0PQHXZZ

of the procedure, as shown in the diagram above of characters from the main section of ICD-10-PCS, called MEDICAL AND SURGICAL. In this diagram the procedure is a closed reduction of a forearm fracture.

Coders need to develop a good working knowledge of anatomy and medical terminology to code in ICD-10-PCS.

As noted above, ICD-10-PCS will be used to report procedures and services in the inpatient hospital setting only and will not be used to report professional services. CPT will continue to be used to report procedures and services in the outpatient setting. This book will not cover ICD-10-PCS and will cover only ICD-10-CM for coding and reporting diagnoses in the inpatient and outpatient settings.

Replacing ICD-9-CM With ICD-10-CM

The need to replace ICD-9-CM was identified more than 10 years ago, when the National Committee on Vital and Health Statistics (NCVHS) reported that ICD-9-CM was rapidly becoming outdated and recommended immediate US commitment to developing a plan for migration to ICD-10 for morbidity and mortality coding. CMS recommended that steps should be taken to improve the flexibility of ICD-9-CM or replace it with a more flexible option sometime after the year 2000. The final date for implementation is October 1, 2013, when all entities covered by the Health Insurance Portability and Accountability Act of 1996 (HIPAA) must convert to ICD-10-CM (diagnosis coding system) and ICD-10-PCS (procedural coding system for inpatient services).

BENEFITS OF REPLACING ICD-9-CM WITH ICD-10-CM

ICD-10 allows for more specificity with the increased number of categories and codes. The increase in the number of codes will allow for more detail on the claim form and allow for more accuracy in coding diagnostic procedures. In order to improve the quality of health care data, the United States is switching to ICD-10 to maintain clinical data comparability with other countries. "The better data provided by ICD-10 will lead to improved patient safety, improved quality of care, and improved public health and bio-terrorism monitoring."[3]

RATIONALE FOR CHANGE

Many organizations support the adoption of ICD-10-CM and ICD-10-PCS, including AHA, AHIMA, and the Federation of American Hospitals (FAH), to name a few. Government and industry leaders cite health care initiatives that rely on data but are in fact compromised by the continued use of ICD-9-CM. These initiatives include quality measurement, performance measures, medical error reduction, public health reporting, actuarial premium setting, cost analysis, and service reimbursement. Adoption of national electronic health records (EHRs) and interoperable health information networks requires improved classification systems for summarizing and reporting data. Conversion to ICD-10-CM and ICD-10-PCS will not only produce better information and support development of computer-assisted coding; it will serve as the necessary foundation for continued improvements and expansion of 21st-century classification systems, nationally and internationally.

HIPAA includes provisions for the standardization of health care information. These administrative simplification provisions include standards for electronic transmission of claims, provider identifiers, privacy, and code sets. A national committee of HHS has worked extensively over the past several years to develop recommendations that meet the HIPAA requirements. Committee discussion of code sets has been lengthy and controversial due to potential costs of the transition to new and revised code sets in terms of infrastructure (computer software), anticipated delays in billing at startup, and costs associated with training and education.

NCHS notes that ICD-10-CM represents a significant improvement over ICD-9-CM and ICD-10 mortality

TABLE 1.1   Comparison of ICD-9-CM and ICD-10-CM

ICD-9-CM	ICD-10-CM
Diagnosis codes are 3-5 characters in length	Diagnosis codes are 3-7 characters in length
Approximately 14 000+ codes	Approximately 69 000+ codes
First character may be alpha (E or V) or numeric; characters 2-5 are numeric	Character 1 is alpha; characters 2 and 3 are numeric; characters 4-7 are alpha or numeric
Limited space for new codes	Flexible for adding new codes
Lacks detail	Very specific
Lacks laterality	Has laterality
Difficult to analyze data due to nonspecific codes	Specificity improves coding accuracy and depth of data for analysis
Codes are nonspecific and do not adequately define diagnoses needed for medical research	Detail improves the accuracy of data used in medical research
Does not support interoperability because it is not used in other countries	Supports interoperability and the exchange of health care data between other countries and the United States

Source: HIPAA administrative simplification: modification to medical data code set standards to adopt ICD-10-CM and ICD-10-PCS. *Fed Regist*. 2008;73(164): 49802.

(cause of death) codes in terms of the increased number of codes in the current draft of ICD-10-CM as compared to the number of codes in ICD-10 and ICD-9-CM. In addition to content and formatting improvements that include the addition of information relevant to ambulatory and managed care encounters, expanded injury codes, and the creation of combination diagnosis/symptom codes to reduce the number of codes needed to fully describe a condition, the addition of alphanumeric subclassifications of up to 7 digits will increase the level of specificity, with the addition of laterality in code assignment. Table 1.1 provides a comparison of ICD-9-CM and ICD-10-CM diagnosis codes.

The Final Rule

THE FINAL RULE FOR THE ADOPTION OF ICD-10-CM AND ICD-10-PCS

On January 16, 2009, HHS published the final regulation, known as the Final Rule, to move from the current ICD-9-CM coding system to the ICD-10-CM/

ICD-10-PCS coding system beginning October 1, 2013. This timeline allowed for time to plan and implement this regulatory change. The final rule to update the current HIPAA Version 4010 electronic administrative transaction standards to the new Version 5010 standards was also published on the same date with an implementation date of January 1, 2012. Version 5010 provides the framework needed to support ICD-10 diagnosis and procedure codes and is the prerequisite to implementing ICD-10.

On January 20, 2009, the White House released a memorandum placing a hold on all regulations that included the ICD-10 rule. In March 2009, a determination was made that the effective date would not be extended and the comment period would not be reopened for the Version 5010 or ICD-10 requirements.

KEY HIGHLIGHTS OF THE FINAL RULE

Highlights of the Final Rule include the following:

- The ICD-10-CM/ICD-10-PCS coding system will replace the current ICD-9-CM coding system on October 1, 2013. This rule includes all inpatient and outpatient facility visits as well as freestanding providers and ancillary services.

- ICD-10-CM diagnosis codes will replace ICD-9-CM diagnosis codes in all settings.

- ICD-10-PCS procedure codes will replace ICD-9-CM procedure codes within the hospital inpatient setting.

- Current Procedural Terminology (CPT) and the Healthcare Common Procedure Coding System (HCPCS) will remain the official coding system for reporting outpatient procedures and services.

- After the implementation of the ICD-10 code set, general acute care inpatient payment for Medicare patients will be based on MS-DRGs using the ICD-10 classification system instead of ICD-9.

The successful transition to ICD-10-CM/ICD-10-PCS is anticipated to meet the increased level of detail required to recognize advancements in medicine and technology, ensure appropriate reimbursement, improve data quality for clinical and financial decision making, support value-based purchasing, and facilitate quality reporting. Mapping files that allow the industry to convert from ICD-9-CM to ICD-10-CM and ICD-10-PCS codes and vice versa have been created and are available on the CMS Web site.

Test Your Knowledge

1. The *International Classification of Diseases, Ninth Revision, Clinical Modification* (ICD-9-CM) was implemented in the United States in the year _____.

2. The ICD has its roots in the _____ when the study of disease began with the work of _____ on the London Bills of Mortality.

3. The ICD is used today not only for disease classification but as the standard for payment justification and supporting _____ for a procedure or service provided to a patient in a health care setting.

4. The act passed by Congress in 1988 that required the use of ICD-9-CM codes for processing Medicare claims is known as the _____.

5. ICD-10 is published by the _____ and was first released in the year _____.

6. Replacing ICD-9-CM with ICD-10-CM will help the United States to maintain clinical data _____ with the rest of the world.

7. ICD-10-PCS is used to report procedures and services in the _____ setting.

8. HHS published the Final Rule for adoption of ICD-10-CM and ICD-10-PCS on _____.

9. The implementation date for the transition to ICD-10-CM and ICD-10-PCS based on the Final Rule is _____.

10. The ICD-10-CM code set is maintained by the _____.

Conclusion

For physicians and other health care providers, ICD-10-CM will enable more precise documentation of clinical care and will potentially ensure more accuracy when reporting medical necessity for services provided. Our health care system faces quality concerns that are attributed to medical errors, poor documentation, lack of support of medical necessity, and fragmented care. The new coding system affords the opportunity for health care providers to code diagnoses and procedures more accurately, which will contribute to health care quality improvement initiatives.

References

1. World Health Organization. International Classification of Diseases (ICD). http://www.who.int/classifications/icd/en/. Accessed June 3, 2011.

2. Centers for Disease Control and Prevention. ICD-10 CM Preface. http://www.cdc.gov/nchs/data/icd9/ICDPreface%202011.pdf. Accessed April 13, 2011.

3. Passport Health Communications Inc. ICD-10 FAQs. http://www.passporthealthcommunications.com/Resources/HIPAA_5010/ICD-10_FAQs.aspx. Accessed June 13, 2011.

Resources

American Health Information Management Association. http://www.ahima.org/ICD10.

American Hospital Association. ICD-10 Overview. http://www.ahacentraloffice.org/ahacentraloffice/html/icd10resources.html.

American Hospital Association. Joint letter from AdvaMed (Advanced Medical Technology Association), American Hospital Association, and Federation of American Hospitals in support of ICD-10 implementation. http://www.ahacentraloffice.org/ahacentraloffice/images/ICD-10McClellanJGLogo.pdf. September 20, 2005.

Centers for Disease Control and Prevention (CDC), National Center for Health Statistics. International Classification of Diseases, Tenth Revision, Clinical

Modification (ICD-10-CM). http://www.cdc.gov/nchs/icd/icd10cm.htm.

Centers for Medicare & Medicaid Services. Final Rule for ICD-10. http://www.cms.gov/ICD10/10a_Statute_Regulations.asp.

Centers for Medicare & Medicaid Services. ICD-10-CM 2011 release. http://www.cms.hhs.gov/ICD10.

Critical Access to Health Information Technology Act of 2007, S 628, 110th Cong (2007). http://thomas.loc.gov/cgi-bin/query/z?c110:S.628.IS:.

National Committee on Vital and Health Statistics. Letter from John Lumpkin, Chair of the National Committee on Vital and Health Statistics, to Tommy G. Thompson, Secretary of the US Department of Health and Human Services, on ICD-10-CM and ICD-10-PCS. http://ncvhs.hhs.gov/031105lt.htm. November 5, 2003.

World Health Organization. International Classification of Diseases (ICD). http://www.who.int/classifications/icd/en/.

CHAPTER 2

Overview of Content and Format

LEARNING OBJECTIVES

- Understand the format of ICD-10-CM
- Understand the Alphabetic Index and the Tabular List
- Understand the level of specificity
- Understand dummy placeholders and the use of the "x"
- Demonstrate knowledge of the ICD-10-CM content and format

Introduction

This chapter covers the structure and function of ICD-10-CM and explains how the content is formatted for coding purposes. Chapter 4 will discuss specific ICD-10-CM coding guidelines.

ICD-10-CM has 21 chapters, and includes separate chapters for the eye and adnexa and for the ear. These chapters are subdivided into blocks or categories consisting of 3 alphanumeric characters.

ICD-10-CM manuals are available from various publishers and are based on the official government version of ICD-10-CM (available at www.cdc.gov/nchs/icd/icd10cm.htm). All publications contain the basic information (eg, codes, guidelines, instructional notes), but some publishers have added enhancements for ease of use such as color coding and unique symbols to help the user find the correct code more quickly and accurately. It would be worthwhile to scan the various editions and select the coding manual with which you are most comfortable.

Medical coders should understand the basic coding principles behind the classification system in order to use ICD-10-CM correctly. An understanding of coding guidelines and conventions is critical to correct diagnosis coding. A good companion tool is the *Coding Clinic* published by the Central Office on ICD-10-CM of the American Hospital Association (AHA) and approved by the Centers for Medicare & Medicaid Services (CMS), the American Health Information Management Association (AHIMA), and the National Center for Health Statistics (NCHS).

Guidance for the use of the classification can be found in the ICD-10-CM Official Guidelines for Coding and Reporting, available at www.cdc.gov/nchs/icd/icd10cm.htm. Many of these guidelines will be discussed in this chapter. ICD-10 is copyrighted by the World Health Organization (WHO) and reproduced by permission for US government purposes.

ICD-10-CM codes are maintained by the ICD-10 Coordination and Maintenance Committee. ICD-10-CM is revised yearly to incorporate changes in new technology, further clarify the Official Guidelines, and add new diseases as they are discovered.

Changes from ICD-9-CM to ICD-10-CM

ICD-10-CM is more comprehensive than ICD-9-CM. Currently in 2011 there are 69 368 diagnosis codes, which will be expanded by 2013. ICD-9-CM has 14 400 diagnosis codes (Volumes 1 and 2) and 3800 procedure codes (Volume 3). ICD-10-PCS (replacing ICD-9-CM Volume 3) has 72 000 procedure codes.

ICD-10-CM further defines the health status of the patient, and the procedure codes in ICD-10-PCS define the institutional procedures that patients may receive to maintain or improve their health state. ICD-10-CM includes major changes in the code structure with the use of up to 7 characters to further explain the condition, changes in terminology (more clinical), and changes in the coding rules.

"The clinical modification represents a significant improvement over ICD-9-CM and ICD-10. Specific improvements include: the addition of information relevant to ambulatory and managed care encounters; expanded injury codes; the creation of combination diagnosis/symptom codes to reduce the number of codes needed to fully describe a condition; the addition of sixth and seventh characters; incorporation of common 4th and 5th digit subclassifications; laterality; and greater specificity in code assignment. The new structure will allow further expansion than was possible with ICD-9-CM."[1]

ICD-10-CM has an alphanumeric structure rather than a numeric structure. Differences between ICD-9-CM and ICD-10-CM are as follows:

1. Some chapters have been rearranged.

2. Some titles have changed.

3. Conditions have been regrouped.

4. ICD-10-CM has almost twice as many categories as ICD-9-CM.

5. Minor changes have been made in the coding rules for mortality.

6. The number of chapters has been expanded from 19 to 21 with the eye and adnexa and the ear now having their own chapters.

7. The external cause of injury codes have been expanded along with codes for injuries and poisonings.

8. Some coding guidelines have changed.

Table 2.1 lists the chapters of ICD-10-CM. Notice that in contrast to ICD-9-CM, diseases of the eye and adnexa and diseases of the ear and mastoid process have their own chapters in ICD-10-CM.

With the expansion of the codes along with expanded disease classifications in ICD-10-CM, it will be imperative to understand the classification at a more clinical level. The highest level of specificity in ICD-9-CM

TABLE 2.1   ICD-10-CM Chapters

CHAPTER NUMBER	CHAPTER TITLE
1	Certain Infectious and Parasitic Diseases
2	Neoplasms
3	Disease of the Blood and Blood-Forming Organs and Certain Disorders Involving the Immune Mechanism
4	Endocrine, Nutritional and Metabolic Diseases
5	Mental and Behavioral Disorders
6	Diseases of the Nervous System
7	Diseases of the Eye and Adnexa
8	Diseases of the Ear and Mastoid Process
9	Diseases of the Circulatory System
10	Diseases of the Respiratory System
11	Diseases of the Digestive System
12	Diseases of the Skin and Subcutaneous Tissue
13	Diseases of the Musculoskeletal System and Connective Tissue
14	Diseases of the Genitourinary System
15	Pregnancy, Childbirth and the Puerperium
16	Certain Conditions Originating in the Perinatal Period
17	Congenital Malformations, Deformations and Chromosomal Abnormalities
18	Symptoms, Signs and Abnormal Clinical and Laboratory Findings, Not Elsewhere Classified
19	Injury, Poisoning and Certain Other Consequences of External Causes
20	External Causes of Morbidity
21	Factors Influencing Health Status and Contact With Health Services

was 5 digits, whereas ICD-10-CM includes sixth- and seventh-character levels of specificity to fully explain the condition. The further explanation may include laterality or the type of encounter, allowing for a more complete explanation when submitting a claim for payment, which in turn may potentially reduce claim denials and carrier scrutiny.

ICD-10-CM Format and Structure

ICD-10-CM is organized in a similar manner as ICD-9-CM. The classification is divided into two main parts:

- Alphabetic Index
- Tabular List

The Tabular List is a list of alphanumeric codes divided into chapters based on condition and/or body system. The Tabular List contains categories, subcategories, and valid codes. All codes in the Tabular List are alphanumeric with the first character a letter. The third and fourth characters and final character of the code may be letters or numbers. Diagnosis codes should be selected from the Tabular List and not from the Alphabetic Index as more information, including instructional notes, is found in the Tabular List.

The Alphabetic Index contains the Index to Diseases and Injuries, which is the listing of conditions, diseases, and circumstances a health care provider may encounter. Using the Alphabetic Index is the first step in selection of the code. The index is similar to a medical dictionary.

The Alphabetic Index is organized alphabetically by disease or condition and is where the user can reference the condition or disease to find the appropriate category to go to in the Tabular List. For example, if the diagnosis is Bronchostenosis, the user would reference this term in the Alphabetic Index. Once the user has referenced the code in the Alphabetic Index, the code is selected in the Tabular List.

The main Index also includes a Table of Neoplasms, a Table of Drugs and Chemicals, and an External Cause of Injuries Index.

CODING TIP Never code from the Alphabetical Index. Always confirm your code choice in the Tabular List to ensure appropriate code selection.

THE TABULAR LIST

The Tabular List is set up in chapters that cover similar conditions and/or diseases. Each chapter contains categories or blocks that are divided into subcategories based on the condition or disease. All categories or blocks are 3 alphanumeric characters. For example, ICD-10-CM code G21 is the classification or category for Secondary parkinsonism. Notice that the first character is a letter. All ICD-10-CM codes begin with a letter, not a number. Codes are further subdivided into subcategories. ICD-10-CM uses an indented format, and each code is listed along with a description of the code. Review the example in Figure 2.1.

FIGURE 2.1 Example of Category and Subcategory Codes

G21   Secondary parkinsonism
   G21.0 Malignant neuroleptic syndrome
   G21.1 Other drug induced secondary parkinsonism

The first 3 characters identify the category:

FIGURE 2.2 Example of 3-Character Category

S06   Intracranial injury

Characters 4 through 6 identify the anatomic site, etiology, or severity:

FIGURE 2.3 Examples of Characters 4 through 6

S06.37   Contusion, laceration, and hemorrhage of cerebellum
   S06.370 Contusion, laceration, and hemorrhage of cerebellum without loss of consciousness

Certain categories have seventh characters available. Character 7 is an extension that provides greater detail.

FIGURE 2.4 Example of Seventh-Character Extension

S06.370A   Contusion, laceration, and hemorrhage of cerebellum without loss of consciousness, **initial encounter**

Since you must code to the highest level of specificity, if a fourth, fifth, sixth, or seventh character is provided you must report the diagnosis at the highest level available.

CODING TIP Make certain that you code to the highest level of specificity.

See Table 2.2 for an overview of the format of the Tabular List.

3-Character Categories

Each ICD-10-CM chapter begins with a list of blocks or 3-character categories. The following are the 3-character categories by chapter in ICD-10-CM.

Chapter 1: Certain Infectious and Parasitic Diseases (A00-B99)

A00-A09	Intestinal infectious diseases
A15-A19	Tuberculosis
A20-A28	Certain zoonotic bacterial diseases
A30-A49	Other bacterial diseases
A50-A64	Infections with a predominantly sexual mode of transmission
A65-A69	Other spirochetal diseases
A70-A74	Other diseases caused by chlamydiae

TABLE 2.2 Format of the ICD-10-CM Tabular List

Chapter	The Tabular List consists of 21 chapters—the main divisions in the ICD-10-CM manual—with code ranges of A00-Z99.
Category	Alphanumeric 3-character categories (also referred to as rubrics) each represent a single condition or disease.
Subcategory	Subcategories of 4 to 6 characters provide a higher level of specificity as compared to the 3-character categories. These additional characters can further define the etiology, anatomical site, and severity of the condition. A fourth, fifth, or sixth character must be used when available. Each level of subdivision after a category is referred to as a subcategory or subclassification. The final character in a code may be either a number or a letter.
Extension	The seventh-character extension provides additional information in the diagnosis.

A75-A79	Rickettsioses
A80-A89	Viral and prion infections of the central nervous system
A90-A99	Arthropod-borne viral fevers and viral hemorrhagic fevers
B00-B09	Viral infections characterized by skin and mucous membrane lesions
B10	Other human herpesviruses
B15-B19	Viral hepatitis
B20	Human immunodeficiency virus [HIV] disease
B25-B34	Other viral diseases
B35-B49	Mycoses
B50-B64	Protozoal diseases
B65-B83	Helminthiases
B85-B89	Pediculosis, acariasis and other infestations
B90-B94	Sequelae of infectious and parasitic diseases
B95-B97	Bacterial and viral infectious agents
B99	Other infectious diseases

Chapter 2: Neoplasms (C00-D49)

C00-C14	Malignant neoplasm of lip, oral cavity and pharynx
C15-C26	Malignant neoplasm of digestive organs
C30-C39	Malignant neoplasm of respiratory and intrathoracic organs
C40-C41	Malignant neoplasm of bone and articular cartilage
C43-C44	Melanoma and other malignant neoplasms of skin
C45-C49	Malignant neoplasms of mesothelial and soft tissue
C50	Malignant neoplasm of breast
C51-C58	Malignant neoplasm of female genital organs
C60-C63	Malignant neoplasms of male genital organs
C64-C68	Malignant neoplasm of urinary tract
C69-C72	Malignant neoplasms of eye, brain and other parts of central nervous system

C73-C75   Malignant neoplasm of thyroid and other endocrine glands

C7A   Malignant neuroendocrine tumors

C7B   Secondary neuroendocrine tumors

C76-C80   Malignant neoplasms of ill-defined, other secondary and unspecified sites

C81-C96   Malignant neoplasms of lymphoid, hematopoietic and related tissue

D00-D09   In situ neoplasms

D10-D36   Benign neoplasms, except benign neuroendocrine tumors

D3A   Benign neuroendocrine tumors

D37-D48   Neoplasms of uncertain behavior, polycythemia vera and myelodysplastic syndromes

D49   Neoplasms of unspecified behavior

Chapter 3: Diseases of the Blood and Blood-Forming Organs and Certain Disorders Involving the Immune Mechanism (D50-D89)

D50-D53   Nutritional anemias

D55-D59   Hemolytic anemias

D60-D64   Aplastic and other anemias and other bone marrow failure syndromes

D65-D69   Coagulation defects, purpura and other hemorrhagic conditions

D70-D77   Other diseases of blood and blood-forming organs

D78   Intraoperative and postprocedural complications of the spleen

D80-D89   Certain disorders involving the immune mechanism

Chapter 4: Endocrine, Nutritional and Metabolic Diseases (E00-E89)

E00-E07   Disorders of thyroid gland

E08-E13   Diabetes mellitus

E15-E16   Other disorders of glucose regulation and pancreatic internal secretion

E20-E35   Disorders of other endocrine glands

E40-E46   Malnutrition

E50-E64   Other nutritional deficiencies

E65-E68   Overweight, obesity and other hyperalimenation

E70-E88   Metabolic disorders

Chapter 5: Mental and Behavioral Disorders (F01-F99)

F01-F09   Mental disorders due to known physiological conditions

F10-F19   Mental and behavioral disorders due to psychoactive substance use

F20-F29   Schizophrenia, schizotypal, delusional, and other non-mood psychotic disorders

F30-F39   Mood [affective] disorders

F40-F48   Anxiety, dissociative, stress-related, somatoform and other nonpsychotic mental disorders

F50-F59   Behavioral syndromes associated with physiological disturbances and physical factors

F60-F69   Disorders of adult personality and behavior

F70-F79   Mental retardation

F80-F89   Pervasive and specific developmental disorders

F90-F98   Behavioral and emotional disorders with onset usually occurring in childhood and adolescence

F99   Unspecified mental disorder

Chapter 6: Diseases of the Nervous System (G00-G99)

G00-G09   Inflammatory diseases of the central nervous system

G10-G14   Systemic atrophies primarily affecting the central nervous system

G20-G26   Extrapyramidal and movement disorders

G30-G32   Other degenerative diseases of the nervous system

G35-G37   Demyelinating diseases of the central nervous system

G40-G47   Episodic and paroxysmal disorders

G50-G59   Nerve, nerve root and plexus disorders

G60-G65   Polyneuropathies and other disorders of the peripheral nervous system

G70-G73   Diseases of myoneural junction and muscle

G80-G83   Cerebral palsy and other paralytic syndromes

G90-G99   Other disorders of the nervous system

Chapter 7: Diseases of the Eye and Adnexa (H00-H59)

H00-H05	Disorders of eyelid, lacrimal system and orbit
H10-H11	Disorders of conjunctiva
H15-H22	Disorders of sclera, cornea, iris and ciliary body
H25-H28	Disorders of lens
H30-H36	Disorders of choroid and retina
H40-H42	Glaucoma
H43-H44	Disorders of vitreous body and globe
H46-H47	Disorders of optic nerve and visual pathways
H49-H52	Disorders of ocular muscles, binocular movement, accommodation and refraction
H53-H54	Visual disturbances and blindness
H55-H59	Other disorders of eye and adnexa

Chapter 8: Diseases of the Ear and Mastoid Process (H60-H95)

H60-H62	Diseases of external ear
H65-H75	Diseases of middle ear and mastoid
H80-H83	Diseases of inner ear
H90-H94	Other disorders of ear
H95	Intraoperative and postprocedural complications and disorders of ear and mastoid process, not elsewhere classified

Chapter 9: Diseases of the Circulatory System (I00-I99)

I00-I02	Acute rheumatic fever
I05-I09	Chronic rheumatic heart diseases
I10-I15	Hypertensive diseases
I20-I25	Ischemic heart diseases
I26-I28	Pulmonary heart disease and diseases of pulmonary circulation
I30-I52	Other forms of heart disease
I60-I69	Cerebrovascular diseases
I70-I79	Diseases of arteries, arterioles and capillaries
I80-I89	Diseases of veins, lymphatic vessels and lymph nodes, not elsewhere classified
I95-I99	Other and unspecified disorders of the circulatory system

Chapter 10: Diseases of the Respiratory System (J00-J99)

J00-J06	Acute upper respiratory infections
J09-J18	Influenza and pneumonia
J20-J22	Other acute lower respiratory infections
J30-J39	Other diseases of upper respiratory tract
J40-J47	Chronic lower respiratory diseases
J60-J70	Lung diseases due to external agents
J80-J84	Other respiratory diseases principally affecting the interstitium
J85-J86	Suppurative and necrotic conditions of the lower respiratory tract
J90-J94	Other diseases of the pleura
J95	Intraoperative and postprocedural complications and disorders of respiratory system, not elsewhere classified
J96-J99	Other diseases of the respiratory system

Chapter 11: Diseases of the Digestive System (K00-K94)

K00-K14	Diseases of oral cavity and salivary glands
K20-K31	Diseases of esophagus, stomach and duodenum
K35-K38	Diseases of appendix
K40-K46	Hernia
K50-K52	Noninfective enteritis and colitis
K55-K63	Other diseases of intestines
K65-K68	Diseases of peritoneum and retroperitoneum
K70-K77	Diseases of liver
K80-K87	Disorders of gallbladder, biliary tract and pancreas
K90-K94	Other diseases of the digestive system

Chapter 12: Diseases of the Skin and Subcutaneous Tissue (L00-L99)

L00-L08	Infections of the skin and subcutaneous tissue
L10-L14	Bullous disorders
L20-L30	Dermatitis and eczema
L40-L45	Papulosquamous disorders
L49-L54	Urticaria and erythema
L55-L59	Radiation-related disorders of the skin and subcutaneous tissue

L60-L75   Disorders of skin appendages

L76   Intraoperative and postprocedural complications of dermatologic procedures

L80-L99   Other disorders of the skin and subcutaneous tissue

Chapter 13: Diseases of the Musculoskeletal System and Connective Tissue (M00-M99)

M00-M02   Infectious arthropathies

M05-M14   Inflammatory polyarthropathies

M15-M19   Osteoarthritis

M20-M25   Other joint disorders

M26-M27   Dentofacial anomalies [including malocclusion] and other disorders of jaw

M30-M36   Systemic connective tissue disorders

M40-M43   Deforming dorsopathies

M45-M49   Spondylopathies

M50-M54   Other dorsopathies

M60-M63   Disorders of muscles

M65-M67   Disorders of synovium and tendon

M70-M79   Other soft tissue disorders

M80-M85   Disorders of bone density and structure

M86-M90   Other osteopathies

M91-M94   Chondropathies

M95   Other disorders of the musculoskeletal system and connective tissue

M96   Intraoperative and postprocedural complications and disorders of musculoskeletal system, not elsewhere classified

M99   Biomechanical lesions, not elsewhere classified

Chapter 14: Diseases of the Genitourinary System (N00-N99)

N00-N08   Glomerular diseases

N10-N16   Renal tubulo-interstitial diseases

N17-N19   Acute kidney failure and chronic kidney disease

N20-N23   Urolithiasis

N25-N29   Other disorders of kidney and ureter

N30-N39   Other diseases of the urinary system

N40-N53   Diseases of male genital organs

N60-N65   Disorders of breast

N70-N77   Inflammatory diseases of female pelvic organs

N80-N98   Noninflammatory disorders of female genital tract

N99   Intraoperative and postprocedural complications and disorders of genitourinary system, not elsewhere classified

Chapter 15: Pregnancy, Childbirth and the Puerperium (O00-O99)

O00-O08   Pregnancy with abortive outcome

O09   Supervision of high-risk pregnancy

O10-O16   Edema, proteinuria and hypertensive disorders in pregnancy, childbirth and the puerperium

O20-O29   Other maternal disorders predominantly related to pregnancy

O30-O48   Maternal care related to the fetus and amniotic cavity and possible delivery problems

O60-O77   Complications of labor and delivery

O80, O82   Encounter for delivery

O85-O92   Complications predominantly related to the puerperium

O94-O9A   Other obstetric conditions, not elsewhere classified

Chapter 16: Certain Conditions Originating in the Perinatal Period (P00-P96)

P00-P04   Newborn affected by maternal factors and by complications of pregnancy, labor and delivery

P05-P08   Disorders related to length of gestation and fetal growth

P10-P15   Birth trauma

P19-P29   Respiratory and cardiovascular disorders specific to the perinatal period

P35-P39   Infections specific to the perinatal period

P50-P61   Hemorrhagic and hematological disorders of newborn

P70-P74   Transitory endocrine and metabolic disorders specific to newborn

P76-P78   Digestive system disorders of newborn

P80-P83   Conditions involving the integument and temperature regulation of newborn

Chapter 20: External Causes of Morbidity (V01-Y99)

V00-X58	Accidents
V00-V99	Transport accidents
V00-V09	Pedestrian injured in transport accident
V10-V19	Pedal cyclist injured in transport accident
V20-V29	Motorcycle rider injured in transport accident
V30-V39	Occupant of three-wheeled motor vehicle injured in transport accident
V40-V49	Car occupant injured in transport accident
V50-V59	Occupant of pick-up truck or van injured in transport accident
V60-V69	Occupant of heavy transport vehicle injured in transport accident
V70-V79	Bus occupant injured in transport accident
V80-V89	Other land transport accidents
V90-V94	Water transport accidents
V95-V97	Air and space transport accidents
V98-V99	Other and unspecified transport accidents
W00-W19	Slipping, tripping, stumbling and falls
W20-W49	Exposure to inanimate mechanical forces
W50-W64	Exposure to animate mechanical forces
W65-W74	Accidental drowning and submersion
W85-W99	Exposure to electric current, radiation and extreme ambient air temperature and pressure
X00-X08	Exposure to smoke, fire and flames
X10-X19	Contact with heat and hot substances
X30-X39	Exposure to forces of nature
X52-X58	Accidental exposure to other specified factors
X71-X83	Intentional self-harm
X02-Y09	Assault
Y21-Y33	Event of undetermined intent
Y35-Y38	Legal intervention, operations of war, military operations and terrorism
Y62-Y69	Misadventures to patients during surgical and medical care

Y70-Y82	Medical devices associated with adverse incidents in diagnostic and therapeutic use
Y83-Y84	Surgical and other medical procedures as the cause of abnormal reaction of the patient, or of later complication, without mention of misadventure at the time of the procedure
Y90-Y99	Supplementary factors related to causes of morbidity classified elsewhere

Chapter 21: Factors Influencing Health Status and Contact With Health Services (Z00-Z99)

Z00-Z13	Persons encountering health services for examination
Z14-Z15	Genetic carrier and genetic susceptibility to disease
Z16	Infection with drug-resistant microorganisms
Z17	Estrogen receptor status
Z18	Retained foreign body fragments
Z20-Z28	Persons with potential health hazards related to communicable diseases
Z30-Z39	Persons encountering health services in circumstances related to reproduction
Z55-Z65	Persons with potential health hazards related to socioeconomic and psycho-social circumstances
Z66	Do not resuscitate (DNR) status
Z67	Blood type
Z68	Body mass index (BMI)
Z69-Z76	Persons encountering health services in other circumstances
Z79-Z99	Persons with potential health hazards related to family and personal history and certain conditions influencing health status

4-Character Subcategories

The 4-character subcategories further define the site, etiology, and manifestation or state of the disease or condition. The 4-character subcategory includes the 3-character category plus a decimal point followed by an additional character to further identify the condition to a higher level of specificity. This example shows 4-character subcategories:

CHECKPOINT EXERCISE 2-1

In what chapter of the Tabular List would you find the following conditions?

1. _____ heart attack

2. _____ schizophrenia

3. _____ pneumonia

4. _____ gastritis

5. _____ abdominal pain

6. _____ femoral hernia

7. _____ diabetes mellitus

8. _____ glaucoma

9. _____ hypertension

10. _____ cystitis

11. _____ HIV

12. _____ bipolar disorder

13. _____ gynecological exam

14. _____ asthma

15. _____ cytopenia

16. _____ contact dermatitis

17. _____ awaiting organ transplant

18. _____ chronic obstructive pulmonary disease (COPD)

19. _____ acute nephritis

20. _____ skull fracture

FIGURE 2.5   Example of 4-Character Subcategories

C15	Malignant neoplasm of esophagus
C15.3	Malignant neoplasm of upper third of esophagus
C15.4	Malignant neoplasm of middle third of esophagus
C15.5	Malignant neoplasm of lower third of esophagus
C15.8	Malignant neoplasm of overlapping sites of esophagus
C15.9	Malignant neoplasm of esophagus, unspecified

Figure 2.6 provides an additional example of 3- and 4-character codes in ICD-10-CM.

FIGURE 2.6   Example of 3 and 4 -Character Categories for Umbilical Hernia

Chapter	→	Diseases of the Digestive System
3-character category	→	K42 Umbilical hernia
4-character subcategory	→	K42.0 Umbilical hernia with obstruction, without gangrene
		K42.1 Umbilical hernia with gangrene
		K42.9 Umbilical hernia without obstruction or gangrene

5- and 6-Character Subcategories

In ICD-9-CM, the fifth digit was the most precise level of specificity. In ICD-10-CM, fifth- or sixth-character subclassifications represent a level of further specificity. Coding to the fifth and sixth character gives more information about the condition or diagnosis. Review the following examples.

FIGURE 2.7a   Examples of 5-Character Subcategories

J10.8	Influenza due to other identified influenza virus with other manifestations
J10.81	Influenza due to other identified influenza virus with encephalopathy
J10.82	Influenza due to other identified influenza virus with myocarditis
J10.83	Influenza due to other identified influenza virus with otitis media
J10.89	Influenza due to other identified influenza virus with other manifestations

FIGURE 2.7b   Example of a 6-Character Subcategory

S55.011	Laceration of ulnar artery at forearm level, right arm

Review the illustration of category F50 for eating disorders, which includes 5-character subcategories.

FIGURE 2.7c   Example of 5-Character Subcategories

3-character category	→	F50 Eating disorders
4-character category	→	F50.0 Anorexia nervosa
5-character subcategories	→	F50.00 Anorexia nervosa, unspecified
		F50.01 Anorexia nervosa, restrictive type
		F50.02 Anorexia nervosa, binge eating/purging type

Note that in the 3-character category in this example, there is not a sixth digit. Not every ICD-10-CM diagnosis code will have fourth- through seventh-character subcategories or extensions.

Review this example of sixth-character subclassifications:

FIGURE 2.8 Use of the Sixth-Character Subclassifications

Chapter	→	Diseases of the Digestive System
3-character category	→	**K50 Crohn's disease [regional enteritis]**
4-character subcategory	→	**K50.0 Crohn's disease of small intestine**
5-character subcategory	→	K50.01 Crohn's disease of small intestine without complications
6-character subclassifications	→	K50.011 Crohn's disease of small intestine with rectal bleeding
		K50.012 Crohn's disease of small intestine with intestinal obstruction
		K50.013 Crohn's disease of small intestine with fistula
		K50.014 Crohn's disease of small intestine with abscess
		K50.018 Crohn's disease of small intestine with other complication
		K50.019 Crohn's disease of small intestine with unspecified complications

Seventh-Character Extension

Some ICD-10-CM categories, such as injuries and poisonings, require a seventh-character extension. Notes in the Tabular List identify codes that require a seventh character on the claim. A dummy placeholder consisting of the letter "x" is used if the code category does not specify a sixth character. Review the following example:

A patient presented to the spine surgeon with back pain. After performing diagnostic x-rays and performing an MRI of the spine, the physician diagnosed the patient with a sprain of the sacroiliac joint.

In this example, the diagnosis code S33.6, Sprain of sacroiliac joint, is only coded to the fourth character, but the notes in the Tabular List require a seventh character. If this is the patient's initial encounter, the letter "A" is the seventh-character extension.

In order to code to the highest level, the dummy placeholder "x" must be used as the fifth and sixth characters to reach the highest level of specificity. The encounter would be reported as S33.6xxA. Now review the following examples:

FIGURE 2.9 Examples of Seventh-Character Extensions

S50.311A	**Abrasion of right elbow, initial encounter**
T23.201D	**Burn of second degree of right hand, unspecified site, subsequent encounter**
T41.5x2A	**Poisoning by therapeutic gases, intentional self-harm, initial encounter**

The seventh character in these examples explains:

A   initial encounter

D   subsequent encounter

S   sequela

Note: The "x" in code T41.5x2A in Figure 2.9 is a dummy placeholder. As discussed earlier, the letter "x" may be used as a dummy placeholder to reach the highest level of specificity when a sixth or seventh character is required. The "x" is used as a fifth- or sixth-character placeholder to allow for future expansion of the code set. Some codes have dummy placeholders built into the code. Review the example:

FIGURE 2.10 Example of Dummy Placeholders

O33.5xx0	**Maternal care for disproportion due to unusually large fetus, not applicable or unspecified**

CODING TIP Always code to the highest level of specificity. If a 6-character code is available, it must be selected. If a 6-character code includes a seventh-character extension, the extension must be used to code to the highest level.

3-Character Complete Codes

A few categories exist that are at the highest level of specificity with just the 3-character code. The following examples are a few of the 3-character code categories without further definition:

FIGURE 2.11 Examples of 3-Character Codes

A35	**Other tetanus**
	Tetanus NOS
E54	**Ascorbic acid deficiency**
N10	**Acute tubulo-interstitial nephritis**

THE ALPHABETIC INDEX

As noted above, the Alphabetic Index is divided into 4 sections and is organized by main term.

Section 1—Index to Diseases and Injuries

Section 2—Table of Neoplasms

Section 3—Table of Drugs and Chemicals

Section 4—External Cause of Injuries Index

The Alphabetic Index in ICD-10-CM is organized in the same manner as in ICD-9-CM. Codes are listed by main term, which describes the disease and/or condition. As in ICD-9-CM, cross-references such as "see" and "see also" are found in ICD-10-CM. Subterms and modifiers are located under the main terms in an indented format. Nonessential modifiers are found in parentheses after the main term. A nonessential modifier does not affect selection of the code and is used as guidance. In the section on external causes of injury, the main term and modifiers identify the type of accident or occurrence, the vehicles(s) involved, the place of occurrence, and so forth.

Notes appear in the Alphabetic Index to

1. Define terms

2. Provide direction

3. Provide coding instructions

Index to Diseases and Injuries

This index contains terms in alphabetical sequence. It is used to reference diseases, symptoms, and conditions included in the Tabular List. The Index to Diseases and Injuries contains terms and the corresponding ICD-10-CM codes. Never code directly from the Alphabetic Index. Always reference the diagnostic categories in the Tabular List.

Review the following examples:

FIGURE 2.12   Identifying the Main Term

EXAMPLE: *The patient was diagnosed with a cardiac **bruit**.*

main term ➡ *bruit*

Alphabetic Index:
Bruit (arterial) R09.89
    cardiac R01.1

FIGURE 2.13   Identifying the Main Term

EXAMPLE: *A patient is diagnosed with a **filling defect** of the bladder found on diagnostic imaging.*

main term ➡ *filling defect*

Alphabetic Index:
Filling defect
    biliary tract R93.2
    bladder R93.4
    duodenum R93.3
    gallbladder R93.2
    gastrointestinal tract R93.3
    intestine R93.3
    kidney R93.4
    stomach R93.3
    ureter R93.4

Table of Neoplasms

The Alphabetic Index contains the Table of Neoplasms (C and D codes). The use of this table will be discussed in detail in Chapter 5.

Table of Drugs and Chemicals

This table classifies drugs and other chemical substances to identify poisoning states and external causes of adverse effects. Poisonings are reported when documentation indicates that a poisoning occurred, a correct substance was taken correctly but affected the patient adversely, an overdose occurred whether intention or unintentional, or a wrong substance was taken. These codes, which begin with the letter "T," are listed in the Table of Drugs and Chemicals for reference and validated in the Tabular List. The table also contains a listing of external causes of adverse effects from the poisoning. These T code listings are divided into the following categories:

- Poisoning (accidental, unintentional)

- Poisoning (intentional, self-harm)

- Poisoning (assault)

- Poisoning (undetermined)

- Adverse effect

- Underdosing

The adverse effect column is used to code drugs, medicinal, and biological substances causing adverse effects in therapeutic use. The adverse effect column is not used in connection with poisoning. The use of this table will be discussed in detail in Chapter 10.

External Cause of Injuries Index

The External Cause of Injuries Index (V to Y codes) is an alphabetical listing of the codes describing external causes of injury and poisoning. This index contains terms that describe an accident or act of violence. It is organized according to the type of violence or accident (eg, assault with a gun or motor vehicle accident).

CHECKPOINT EXERCISE 2-2

List the code range you would find the following conditions

1. _____ Malignant Neoplasm of the bone and articular cartridge

2. _____ Disorders of the conjunctiva

3. _____ Viral hepatitis

4. _____ Ischemic heart diseases

Reference

1. Centers for Disease Control and Prevention (CDC), National Center for Health Statistics. International Classification of Diseases, Tenth Revision, Clinical Modification (ICD-10-CM). http://www.cdc.gov/nchs/icd/icd10cm.htm. Accessed June 16, 2011.

Resources

Centers for Disease Control and Prevention (CDC), National Center for Health Statistics. International Classification of Diseases, Tenth Revision, Clinical Modification (ICD-10-CM) [2011 revision available for download]. http://www.cdc.gov/nchs/icd/icd10cm.htm.

Centers for Medicare & Medicaid Services. ICD-10-CM Official Guidelines for Coding and Reporting. 2010. http://www.cms.gov/ICD10/Downloads/7_Guidelines10cm2010.pdf.

Test Your Knowledge

Matching

1. _____ Dummy placeholder   S

2. _____ Sequela   A

3. _____ Subsequent encounter   X

4. _____ Initial encounter   D

Fill in the blanks with the number of the chapter in the Tabular List in which you would find each code or disease.

5. _____ J45.90

6. _____ Obstructed labor due to breech presentation

7. _____ S83.001A

8. _____ Type 2 diabetes mellitus with other skin complications

9. _____ Conductive hearing loss, unilateral, right ear, with unrestricted hearing on the contralateral side

10. _____ K71.1

11. _____ Benign neoplasm of peritoneum

12. _____ M67.91

13. _____ Phonological disorder

14. _____ T50.8x1A

15. _____ Encounter for examination of ears and hearing with abnormal findings

CHAPTER 3

Conventions and Terminology

LEARNING OBJECTIVES

- Understand the use of the ICD-9-CM conventions
- Review the ICD-10-CM Official Guidelines for Coding and Reporting
- Recognize symbols and abbreviations used in the ICD-10-CM code set
- Understand the terminology unique to ICD-10-CM coding
- Demonstrate understanding of ICD-10-CM conventions and terminology

Introduction

In order to select the appropriate ICD-10-CM code, it is necessary to understand the ICD-10-CM Official Guidelines for Coding and Reporting as well as the various conventions and terminology used throughout the ICD-10-CM manual. Accurate coding depends on understanding the meaning of the Official Guidelines, conventions, and terms.

ICD-10-CM Official Guidelines

Diagnoses reported in the medical record remain the responsibility of the rendering provider. A joint effort between the provider and the coder is essential in ensuring accurate diagnosis and code selection. Guidelines were developed to assist the provider and coder in assigning the appropriate diagnosis in ICD-10-CM.

The ICD-10-CM Official Guidelines are organized into sections. The format and structure of ICD-10-CM, conventions for use, and general guidelines for coding are found in Section 1, which applies to the entire classification and is used in both inpatient and outpatient settings, unless specified otherwise. This section also includes chapter-specific guidelines arranged by disease classification. Chapter-specific guidelines are sequenced in the order in which the chapters appear in the Tabular List and will be covered beginning in Chapter 5 of this book. Section 2 of the guidelines is applicable for coding and reporting diagnoses in the outpatient setting and is used in all outpatient settings including physicians' offices, hospital outpatient settings, and other outpatient health care entities. Section 2 also includes guidelines for reporting diagnoses in a inpatient setting. Section 3 of the guidelines is used for reporting the principal diagnosis in a inpatient setting.

Section 4 includes guidelines for reporting outpatient services. To understand the rules and instructions for coding in ICD-10-CM, it is necessary to review all sections of the guidelines before selection of a diagnosis code.

Note that the term *principal diagnosis code* is typically used in the inpatient setting. The term *first-listed diagnosis* is typically used in the outpatient setting.

The ICD-10-CM Official Guidelines are located at www.cdc.gov/nchs/icd/icd10cm.htm. The Official Guidelines should be referenced frequently to avoid diagnosis coding errors. Many of these guidelines will be discussed in this chapter.

CODING TIP It is important to have a good understanding of the ICD-10-CM Official Guidelines as well as the conventions of ICD-10-CM.

Conventions of ICD-10-CM

The conventions of ICD-10-CM are the general rules for use of the classification independent of the chapter-specific guidelines. The conventions are located in both the Tabular List and the Alphabetic Index of ICD-10-CM. The conventions take precedence over the specific guidelines. Coding conventions include instructional notes, abbreviations, punctuation, symbols, formatting, typefaces, and rules.

INSTRUCTIONAL NOTES

Instructional notes that further define or provide examples can apply to the chapter, section, or category of ICD-10-CM. Notes are used to define terms and give additional instructions. For example, instructional notes are used in ICD-10-CM to indicate diagnoses that are to be coded elsewhere. They can be located at the beginning of a chapter or section, below a category or subcategory, or under a code. Instructional notes such as "Includes," "Excludes1," "Excludes2," "Use additional code," and some others appear only in the Tabular List. Never code from the Alphabetic Index because important instructional notes may be missed.

Review the following and pay attention to the note after the code and description:

FIGURE 3.1 Excerpt from Tabular List Showing an Instructional Note

> **M80 Osteoporosis with current pathological fracture**
>   **Note:** fragility fracture is defined as a fracture sustained with trauma no more than a fall from a standing height or less that occurs under circumstances that would not cause a fracture in a normal healthy bone

Following are some instructional notes and abbreviations found in ICD-10-CM.

"Includes"

An "includes" note further defines or clarifies the content of the chapter, subchapter, category, subcategory, or subclassification. This note may appear immediately under a 3-character code title to give examples of the content of the category. These terms are some of the conditions for which that code number is to be used. "Includes" notes are also found under certain 4- to 6-character codes. "Includes" notes indicate modifying conditions or diseases and further define or give examples of the content of the category. The terms may be synonyms of the code title or, in the case of "other specified" codes, may be a list of conditions assigned to that code. Review Figure 3.2.

FIGURE 3.2 Excerpt from Tabular List Showing an "Includes" Note

> **I10 Essential (primary) hypertension**
>   **INCLUDES** high blood pressure
>   hypertension (arterial) (benign) (essential) (malignant) (primary) (systemic)

"Excludes"

"Excludes" notes indicate that a category, subcategory, or subclassification is excluded from the category. The two types of "Excludes" notes are "Excludes1" and "Excludes2," each having a different definition for use.

"Excludes1" "Excludes1" indicates that the excluded code should never be used at the same time as the code above the "Excludes1" note. "Excludes1" is used when two conditions cannot occur together, such as a congenital form and an acquired form of the same

condition. Conditions listed with "Excludes1" are mutually exclusive; therefore, they would never be reported together. Review Figure 3.3.

FIGURE 3.3   Excerpt from Tabular List Showing an "Excludes1" Note

> **E11   Type 2 diabetes mellitus**
> **EXCLUDES 1**   gestational diabetes (O24.4-)
>   type 1 diabetes mellitus (E10.-)

In the example, "Excludes1" instructs the user to go to another code for the excluded condition. If the patient is pregnant and the reason for the type 2 diabetes is gestational, it is coded only as gestational diabetes and not in category E11.

"Excludes2"   The "Excludes2" note represents "Not included here." "Excludes2" indicates that the condition excluded is not part of the condition represented by the code, but the patient may have both conditions at the same time. When an "Excludes2" note appears under a code, it is acceptable to use both the code and the excluded code together when the medical documentation reflects that both conditions exist. See Figure 3.4.

FIGURE 3.4   Excerpt from Tabular List Showing an "Excludes2" Note

> **I10   Essential (primary) hypertension**
> **EXCLUDES 2**   essential (primary) hypertension involving
>   vessels of brain (I60-I69)
>   essential (primary) hypertension involving
>   vessels of eye (H35.0)

In Figure 3.4, "Excludes2" instructs the user that hypertension involving vessels of the eye has a different code than essential hypertension without further specification. If the patient has both systemic hypertension and primary hypertension of the eye, then it would be appropriate to assign a code for both conditions.

"Code first underlying condition or disease"

This instruction is used in categories not intended for use as a principal diagnosis for a disease. These codes, called manifestation codes, may never be used alone or as the principal diagnosis (sequenced first). They must always be preceded by another ICD-10-CM code.

The code and its descriptor appear in brackets in the Alphabetic Index. "Code first underlying disease" is usually followed by the code or code(s) for the etiology (underlying disease). Record the etiology as the principal diagnosis and then record the italicized manifestation codes in the secondary position.

Etiology/manifestation paired codes have a specific index entry structure. In the Alphabetic Index, both conditions are listed together, with the etiology code first followed by the manifestation codes in brackets. The code in brackets is always to be sequenced second.

CODING TIP   When a code appears in brackets next to another code in the Alphabetic Index, report both codes. The italicized code is reported as a secondary diagnosis.

Review the example and Figure 3.5.

> **EXAMPLE:** *A glaucoma patient was diagnosed with Lowe's syndrome*
>
> **Alphabetic Index:**
>   Glaucoma ➡ with ➡ Lowe's syndrome E72.03 [H42]
>
> **Tabular List:**
>   H42 ➡ Code first underlying condition as E72.03

FIGURE 3.5   Excerpt from Tabular List

> **H42   Glaucoma in diseases classified elsewhere**
>   **Code first**   underlying condition, such as:
>   amyloidosis (E85.-)
>   aniridia (Q13.1)
>   Lowe's syndrome (E72.03)
>   Reiger's anomaly (Q13.81)
>   specified metabolic disorder (E70-E88)

CODING TIP   The code in brackets in the Alphabetic Index is always sequenced as the secondary diagnosis.

"Use additional code"

This instruction indicates that an additional code should be used to represent the etiology and/or manifestation (when the information is available) to provide a more complete description of the diagnosis. Certain conditions have an underlying etiology affecting multiple body systems, or a single condition may require reporting of more than one code. Whenever a combination exists, there is an instructional note, "use additional code," at the etiology code. This instruction indicates that an additional or secondary diagnosis is required for the category, subcategory, or subclassification to further identify the disease when it is manifested. This instructional note indicates the proper sequencing in which the codes must be listed. See Figure 3.6.

FIGURE 3.6   Excerpt from Tabular List Including Note Indicating Secondary Diagnosis is Required

> **Chapter 1**
> **Certain infectious and parasitic diseases (A00–B99)**
> [INCLUDES]   diseases generally recognized as communicable or transmissible
> **Use additional**   code for any associated drug resistance (Z16)

"And"

The word "and" should be interpreted to mean either "and" or "or" when it appears in a code title.

"See"

The instruction "See" in the Alphabetic Index acts as a cross-reference and directs the user to look elsewhere. This instruction is often found when the term or condition may not be the appropriate term. This is a mandatory instruction and must be followed for proper code selection.

"See also"

"See also" is a reference note in the Alphabetic Index directing the user to see a specific category, subcategory, or subclassification before making a code selection. A "see also" instruction following a main term in the index indicates that another main term may also be referenced that may provide additional useful index entries. "See also" notes may be helpful if you cannot find the diagnosis code listed under a main term in the Alphabetic Index. Differing from the "see" instruction, "see also" instructions are not required should the main term provide the necessary code to describe the condition. See the example in Figure 3.7.

FIGURE 3.7   Excerpt from the Alphabetic Index for Amentia

> Amentia—*see also* Retardation, mental
>   Meynert's (nonalcoholic) F04

"Code also"

The instruction "code also" alerts the user that more than one code may be required to describe the condition fully. Determining sequencing depends on the reason for the encounter and the severity.

"With"/"Without"

The terms "with" and "without" are found in the Alphabetic Index and the Tabular List. "With" is sequenced immediately following the main term in the Alphabetic Index when the final character of the diagnosis code can indicate that a diagnosis is "with" or "without" a related condition. When "with" and "without" are the two options for the final character of a set of codes, the default is always "without." In 5-character codes, "1" as the fifth character represents "with" and "0" as the fifth character represents "without." In 6-character codes, "1" as the sixth character represents "with" and "9" as the sixth character represents "without." Review the excerpt from the Tabular List in Figure 3.8.

FIGURE 3.8   Excerpt from the Tabular List

> **G40.501**   **Special epileptic syndromes, not intractable, with status epilepticus**
> **G40.519**   **Special epileptic syndromes, intractable, without status epilepticus**

"NEC" (not elsewhere classifiable)/"Other specified"

Use the "not elsewhere classifiable" code assignment when the information at hand specifies a condition but no separate code for that condition is provided. When a specific code is not available for a condition, the Alphabetic Index directs the coder to the "other specified" code in the Tabular List. The fourth or sixth character is "8" or "z," and the fifth character is always "9." Review the Alphabetic Index entry shown in Figure 3.9.

FIGURE 3.9   Excerpt from the Alphabetic Index

> **Abruptio placentae** O45.9-
>   with
>   afibrinogenemia O45.01-
>   coagulation defect O45.00-
>   specified NEC O45.09-
>   disseminated intravascular coagulation O45.02-
>   hypofibrinogenemia O45.01-

"NOS" (not otherwise specified)/"Unspecified"

Codes in the Tabular List with "Unspecified . . ." in the title are for use when the information in the medical record is insufficient to assign a more specific code. The abbreviation NOS, "Not otherwise specified," in the Tabular List is the equivalent of unspecified which is typically a fourth or sixth character of "9" and a fifth character "0". These codes are used when information in the medical record is insufficient to assign a more specific code.

Do not assign these codes when a more specific diagnosis has been determined. See the example in Figure 3.10.

FIGURE 3.10   Excerpt from the Tabular List

A04.9   **Bacterial intestinal infection, unspecified**
   Bacterial enteritis NOS
A25.9   **Rat-bite fever, unspecified**

Other Specified

Codes in the Tabular List with "Other . . ." or "Other specified . . ." are for use when the information in the medical record provides detail for which a specific code does not exist. The abbreviation NEC, "Not elsewhere classifiable" represents "other specified." An index entry that states NEC directs the coder to an "other specified" code in the Tabular List.

DEFAULT CODES

A code listed next to a main term in the ICD-10-CM Alphabetic Index is referred to as a default code. The default code represents the condition that is most commonly associated with the main term. It is the unspecified code for the condition. If a condition is documented in a medical record without any additional information, such as whether the condition is acute or chronic, the default code should be assigned.

> **EXAMPLE:** *A simple statement of "appendicitis" without further documentation would be coded K37 for Unspecified appendicitis.*

SYNDROMES

In the absence of guidance in the Alphabetic Index, assign codes for the documented manifestations of the syndrome.

LATERALITY

For bilateral sites, the final character of the ICD-10-CM code indicates laterality. The right side is always "1," and the left side is "2." In cases where a bilateral code is provided, the bilateral character is always "3." A code for an unspecified side is also provided for use should the side not be identified in the medical record. The character indicating the unspecified side is either "0" or "9" depending on whether it is the fifth or sixth character in the code.

CODING TIP   Even though a bilateral condition is present, when there is no distinct code(s) identifying laterality of that condition, the ICD-10-CM diagnosis code is reported only once.

> **Review the example.**
> *A patient is treated for an abscess of a bursa on the left wrist in the hospital emergency department.*

When reviewing Figure 3.11, notice the laterality in the code descriptors and the final character of the code. The correct code for this patient encounter is M71.032.

FIGURE 3.11   Excerpt from the Tabular List for M71.03

M71.03   **Abscess of bursa, wrist**
   M71.031   **Abscess of bursa, right wrist**
   M71.032   **Abscess of bursa, left wrist**
   M71.039   **Abscess of bursa, unspecified wrist**

ITALICS

In some versions of ICD-10-CM, italicized type is used for all exclusion notes and in the Alphabetic Index to identify manifestation codes that are not reported as the first-listed diagnosis code but are reported secondarily to the first-listed code.

PUNCTUATION

Brackets

Brackets ("[ ]") have two usages. In the Tabular List, brackets are used to enclose synonyms, alternative wording, or explanatory phrases. In the Alphabetic Index, brackets identify manifestation codes. ICD-10-CM codes in brackets in the Alphabetic Index can never be sequenced as a principal diagnosis. The brackets ("[ ]") are used to indicate that a principal diagnosis is required.

Coding directives require that codes in brackets be sequenced in the order in which they appear in the Alphabetic Index. In Figure 3.12, you must use both the code for the diagnosis of dementia with Lewy bodies (G31.83) as the principal diagnosis and F02.80 as the secondary diagnosis to report the dementia.

FIGURE 3.12   Excerpt from the Alphabetic Index

> **Dementia** (degenerative (primary)) (old age) (persisting) F03
>   with
>   Lewy bodies G31.83 *[F02.80]*

Colon

A colon (":") is used after an incomplete term that needs one or more of the modifiers that follow to make it assignable to a given category. Open the ICD-10-CM codebook to the Tabular List and review the following. The use of the colon in the Tabular List in Figure 3.13 indicates that in order to code the aortic valve disorder, an additional modifier is needed.

FIGURE 3.13   Excerpt from the Tabular List for T36–T50

> **Code first**   (T36-T50) to identify drug, if drug-induced
> **Use additional**   code to identify associated manifestations,
>   such as:
>   arthropathy associated with dermatological disorders
>   (M14.8-)
>   conjunctival edema (H11.42)
>   conjunctivitis (H10.22-)
>   corneal scars and opacities (H17.-)
>   corneal ulcer (H16.0-)
>   edema of eyelid (H02.84)
>   inflammation of eyelid (H01.8)
>   keratoconjunctivitis sicca (H16.22-)
>   mechanical lagophthalmos (H02.22-)
>   stomatitis (K12.-)
>   symblepharon (H11.23-)

Parentheses

Parentheses ("( )") are used in both the Alphabetic Index and Tabular List to enclose supplementary words that may not affect the selection of the diagnosis code. The terms within the parentheses are referred to as non-essential modifiers. Review the example in Figure 3.14.

FIGURE 3.14   Excerpt from the Alphabetic Index

> Valve, valvular (formation)
>   ureter (pelvic junction) (vesical orifice) Q62.39

Dash

A dash ("-") at the end of a code indicates that additional digits are required to complete the diagnostic statement. Review Figure 3.15.

FIGURE 3.15   Excerpt from the Alphabetic Index

> Injury → muscle → hip → strain → S76.01-

Comma

The words following a comma (",") are essential modifiers. The term(s) following the comma must be present in the diagnostic statement to for the code to be used.

Terminology

Table 3.1 contains terminology that a coder may encounter when selecting diagnosis codes.

TABLE 3.1   Terminology Related to Diagnosis Code Selection

TERM	DEFINITION
acute	having rapid onset, severe symptoms, and a short course
chronic	of long duration; denotes a disease showing little change or slow progression
diagnosis	a decision determining the cause and/or nature of a condition
eponym	a name for a disease, organ, function, or bodily location adapted from the name of a particular person or a geographic location; example: Hodgkin's disease
etiology	the cause(s) or origin of a disease
manifestation	sign or symptom of an underlying disease, condition, or cause
recurrent	returning after a remission; reappearing; relapse

Resource

Centers for Medicare & Medicaid Services. ICD-10-CM Official Guidelines for Coding and Reporting. 2010. http://www.cms.gov/ICD10/Downloads/7_Guidelines10cm2010.pdf.

Test Your Knowledge

Answer the following questions using both the Alphabetic Index and Tabular List of ICD-10-CM.

1. What does the note say that is listed immediately after category S25?

2. What does category K71 include?

3. What does code category M71 exclude?

4. What coding order does the index indicate for the diagnosis "neuropathy with anemia"?

5. When coding congenital syphilitic endarteritis, which code is listed first and which is second?

6. What instruction is given immediately following the main term *scratch*?

7. The listing for gluteal tendinitis under the main term *enthesopathy* directs you to see what main term?

8. What does the instruction "Use additional code to identify manifestations, such as" mean?

9. What does the note under code category E27.3 instruct the coder to do?

10. What does code category G45 exclude?

11. What does the symbol "[ ]" indicate?

12. When is the abbreviation "NOS" used?

13. What does "See also" direct the coder to do?

14. What does the instructional note "Excludes2" mean?

15. When a code cannot be used as the first listed or principal diagnosis, it is identified in the Alphabetic Index with what symbol?

CHAPTER 4

The Coding Process

LEARNING OBJECTIVES

- Describe the ICD-10-CM coding process

- Apply the steps to correctly select a diagnosis code

- Demonstrate the ability to code to the highest level of specificity

Now that you have been introduced to the content and format of ICD-10-CM, it is time to look at the coding process. This chapter reviews 6 essential steps in the coding process and discusses the various notes and conventions that help in identifying the appropriate code(s). Also included in this chapter are discussions on how to code for more than one diagnosis, how to code when the diagnosis is uncertain, and how to code for chronic conditions and surgical procedures.

The Coding Process

The ICD-10-CM codes are composed of up to 6 characters with a seventh-character extension in some diagnosis codes. Not all codes have 7 characters. A 3-digit code can be used only if no more specificity is available. For example, if a diagnosis code has up to 5 characters, you must code to the highest level. A 3-character code would not be acceptable if a 5-character code is available. Review the following example.

FIGURE 4.1 Example from the Tabular List

E10.3	Type 1 diabetes mellitus with ophthalmic complications	
	E10.31	Type 1 diabetes mellitus with unspecified diabetic retinopathy
		E10.311 Type 1 diabetes mellitus with unspecified diabetic retinopathy with macular edema
		E10.319 Type 1 diabetes mellitus with unspecified diabetic retinopathy without macular edema

In this example, since a 6-character code is available, the diagnosis must be coded to the highest level of specificity.

When locating a code in ICD-10-CM, locate the term in the Alphabetic Index, then verify the code in the Tabular List. Relying on only the Alphabetic Index or the Tabular List leads to errors in code assignments and less specificity in code selection. Make sure to read all instructional notes in both the Alphabetic Index and Tabular List and verify that the documentation in the medical record supports the code assigned. Keep in mind that the Alphabetic Index does not always provide the complete code. Selection of a diagnosis code includes laterality and further extensions, which are found in the Tabular List. In the Alphabetic Index, a dash ("-") at the end of an entry indicates that additional characters are required. Even if a dash is not included in the Alphabetic Index, one should never code from this volume and should always reference the Tabular List for the final code selection.

STEPS IN THE CODING PROCESS

Following are the 6 essential steps used in determining a correct code.

Step 1: Identify the Main Term in the Diagnostic Statement

The main term is the key word that will be used to locate the correct diagnosis code. The primary arrangement of the Alphabetic Index is by condition. The main term should be the term that describes the condition or disease process that is occurring. Review the following list as an example:

Chronic renal failure

Acute pharyngitis

Generalized convulsive epilepsy

Allergic rhinitis

Ankylosis of the spine

Tension headache

Diaphragmatic hernia

In each phrase, the underlined term will be the main term or key word used to locate the correct diagnosis code for each statement.

Step 2: Locate the Main Term in the Alphabetic Index

Once the main term has been identified, refer to the Alphabetic Index for the specific condition for which you are looking. To locate the correct diagnosis code, follow this sequence:

- Condition (eg, failure, attack, inflammation)

- Organ or anatomic site (eg, renal, heart, skin)

- Manifestations (when applicable)

- Modifiers (eg, acute or chronic)

- Laterality

The following example illustrates how to locate the main term in the Alphabetic Index that will drive coding.

CODING TIP If you are uncertain which term is the main term, circle the body part and terms such as *acute* or *chronic* to eliminate them as options.

> **EXAMPLE:** *chronic renal failure*
>
> **Alphabetic Index:**
> main term ➡ *failure*
>
> organ or anatomic site ➡ *renal (kidneys)*
>
> modifier ➡ *chronic*

The Alphabetic Index refers the coder to chronic renal failure, N18.9 (see Figure 4.2).

FIGURE 4.2 Alphabetic Index Entry for Chronic Renal Failure

Failure, failed
  renal N19
    chronic N18.9

> **EXAMPLE:** *hip contraction*
>
> **Alphabetic Index:**
> main term ➡ *contraction*
>
> organ or anatomic site ➡ *joint*
>
> joint ➡ *hip*

The Alphabetic Index refers the coder to M24.55- for "contraction, joint, hip" (Figure 4.3).

In this example, the dash ("-") indicates that an additional digit is required. Review Figure 4.3.

FIGURE 4.3 Excerpt from the Tabular List for Hip Contracture

M24.55	Contracture, hip
M24.551	Contracture, right hip
M24.552	Contracture, left hip
M24.559	Contracture, unspecified hip

In this example, laterality (right versus left) is important information in selecting the code.

CODING TIP Use caution when selecting unspecified codes when laterality is part of the code description. Some insurance contractors/carriers may deny payment for a procedure or service based on the lack of specificity.

CODING TIP Keep in mind medical necessity is the overarching criterion for selecting a procedure or service. Medical necessity for a procedure or service is supported with a diagnosis code.

Step 3: Refer to Any Cross-References and Notes Under the Main Term

In order to code to the highest level of specificity, refer to any cross-references under the main term in the Alphabetic Index. Four types of cross-references that are important in the code selection process are as follows:

- See: directs the coder to a more specific term where the code may be found.

   EXAMPLE: Broken bone—see Fracture

- See also: indicates that additional information is available that may provide an additional diagnosis code. Always follow the instructions to ensure correct coding.

   EXAMPLE: Painful—see also Pain

- See also category: directs the coder to review the 3-digit category and any applicable notes in the Tabular List before assigning a code. Review Figure 4.4.

FIGURE 4.4   Excerpt from the Alphabetic Index Showing "see also" Category

---

Arthritis, arthritic (acute) (chronic) (nonpyogenic) (subacute)
   M19.90
   allergic —*see* Arthritis, specified form NEC
   ankylosing (crippling) (spine) —*see* also Spondylitis,
      ankylosing
         sites other than spine —*see* Arthritis, specified form NEC
   atrophic —*see* Osteoarthritis
      spine —*see* Spondylitis, ankylosing
   back —*see* Spondylopathy, inflammatory
   blennorrhagic (gonococcal) A54.42
   Charcot's —*see* Arthropathy, neuropathic
      diabetic —*see* Diabetes, arthropathy, neuropathic
      syringomyelic G95.0
   chylous (filarial) (*see also* category M01) B74.9
   climacteric (any site) NEC —*see* Arthritis, specified form NEC
   crystal(-induced) —*see* Arthritis, in, crystals
   deformans —*see* Osteoarthritis
   degenerative —*see* Osteoarthritis
   due to or associated with
      acromegaly E22.0
      brucellosis —*see* Brucellosis
      caisson disease T70.3
      diabetes —*see* Diabetes, arthropathy
   dracontiasis (*see also* **category M01**) **B72**
   enteritis NEC
      regional —*see* Enteritis, regional

---

erysipelas A46
erythema
   epidemic A25.1
   nodosum L52
filariasis NOS B74.9
glanders A24.0
helminthiasis (*see also* category M01) **B83.9**

- **Notes:** Notes in the Tabular List further define terms, clarify notes, or indicate requirement of a seventh-character extension.

   EXAMPLE: See note for category S04, Injury of cranial nerve (Figure 4.5).

FIGURE 4.5   Excerpt from the Tabular List for Category S04

S04 Injury of cranial nerve
   The appropriate seventh character is to be added to each code from category S04
      A - initial encounter
      D - subsequent encounter
      S - sequela

CODING TIP Make sure to review all instructional notes.

Step 4: Refer to Any Modifiers of the Main Term

Two types of modifiers appear within the Alphabetic Index: essential modifiers and nonessential modifiers.

Essential modifiers are subterms that are listed below the main term in alphabetical order (eg, "with," "with the exception of," and "without"). Essential modifiers are indented 2 spaces. An essential modifier that clarifies the previous one is indented 2 more spaces. When only 1 subterm is listed, a comma separates the subterm from the main listing (see Figure 4.6).

FIGURE 4.6   Excerpt from the Alphabetic Index

Infarct, infarction
   adrenal (capsule) (gland) E27.49
   appendices epiploicae K55.0
   bowel K55.0
   brain (stem) —*see* Infarct, cerebral
   breast N64.89
   brewer's (kidney) N28.0
   cardiac —*see* Infarct, myocardium
   cerebellar —*see* Infarct, cerebral
   cerebral (*see also* Occlusion, artery cerebral or precerebral,
      with infarction) I63.9

Nonessential modifiers are terms enclosed in parentheses following the main term. Nonessential modifiers may clarify the diagnosis; however, they are not required in the coding statement. They do not affect the selection of the diagnosis code. They serve as examples to help translate terminology into numeric codes (see Figure 4.7).

FIGURE 4.7   Excerpt from the Alphabetic Index

Pneumonia (acute) (Alpenstich) (benign) (bilateral) (brain) (cerebral) (circumscribed) (congestive) (creeping) (delayed resolution) (double) (epidemic) (fever) (flash) (fulminant) (fungoid) (granulomatous) (hemorrhagic) (incipient) (infantile) (infectious) (infiltration) (insular) (intermittent) (latent) (migratory) (organized) (overwhelming) (primary) (atypical) (progressive) (pseudolobar) (purulent) (resolved) (secondary) (senile) (septic) (suppurative) (terminal) (true) (unresolved) (vesicular) J18.9

Step 5: Verify the Code Number in the Tabular List

After the main term has been found and the cross-references and notes have been verified, proceed to the Tabular List. The Tabular List is the authoritative ICD-10-CM coding reference. It contains diagnosis codes, full descriptions, additional instructional notes, and examples of conditions assigned to each code. Review the following to see the importance of using the Tabular List to verify the code selection from the Alphabetic Index.

> **EXAMPLE:** *Diagnosis: Urinary tract infection caused by E. coli*

Alphabetic Index:
> *Infection* ➡ *Urinary (tract)*
>
> *Because the site is unknown, the index directs the coder to use N39.0.*
>
> *Correct code based on diagnostic statement: N39.0, Urinary tract infection, site not specified*

Tabular List:
> *Confirms the code N39.0, but an instructional note directs the coder to use an additional code to identify the infectious agent (B95-B97). When coding, make sure the infectious agent, in this case E. coli (B96.2), is identified in the medical record documentation. This note appears only in the Tabular List, not in the Alphabetic Index. Without confirming the code in the Tabular List, the coder would miss valuable coding instructions designed to provide additional information necessary to support medical necessity.*

Correct codes:
> N39.0   *Urinary tract infection (first listed)*
>
> B96.2   *E. coli (secondary)*

Step 6: Code to the Highest Level of Specificity

When choosing a diagnosis code from the Tabular List, always code to the highest level of specificity. Use fourth, fifth, and sixth characters when available. For certain conditions such as injuries and/or poisonings, a seventh-character extension is required.

As stated in Chapter 2 of this book, the first 3 characters describe the category and identify the main condition or disease. The fourth through sixth characters further specify the diagnosis. Follow these guidelines:

1. Assign 3-character codes only if there are no 4-character codes within that code category.

2. Assign a 4-character code only if there is not a fifth-character subclassification within that category.

3. Assign the fifth- or sixth-character subclassification code for those categories where it exists.

4. Don't forget to assign the seventh-character extension that further identifies the condition, if available, and use the dummy placeholder "x" when a fifth or sixth character is not defined in the code.

A code is invalid if it has not been coded to the full number of characters available for that code. Review the following example and Figure 4.8.

FIGURE 4.8   Excerpt from the Tabular List

H04.53 **EXCLUDES 1**	**Neonatal obstruction of nasolacrimal duct** congenital stenosis and stricture of lacrimal duct (Q10.5)
H04.531	Neonatal obstruction of right nasolacrimal duct
H04.532	Neonatal obstruction of left nasolacrimal duct
H04.533	Neonatal obstruction of bilateral nasolacrimal duct
H04.539	Neonatal obstruction of unspecified nasolacrimal duct

---

> **EXAMPLE:** *A patient has a neonatal nasolacrimal duct obstruction of the left side.*
>
> *Diagnosis: Neonatal obstruction of the left nasolacrimal duct*

CHECKPOINT EXERCISE 4-1

Underline the main term for each of the following diagnostic statements.

Example: chronic renal failure

1. typhoid fever

2. chest pain

3. gastroesophageal reflux

4. otitis media

5. atrial flutter

6. tension headache

7. ectopic pregnancy

8. rheumatoid arthritis of the knee

9. aortic stenosis with mitral valve disease

10. diaphragmatic hernia with gangrene

Alphabetic Index:
  obstruction ➙ lacrimal (passages) (ducts) ➙ neonatal ➙ H04.53-

The index indicates with the dash ("-") that this category needs a sixth-character subclassification to indicate laterality.

Tabular List:
  The appropriate sixth character for the left side is "2" (see Figure 4.8).

  H04.532 Neonatal obstruction of the left nasolacrimal duct

Correct code:
  H04.532

CODING TIP Make certain you reference the Tabular List when selecting the diagnosis code. The Alphabetic Index does not list the sixth- and seventh-character subclassification or extension in many cases. Coding from the Alphabetic Index may result in miscoding the patient encounter.

General Coding Principles

CODING TO THE HIGHEST LEVEL OF SPECIFICITY

It is important to always code to the highest level of specificity. ICD-10-CM diagnosis codes are composed of 3 to 7 characters. Every classification has a category

consisting of 3 alphanumeric characters. Many categories are further subdivided by the use of fourth, fifth, and/or sixth characters, which provide greater detail. Use a 3-character code only if it cannot be further subdivided. Review Example 1, which shows a 3-character code that cannot be further subdivided. Example 2 illustrates a code that is further subdivided with the use of 6 characters.

> **EXAMPLE 1:** C23   *Malignant neoplasm of gallbladder*

> **EXAMPLE 2:** H40.121   *Low-tension glaucoma, right eye*

Some code categories require a seventh-character extension, which adds more information about the condition. Review this example of a code classification with a seventh-character extension.

> **EXAMPLE:** S92.011A   *Displaced fracture of body of right calcaneus, initial encounter for closed fracture*

The seventh character, "A," identifies the code as being for the initial encounter for a closed fracture.

If the seventh character is required and the code can be subdivided only to the fifth-character level of specificity, the dummy placeholder "x" must be used as the sixth character when the seventh character is necessary. Review this example of a code using a dummy placeholder.

> **EXAMPLE:** T83.32   *Displacement of intrauterine contraceptive device*

In this example there only 5 characters, but a seventh character is required in category T83 (see Figure 4.9). The code will be reported as T83.32xA to report the initial encounter for the displacement of the intrauterine contraceptive device.

FIGURE 4.9   Excerpt from the Tabular List for Category T83

The appropriate seventh character is to be added to each code from category T83
  A - initial encounter
  D - subsequent encounter
  S - sequela

CODING TIP A dummy placeholder "x" is used only when a subclassification has 4 or 5 characters and a seventh character is required based on the instructional notes in the Tabular List.

COMBINATION CODING

A combination code is a single code to classify 2 diagnoses that consist of a diagnosis with an associated sign/symptom or a complication. Combination codes are identified by subterm entries in the Alphabetic Index and by the "Includes" and "Excludes" notes in the Tabular List.

Many combination codes include both the etiology and manifestation, in which case the single combination code is assigned as the principal or first-listed diagnosis and no sequencing decision is necessary.

Assign only the combination code when that code fully identifies the diagnostic condition(s) involved or when the Alphabetic Index so directs. Multiple codes should not be used when the classification provides a combination code that clearly identifies all of the elements documented in the diagnosis. When the combination code lacks the necessary specificity to fully describe all elements of a diagnosis, an additional code or codes may be used.

> **EXAMPLE:** *A physician diagnosed a patient with rheumatoid arthritis of the right ankle and foot. The patient also has rheumatoid polyneuropathy.*

> **Tabular List:**
> *The condition is coded in ICD-10-CM using a combination code. In ICD-9-CM, there is not a combination code to fully describe the condition, and 2 codes must be used when reporting this diagnosis. In ICD-10-CM, a combination code is available, so only one code is reported. Review Figure 4.10.*

FIGURE 4.10   Excerpt from the Tabular List

M05.57	**Rheumatoid polyneuropathy with rheumatoid arthritis of ankle and foot**
	Rheumatoid polyneuropathy with rheumatoid arthritis, tarsus, metatarsus and phalanges
M05.571	**Rheumatoid polyneuropathy with rheumatoid arthritis of right ankle and foot**
M05.572	**Rheumatoid polyneuropathy with rheumatoid arthritis of left ankle and foot**
M05.579	**Rheumatoid polyneuropathy with rheumatoid arthritis of unspecified ankle and foot**

> **Correct code:**
> *M05.571   Rheumatoid polyneuropathy with rheumatoid arthritis of right ankle and foot*

USE OF MULTIPLE CODING FOR MULTIPLE DIAGNOSES (ETIOLOGY/MANIFESTATIONS)

The etiology/manifestation convention in the ICD-10 Official Guidelines requires 2 codes to fully describe a single condition that affects multiple body systems. There are other single conditions that also require more than 1 code. "Use additional code" notes are found in the Tabular List and indicate codes that are not part of an etiology/manifestation pair (combination code) that must be used where a secondary code is necessary to fully describe a condition. The sequencing rule is the same as for the etiology/manifestation pair: "use additional code" indicates that a secondary code should be added.

"Code first" notes are also found under certain codes that are not specifically manifestation codes but may be due to an underlying cause. When a "code first" note is present and an underlying condition is present, the underlying condition should be sequenced first.

"Code, if applicable, any causal condition first" notes indicate that this code may be assigned as a principal diagnosis when the causal condition is unknown or not applicable. If a causal condition is known, then the code for that condition should be sequenced as the principal or first-listed diagnosis.

Multiple codes may be needed for late effects, complication codes, and obstetric codes to more fully describe a condition. See the specific guidelines for these conditions for further instruction.

Review the following example:

> *A patient visited his family physician for a follow up examination. The patient has type 1 diabetes, which is currently not well controlled with a blood sugar of 385. The physician performed a detailed history and examination, noting that the patient has a foot ulcer of the right heel and midfoot with muscle necrosis, which is documented as chronic. The physician determined that this condition is related to the diabetes. The physician determined that the patient would need to go to the wound care center to treat the foot ulcer. The physician adjusted the patient's insulin to attempt to get the patient's diabetes under proper control.*

> *In this example, the physician is diagnosing the foot ulcer with necrosis of the muscle, which is a manifestation of the diabetes, and also treating the type 1 diabetes mellitus. The manifestation is the gangrene and the etiology is the diabetes mellitus.*

> *How do you find the code to report?*

Alphabetic Index:

Start with the Alphabetic Index and reference "ulcer" (main term) and "diabetes" (see Figure 4.11).

FIGURE 4.11   Excerpt from the Alphabetic Index

Ulcer
  diabetes, diabetic —*see* Diabetes, ulcer

In this example, under the terms "ulcer" and "diabetes," the Alphabetic Index instructs the user to see "Diabetes, ulcer."

Now look up "Diabetes" (see Figure 4.12).

FIGURE 4.12   Excerpt from the Alphabetic Index

Diabetes, diabetic (mellitus) (sugar)
    type 1 E10.9
      with
          amyotrophy E10.44
          arthropathy NEC E10.618
          autonomic (poly)neuropathy E10.43
          cataract E10.36
          Charcot's joints E10.610
          chronic kidney disease E10.22
          circulatory complication NEC E10.59
          complication E10.8
              specified NEC E10.69
          dermatitis E10.620
          foot ulcer E10.621

The reference "Diabetes, type 1, with foot ulcer" points the user to the code E10.621 in the Tabular List. Now review the Tabular List for E10.621 (Figure 4.13).

FIGURE 4.13   Excerpt from the Tabular List

E10.621   Type 1 diabetes mellitus with foot ulcer
  Use additional code to identify site of ulcer
  (L97.4-, L97.5-)

CODING TIP   When referencing diabetes mellitus in the Alphabetic Index, it is important to identify whether the patient has diabetes mellitus due to an underlying condition (E08), drug- or chemical-induced diabetes (E09), type 1 diabetes (E10), type 2 diabetes (E11), or other specified diabetes (E13).

Since the instructional notes indicate that an additional code must be reported to identify the site of the foot ulcer, reference L97.4- to L97.5- in the Tabular List (Figure 4.14).

FIGURE 4.14   Excerpt from the Tabular List

L97.4   **Non-pressure chronic ulcer of heel and midfoot**
          Non-pressure chronic ulcer of plantar surface of midfoot
    L97.40   **Non-pressure chronic ulcer of unspecified heel and midfoot**
        L97.401   **Non-pressure chronic ulcer of unspecified heel and midfoot limited to breakdown of skin**
        L97.402   **Non-pressure chronic ulcer of unspecified heel and midfoot with fat layer exposed**
        L97.403   **Non-pressure chronic ulcer of unspecified heel and midfoot with necrosis of muscle**
        L97.404   **Non-pressure chronic ulcer of unspecified heel and midfoot with necrosis of bone**
        L97.409   **Non-pressure chronic ulcer of unspecified heel and midfoot with unspecified severity**
    L97.41   **Non-pressure chronic ulcer of right heel and midfoot**
        L97.411   **Non-pressure chronic ulcer of right heel and midfoot limited to breakdown of skin**
        L97.412   **Non-pressure chronic ulcer of right heel and midfoot with fat layer exposed**
        L97.413   **Non-pressure chronic ulcer of right heel and midfoot with necrosis of muscle**
        L97.414   **Non-pressure chronic ulcer of right heel and midfoot with necrosis of bone**
        L97.419   **Non-pressure chronic ulcer of right heel and midfoot with unspecified severity**
    L97.42   **Non-pressure chronic ulcer of left heel and midfoot**
        L97.421   **Non-pressure chronic ulcer of left heel and midfoot limited to breakdown of skin**
        L97.422   **Non-pressure chronic ulcer of left heel and midfoot with fat layer exposed**
        L97.423   **Non-pressure chronic ulcer of left heel and midfoot with necrosis of muscle**
        L97.424   **Non-pressure chronic ulcer of left heel and midfoot with necrosis of bone**
        L97.429   **Non-pressure chronic ulcer of left heel and midfoot with unspecified severity**

Since the right foot is affected, select the code category L97.41-.

Correct codes:

First-listed diagnosis: E10.621   Type 1 diabetes
mellitus with foot ulcer

Secondary diagnosis: L97.413   Non-pressure chronic
ulcer of right heel and midfoot with necrosis of muscle

CODING UNCERTAIN DIAGNOSES

In the outpatient setting, do not code diagnoses listed as
"probable," "possible," "suspected," "questionable," or "rule
out." Instead, code the signs, symptoms, and abnormal
test result(s) or other reason for the visit. This is contrary
to the coding practices used by hospitals and medical
record departments for coding hospital inpatient diagnoses. Manifestations are characteristic signs or symptoms
of an illness. Signs and symptoms that point rather definitely to a given diagnosis are assigned to the appropriate
ICD-10-CM code. Those manifestations may suggest 2
or more diseases or may point to 2 or more systems of
the body. They are used in cases lacking the necessary
study to make a final diagnosis and are assigned codes
from Chapter 18 of the Tabular List, "Symptoms, Signs,
and Abnormal Clinical and Laboratory Findings, Not
Elsewhere Classified." This topic will be discussed in
more detail in Chapter 10 of this book.

Review the following examples.

> **EXAMPLE 1:** *A female patient is seen in the office with
> complaints of fatigue. The physician suspects that the
> patient may have iron-deficiency anemia and orders the
> appropriate lab tests to determine if this is the reason for
> the patient's fatigue.*
>
> *Since there is no definitive diagnosis, the user would
> assign the correct code for the sign and/or symptom,
> which in this case is the fatigue.*

Alphabetic Index:

fatigue ➝ R53.83

Tabular List:

R53.83 ➝ Other fatigue ➝ Fatigue NOS

Correct code:

Since we have no further details of the fatigue, the
correct code is R53.83.

> **EXAMPLE 2:** *A patient is admitted to observation care
> from the emergency room with precordial (chest) pain. The
> ER physician decides to keep the patient overnight to rule
> out a myocardial infarction.*
>
> *Since the physician cannot specifically diagnose the
> condition when the patient is admitted to observation
> care, the encounter is coded using signs and/or symptoms
> the patient is experiencing.*

Alphabetic Index:

pain ➝ precordial (region) ➝ R07.2

Tabular List:

R07.2 ➝ Precordial pain

Correct code:

R07.2

SIGNS AND SYMPTOMS

Coding of signs and symptoms should not be reported
with a confirmed diagnosis if the symptom is integral to
the diagnosis. For example, if the patient is experiencing ear pain and the diagnosis is otitis media, the ear
pain would be integral to the otitis media and would
not be reported. A symptom code is used together with
a confirmed diagnosis only when the symptom is not
associated with the confirmed diagnosis.

> **EXAMPLE:** *A patient is diagnosed with epigastric pain.
> The physician referred the patient to a gastroenterologist
> to rule out an ulcer.*

Alphabetic Index:

Review the Alphabetic Index entry for epigastric pain
(Figure 4.15).

FIGURE 4.15   Excerpt from the Alphabetic Index

Pain(s) (*see also* Painful) R52
   abdominal R10.9
     colic R10.83
     generalized R10.84
       with acute abdomen R10.0
     lower R10.30
       left quadrant R10.32
       pelvic or perineal R10.2
       periumbilical R10.33
       right quadrant R10.31
     rebound —*see* Tenderness, abdominal, rebound
     severe with abdominal rigidity R10.0
     tenderness —*see* Tenderness, abdominal
     upper R10.10
       epigastric R10.13

Notice that for the main term "pain" and subterm "epigastric," the Alphabetic Index refers the user to R10.13.
Open the ICD-10-CM codebook to R10.0 to reference
this category in the Tabular List.

Tabular List:

Review Figure 4.16.

Correct code:

R10.13   Epigastric pain

FIGURE 4.16 Excerpt from the Tabular List

R10.0 **Acute abdomen**
Severe abdominal pain (generalized) (with abdominal rigidity)
EXCLUDES 1 abdominal rigidity NOS (R19.3)
generalized abdominal pain NOS (R10.84)
localized abdominal pain (R10.1-R10.3-)
R10.1 **Pain localized to upper abdomen**
R10.10 **Upper abdominal pain, unspecified**
R10.11 **Right upper quadrant pain**
R10.12 **Left upper quadrant pain**
R10.13 **Epigastric pain**
Dyspepsia
EXCLUDES 1 functional dyspepsia (K30)

FIGURE 4.17 Code J01 for Acute Sinusitis in the Tabular List

J01 **Acute sinusitis**
INCLUDES acute abscess of sinus
acute empyema of sinus
acute infection of sinus
acute inflammation of sinus
acute suppuration of sinus
Use additional code (B95-B97) to identify infectious agent.
EXCLUDES 1 sinusitis NOS (J32.9)
EXCLUDES 2 chronic sinusitis (J32.0-J32.8)
J01.0 **Acute maxillary sinusitis**
Acute antritis
J01.00 **Acute maxillary sinusitis, unspecified**
J01.01 **Acute recurrent maxillary sinusitis**

Signs and symptoms are generally located in Chapter 18 of ICD-10-CM but may also be located in the body system chapters. Signs and symptoms are not to be used when a definitive diagnosis related to the signs and symptoms can be reported.

CODING TIP A sign or symptom is only to be used if no definitive diagnosis is established at the time the patient encounter is coded. When the diagnosis is confirmed prior to coding the encounter, the confirmed diagnosis is reported.

ACUTE, SUBACUTE, AND CHRONIC CONDITIONS

The ICD-10-CM Official Guidelines state: "If the same condition is described as both acute (subacute) and chronic, and separate subentries exist in the Alphabetic Index at the same indentation level, code both and sequence the acute (subacute) code first." [1(p13)]

EXAMPLE: A patient was diagnosed with acute maxillary sinusitis that is chronic. The physician examined the patient and prescribed medication for the condition and asked the patient to return for follow-up in one week.

In ICD-10-CM, codes for the acute and chronic condition are reported. Review code categories J01 for acute sinusitis and J32 for chronic sinusitis (Figures 4.17 and 4.18).

FIGURE 4.18 Code J32 for Chronic Sinusitis in the Tabular List

J32 **Chronic sinusitis**
INCLUDES sinus abscess
sinus empyema
sinus infection
sinus suppuration
Use additional code to identify:
exposure to environmental tobacco smoke (Z77.22)
exposure to tobacco smoke in the perinatal period (P96.81)
history of tobacco use (Z87.82)
infectious agent (B95-B97)
occupational exposure to environmental tobacco smoke (Z57.31)
tobacco dependence (F17.-)
tobacco use (Z72.0)
EXCLUDES 2 acute sinusitis (J01.-)
J32.0 **Chronic maxillary sinusitis**
Antritis (chronic)
Maxillary sinusitis NOS

Correct codes:
J01.00 *Acute maxillary sinusitis, unspecified*
J32.0 *Chronic maxillary sinusitis*

In the example above, there is an Excludes 2 note indicating conditions that are not included in a code but may be coexistent and, if present, should be coded also. Based on the ICD-10-CM Official Guidelines, if acute (subacute) and chronic forms of a condition are documented in the medical record, it would be appropriate to report both codes.

LATERALITY

As noted in Chapter 3, for bilateral sites the final character of the ICD-10-CM code indicates laterality. The right side is typically "1"; the left side, "2." In cases where a bilateral code is provided, the bilateral character is typically "3." An unspecified side code is also provided for use when the side is not identified in the medical record. The character indicating unspecified side is either "0" or "9" depending on whether it is the fifth or sixth character in the code.

> **EXAMPLE:** *The patient sees Dr. Thompson for follow up for an abscess of a bursa on the left wrist.*

Alphabetic Index:

> *The first step in coding this patient encounter using ICD-10-CM is to identify the main term. The main term is "abscess." Notice in this example that the code selection for abscess of the bursa is based on laterality and affected area. Also note the dashes ("-") after the codes, which indicate that additional characters are required. In the example, the abscess of the bursa is on the left wrist. Review Figure 4.19.*

FIGURE 4.19   Excerpt from the Alphabetic Index

Abscess (connective tissue) (embolic) (fistulous) (infective) (metastatic) (multiple) (pernicious) (pyogenic) (septic) L02.91
   bursa M71.00
      ankle M71.07-
      elbow M71.02-
      foot M71.07-
      hand M71.04-
      hip M71.05-
      knee M71.06-
      multiple sites M71.09
      pharyngeal J39.1
      shoulder M71.01-
      specified site NEC M71.08
      wrist M71.03-

> *When looking up "abscess" in the Alphabetic Index, you will find a selection for wrist (M71.03-). As a reminder, the dash indicates that additional digits, which can only be determined in the Tabular List, are required.*

Tabular List:

> *Now review Figure 4.20 from the Tabular List.*
>
> *When reviewing code M71.03 for abscess of the bursa of the wrist, you will notice that laterality is important. Code M71.03 requires the sixth character to identify the laterality of the bursa.*

Correct code:

> *M71.032*

CODING TIP   When coding laterality, the right side is typically "1," the left side is typically "2," and a bilateral condition is typically "3." The character indicating unspecified side is either "0" or "9."

FIGURE 4.20   Excerpt from the Tabular List

M71 Other bursopathies
   EXCLUDES 1   bunion (M20.1)
         bursitis related to use, overuse or pressure (M70.-)
         enthesopathies (M76-M77)
  M71.0 **Abscess of bursa**
     Use additional code (B95.-, B96.-) to identify causative organism
    M71.00 Abscess of bursa, unspecified site
    M71.01 Abscess of bursa, shoulder
        M71.011 Abscess of bursa, right shoulder
        M71.012 Abscess of bursa, left shoulder
        M71.019 Abscess of bursa, unspecified shoulder
    M71.02 Abscess of bursa, elbow
        M71.021 Abscess of bursa, right elbow
        M71.022 Abscess of bursa, left elbow
        M71.029 Abscess of bursa, unspecified elbow
    M71.03 Abscess of bursa, wrist
        M71.031 Abscess of bursa, right wrist
        M71.032 Abscess of bursa, left wrist
        M71.039 Abscess of bursa, unspecified wrist
    M71.04 Abscess of bursa, hand
        M71.041 Abscess of bursa, right hand
        M71.042 Abscess of bursa, left hand
        M71.049 Abscess of bursa, unspecified hand
    M71.05 Abscess of bursa, hip
        M71.051 Abscess of bursa, right hip
        M71.052 Abscess of bursa, left hip
        M71.059 Abscess of bursa, unspecified hip
    M71.06 Abscess of bursa, knee
        M71.061 Abscess of bursa, right knee
        M71.062 Abscess of bursa, left knee
        M71.069 Abscess of bursa, unspecified knee
    M71.07 Abscess of bursa, ankle and foot
        M71.071 Abscess of bursa, right ankle and foot
        M71.072 Abscess of bursa, left ankle and foot
        M71.079 Abscess of bursa, unspecified ankle and foot
    M71.08 Abscess of bursa, other site
    M71.09 Abscess of bursa, multiple sites

Indicate whether each of the following statements is true or false.

1. _____ A combination code is used to fully identify an instance where 2 diagnoses or a diagnosis with an associated secondary process (manifestation) or complication is included in the description of a single code number.

2. _____ Coding to the highest level of specificity means using a fifth or sixth character if available.

3. _____ Code category L60-L75, Disorders of skin appendages, includes congenital malformations of integument (Q84.-).

4. _____ "Code first the underlying condition" means that the underlying condition should not be identified as a first-listed diagnosis.

5. _____ Nonessential modifiers are terms enclosed in brackets following the main term and are required in the diagnosis statement.

6. _____ It is necessary to always verify the correct code in the Tabular List.

7. _____ The coder should always refer to any cross-references under the main term in the Alphabetic Index.

8. _____ Main terms are found in the Tabular List.

9. _____ Using a combination of more than 1 code when more than 1 diagnosis describes the condition and/or disease is referred to as multiple coding.

10. _____ When the note "Use additional code" is listed, the use of an additional code is optional when both the etiology and manifestation exist.

SELECTION OF PRINCIPAL OR FIRST-LISTED DIAGNOSIS

The code sequenced first is most important because it defines the main reason for the encounter as determined in the medical record documentation. In the inpatient setting, the first code listed on a medical record is referred to as the principal diagnosis. In all other health care settings, it is referred to as the first-listed diagnosis.

The Uniform Hospital Discharge Data Set (UHDDS) defines *principal diagnosis* as "that condition established after study to be chiefly responsible for occasioning the admission of the patient to the hospital for care." [1(p92)]

Selection of principal/first-listed diagnosis is based first on the conventions in the classification that provide sequencing instructions. If no sequencing instructions apply, then sequencing is based on the condition(s) that brought the patient into the hospital or physician's office and the condition that was the primary focus of treatment.

Conditions present on admission that receive treatment but do not meet the definition of principal diagnosis should be coded as additional diagnoses.

Acute Manifestation Versus Underlying Condition

With the UHDDS definition of *principal diagnosis* in mind, it is generally an underlying condition that precipitates the need for an admission since treatment of the underlying condition generally resolves any associated acute manifestations and is the primary focus of treatment. If the acute manifestation is immediately life threatening and primary treatment is directed at the acute manifestation, the acute manifestation should be sequenced before the underlying condition. If the acute manifestation is not the primary focus of treatment, the underlying condition should be sequenced first.

> **EXAMPLE:** *A patient is treated by his primary care physician for impetigo due to otitis externa.*
>
> *In this example, the underlying condition is the impetigo and the manifestation is the otitis externa. This guideline is also based on the etiology/manifestation convention, which requires that the underlying etiology take sequencing precedence over the acute manifestation.*

CODING TIP If the acute manifestation is not the primary focus of treatment, the underlying condition should be sequenced first.

> *Code L01.00 is selected as the first-listed diagnosis because the type of impetigo is not specified in the documentation. The secondary diagnosis that should be reported is H62.41, Otitis externa. Review Figures 4.21 and 4.22.*

FIGURE 4.21   Excerpt from the Tabular List

L01   **Impetigo**
      EXCLUDES 1   impetigo herpetiformis (L40.1)
      L01.0   **Impetigo**
              Impetigo contagiosa
              Impetigo vulgaris
              L01.00   **Impetigo, unspecified**
                       Impetigo NOS
              L01.01   **Non-bullous impetigo**
              L01.02   **Bockhart's impetigo**
                       Impetigo follicularis
                       Perifolliculitis NOS
                       Superficial pustular perifolliculitis
              L01.03   **Bullous impetigo**
                       Impetigo neonatorum
                       Pemphigus neonatorum
              L01.09   **Other impetigo**
                       Ulcerative impetigo

FIGURE 4.22   Excerpt from the Tabular List

H62   **Disorders of external ear in diseases classified elsewhere**
      H62.4   **Otitis externa in other diseases classified**
              H62.40   **Otitis externa in other diseases classified elsewhere, unspecified ear**
              H62.41   **Otitis externa in other diseases classified elsewhere, right ear**
              H62.42   **Otitis externa in other diseases classified elsewhere, left ear**
              H62.43   **Otitis externa in other diseases classified elsewhere, bilateral**

Correct codes:

L01.00   *Impetigo, unspecified*

H62.41   *Otitis externa in other diseases classified elsewhere, right ear*

Two or More Diagnoses That Equally Meet the Definition of Principal/First-Listed Diagnosis

There may be instances when 2 or more confirmed diagnoses equally meet the criteria for principal/first-listed diagnosis as determined by the circumstances of admission, diagnostic workup, and/or therapy provided, and the Alphabetic Index, Tabular List, and coding guidelines do not provide sequencing direction. In this situation, any one of the diagnoses may be sequenced first. This rule applies to the inpatient and outpatient settings.

Complications of Surgery and Other Medical Care

When the admission is for treatment of a complication resulting from surgery or other medical care, the complication code is sequenced first.

> **EXAMPLE:** *Dr. Smith performed a spinal puncture on Mr. Cartwright. The patient was doing well following surgery, but later in the evening, the patient was experiencing weakness and a loss of consciousness. The patient was rushed to the emergency room where Dr. Smith met the patient. The physician examined the patient and determined that cerebrospinal fluid (CFS) was leaking from the puncture site. The physician took the patient into a surgery suite and stopped the leak.*
>
> *Open the ICD-10-CM codebook to the Alphabetic Index and locate the main term. The main term in this diagnosis is "leak."*

Alphabetic Index:
   leak ➝ *cerebrospinal fluid* ➝ *from spinal (lumbar) puncture* ➝ *G97.0*

   Now verify the code in the Tabular List.

Tabular List:
   G97.0   *Cerebrospinal fluid leak from spinal puncture*

Correct code:
   G97.0

SELECTION OF SECONDARY DIAGNOSES

In most cases, more than 1 code is necessary to fully explain a health care encounter. Though a patient has an encounter for a primary reason (the principal/first-listed diagnosis), the additional conditions or reasons for the encounter also need to be coded. These codes are referred to as secondary, additional, or other diagnoses.

For reporting purposes, the definition of "other diagnoses" is interpreted as conditions affecting patient care requiring:

- Clinical evaluation

- Therapeutic treatment

- Diagnostic procedures

- Extended length of hospital stay

- Increased nursing care and/or monitoring

The UHDDS defines other diagnoses as "all conditions that coexist at the time of admission, that develop subsequently, or that affect the treatment received and/or the length of stay. Diagnoses that relate to an earlier episode that have no bearing on the current hospital stay are to be excluded." [1(p94)] UHDDS definitions apply to inpatients in an acute care, short-term, hospital setting. This definition also applies to outpatient encounters.

CODING TIP When the attending physician includes a diagnosis in the discharge summary or face sheet, it is ordinarily coded unless the condition does not meet the "other diagnosis" definition.

PREVIOUS CONDITIONS

Some physicians include in the diagnostic statement resolved conditions or diagnoses and previous procedures that have no bearing on the current treatment. Such conditions are not to be reported and are coded only if required by the hospital or provider office policy.

For example, if the patient is being treated for hypertension and diabetes during the patient encounter and the patient previously had pneumonia, which was resolved 3 months ago and has no bearing on the services rendered at the current visit, the pneumonia would not be reported.

ABNORMAL TEST FINDINGS

Abnormal test findings (laboratory, x-ray, pathologic, and other diagnostic results) are *not* coded and reported unless the physician indicates their clinical significance. If the findings are outside the normal range and the physician has ordered other tests to evaluate the condition or prescribed treatment, it is appropriate to ask the physician whether the abnormal finding should be added.

If the abnormal test finding corresponds to a confirmed diagnosis, it should not be coded in addition to the confirmed diagnosis. A sign or symptom code is to be used as the principal/first-listed code if no definitive diagnosis is established at the time of coding. If the diagnosis is confirmed (eg, an x-ray confirms a fracture, a pathology or laboratory report confirms a diagnosis) prior to coding the encounter, the confirmed diagnosis code should be reported.

CODING CHRONIC CONDITIONS

Chronic conditions treated on an ongoing basis may be coded as many times as required for treatment and care of the patient or when applicable to the patient's plan of care. Do not code conditions previously treated or those that no longer exist, although a history of previous conditions should be coded if it affects patient

care or provides the need for a patient to seek medical care (eg, history of lung cancer). Review the following examples of coding for chronic conditions.

> **EXAMPLE 1:** *A woman is seen today for acute cystitis. The patient's hypertension is well controlled. Blood pressure appears well controlled on current medications. No other problems were managed at this visit. Her problem list includes the following conditions: history of fibrocystic breast disease, hypertension, chronic sinusitis, and viral syndrome (resolved in January 2011).*

> **Correct codes:**
>
> First-listed diagnosis: N30.00   Acute cystitis without hematuria
>
> Secondary diagnosis (managed at this visit):   I10 Hypertension
>
> *The remainder of the diagnoses documented in the medical record either were not managed or have no impact on the medical management of the first-listed diagnosis.*

> **EXAMPLE 2:** *A patient who has type 1 diabetes mellitus is treated for a second-degree burn on her left knee that radiated down to her ankle. The patient was burned when a hot skillet fell and hit her left knee causing the burn. She was in her kitchen when the injury occurred.*

> *Open the ICD-10-CM codebook. The main term is "burn." Review the following:*

> **Alphabetic Index:**
> Burn → knee → left → second degree → T24.222

> **Tabular List:**
> T24.222-   Burn of second degree of left knee

> *The Tabular List instructions indicate a seventh character is required. The choices in category T24 are shown in Figure 4.23.*

FIGURE 4.23   Excerpt from the Tabular List for Category T24

The appropriate 7th character is to be added to each code from category T24

    A - initial encounter

    D - subsequent encounter

    S - sequela

In addition, the instructional notes instruct the user to select a code to identify the source, place, and intent of the burn. Since the patient was injured by a skillet that fell on her knee while she was cooking in the kitchen at home, this information also needs be reported.

The external cause codes have their own alphabetic index in ICD-10-CM. Open the ICD-10-CM codebook to the External Cause of Injuries Index and review the following:

External Cause of Injuries Index:
Contact → with → hot → skillet → X15.3

Tabular List:
X15.3   Contact with hot saucepan or skillet

Since the length of this category is 4 characters and a seventh character is required, 2 dummy placeholders ("x") must be appended to reach the seventh character. Figure 4.24 shows the seventh-character extension required.

FIGURE 4.24   Excerpt from the Tabular List for Category X15

The appropriate seventh character is to be added to each code from category X15
  A - initial encounter
  D - subsequent encounter
  S - sequela

The correct code to report for the cause of the burn is X15.3xxA.

You are not finished yet. The place of occurrence must be reported as well. Since the place of occurrence is the patient's kitchen, this will also be coded. Open the ICD-10-CM codebook to the External Cause of Injuries Index and find the appropriate code.

External Cause of Injuries Index:
Place of occurrence → residence (noninstitutional) (private) → house, single family → kitchen → Y92.010

Tabular List:
Y92.010 → Kitchen of single-family (private) house as the place of occurrence of the external cause

Correct codes:

First-listed diagnosis:	T24.222, Burn of second degree of left knee
Secondary diagnosis:	X15.3xxA, Contact with hot saucepan or skillet
Tertiary diagnosis:	Y92.010, Kitchen of single-family (private) house as the place of occurrence of the external cause
Final diagnosis:	E10.69, Type1 diabetes mellitus with other specified complication

In this example, although the physician may not have actively managed the diabetes at the visit, it is appropriate to report the diabetes in addition to the diagnoses for the treatments because it will impact the management of the burn. Since we do not know if there are any manifestations from the diabetes, the only choice is to use the "other specified" code.

ACUTE AND CHRONIC MANIFESTATIONS

Some diseases have both acute and chronic manifestations. These manifestations may exist alone or together. Use only one code when the code description includes both the acute (subacute) and chronic conditions. See the following example:

EXAMPLE: *Acute and chronic cholecystitis*

Alphabetic Index:
Cholecystitis → acute → with → chronic cholecystitis → K81.2

Tabular List:
K81.2   Acute cholecystitis with chronic cholecystitis

Correct code:
K81.2

When the medical record states that the patient has both acute and chronic forms of a disease and no single code exists for the combined acute and chronic disease, observe the following rules:

- The acute condition is listed as the first-listed diagnosis.

- The chronic condition is listed as the secondary diagnosis.

EXAMPLE: *Acute and chronic tonsillitis*

Alphabetic Index:
Tonsillitis → acute → J03.90

Tabular List:
When referencing the Tabular List, note that there are two choices:

J03.90   Acute tonsillitis, unspecified

J03.91   Acute recurrent tonsillitis, unspecified

If the documentation does not specify recurrent, J03.90 is reported.

Since a combination code to report chronic tonsillitis does not exist, the chronic condition is reported as the secondary diagnosis. ICD-10-CM coding guidelines indicate that the acute condition is reported as the first-listed diagnosis with the chronic condition reported secondarily.

CHECKPOINT EXERCISE 4-3

Underline the condition you would code for in each of the following diagnostic statements.

Example: <u>fatigue</u>, suspect iron-deficiency anemia

1. nausea and vomiting, suspect viral gastroenteritis

2. chest pain, possible myocardial infarction

3. headache, rule out viral meningitis

4. diarrhea, probable infectious colitis

5. shortness of breath, possible bronchiectasis

6. burning on urination, suspect UTI

7. vertigo, rule out Ménière's disease

8. rule out diabetes mellitus, abnormal glucose tolerance test

9. abdominal pain, rule out gastric ulcer

10. convulsions, probable seizure disorder

Alphabetic Index:
Tonsillitis → chronic → J35.01

Tabular List:
J35.01   Chronic tonsillitis

Correct codes:
J03.90   Acute tonsillitis, unspecified (first-listed diagnosis)

J35.01   Chronic tonsillitis (secondary diagnosis)

CODING DIAGNOSES FOR SURGICAL PROCEDURES

For surgical procedures, code the diagnosis that is applicable to the procedure. If at the time the claim is filed the postoperative diagnosis is different from the preoperative diagnosis, report the postoperative diagnosis since it is the most definitive. Keep in mind you must read the entire operative note as sometimes the detail in the note indicates a different postoperative diagnosis. These guidelines are applicable to physicians' and nonphysician practitioners' professional services.

EXAMPLE 1: *Operative Note*

Preoperative diagnosis: Chronic cholecystitis

Postoperative diagnosis: Cholelithiasis with chronic cholecystitis

Procedure: Laparoscopic cholecystectomy

Anesthesia: General endotracheal anesthesia

Description of procedure: Under general endotracheal anesthesia with the patient in the supine position, the abdomen was prepped with Betadine and draped. The oral gastric tube and Foley catheter were inserted. An infraumbilical incision was made. A versus needle was inserted and the abdomen was insufflated to 15 mm Hg with carbon dioxide. A 10- to 11-mm trocar was inserted and zero-degree laparoscope was inserted. A 5-mm trocar was placed 3 finger breadths below the right costal margin in the anterior axillary line 2 finger breadths below the right costal margin in the midclavicular line and 3 finger breadths below the xiphoid in the midline. The gallbladder was elevated superiorly and adhesions from the gallbladder to the hepatic flexure and omentum were reflected inferiorly. Dissection was carried out at the neck of the gallbladder and cystic duct. A silver clip was placed on the neck of the gallbladder to prevent stones from migrating down the cystic duct. The cystic duct was ligated times two with #0 chromic Endoloop approximately 4 mm from its junction with the common duct, and a silver clip was placed between these two loops. The cystic artery was doubly silver clipped and divided. The gallbladder was removed from the liver fossa by means of a hook cautery, placed in an Endopouch, and retrieved through the umbilicus. During the procedure, the abdomen was copiously irrigated with a solution of heparinized saline and Ancef. Once hemostasis was ensured, air was evacuated and trocars were removed. The umbilical fascial defect was closed with a figure-of-eight suture of #0 Vicryl. The skin was closed with subcuticular #3-0 Vicryl. Steri-Strips were applied. The patient tolerated the procedure well. The patient was transferred to the recovery room in satisfactory condition.

Preoperative diagnosis: Chronic cholecystitis

Postoperative diagnosis: Cholelithiasis with chronic cholecystitis

Correct code:
K80.12   Calculus of gallbladder with acute and chronic cholecystitis without obstruction

EXAMPLE 2: *Operative Note*

Preoperative diagnosis: Nodular basal cell carcinoma, right lower lip and chin

Postoperative diagnosis: Same

Description of procedure: With the patient in the supine position, the face was prepared with Chlorhexidine and draped in the usual manner. The tumor measured 1.5 cm × 1.0 cm arising in the right lateral lower lip skin *and adjacent chin. Just medial and slightly superior to the tumor was an atrophic scar from a previous basal cell cancer removed 9 years earlier. Proposed lines of excision were drawn around the tumor to include the adjacent scar and the area was anesthetized with 1% Xylocaine with 1:100,000 epinephrine, buffered with sodium bicarbonate. The tumor was excised down to the orbicularis oris muscle, resulting in a defect measuring 2.1 cm wide × 3.0 cm high in the shape of an inverted teardrop. Bleeding vessels were controlled with bipolar electrocoagulation. Adjacent skin was undermined at the deep subcutaneous level medially and laterally. Consideration was given to a rotation flap repair versus a complex linear repair. It was elected to repair the deficit extending to the vermillion border to convert the original defect to a lazy-S ellipse. Additional undermining was accomplished and the defect was approximated with layers of 5-0 Polyglactin suture deep. Final skin repair was accomplished and the defect was approximated 6-0 Nylon sutures, supported by sterile strips over surgical adhesive followed by sterile occlusive dressing. The specimen was submitted to pathology, after staining its superior margin red, its medial and deep margin black, and its lateral margin blue for pathologic orientation. The patient tolerated the procedure well and received 1 g of acetaminophen postoperatively. The pathology report confirms nodular basal cell carcinoma of the right lower lip and chin.*

Correct codes:

C44.39   *Malignant neoplasm of skin of other parts of face*

C44.0   *Malignant neoplasm of skin of lip*

In this example, the preoperative and postoperative diagnoses are the same. Since there does not exist a single code or a combination code that describes the diagnosis, each area (chin and lower lip) is reported separately.

ICD-10-CM and Medical Necessity

ICD-10-CM codes form a crucial partnership with CPT procedural codes by supporting the medical necessity of the CPT procedure or service performed.

Diagnosis codes identify the medical necessity of services provided by describing the circumstances of the patient's condition. Most third-party payers employ claims "edits" or automatic denial/review commands within the computer software to review claims. These edits ensure that payment is made for specific procedure codes when provided for a patient with a specific diagnosis code or a diagnosis in a predetermined range of ICD-10-CM codes. An important point to realize when filing claims is that neither the CPT codes nor the ICD-10-CM codes can stand alone.

Apply the following principles to diagnosis coding to properly demonstrate medical necessity for physician or outpatient services:

1. List the principal/first-listed diagnosis, condition, problem, or other reason for the medical service or procedure.

2. Assign the code to the highest level of specificity.

3. Never code a "rule-out," "probable," "possible," or "suspect" statement; this could label the patient with a condition that does not exist. Code signs, symptoms, abnormal test results, or other reason for the visit if no definitive diagnosis is determined.

4. Be specific in describing the patient's condition, illness, or disease.

5. Distinguish between acute and chronic conditions, when appropriate.

6. Identify the acute condition of an emergency situation (eg, coma, loss of consciousness, hemorrhage).

7. Identify chronic complaints, or secondary diagnoses, only when treatment is provided for them or when they impact the overall management of the patient's care.

8. Identify how injuries occur.

These facts must be substantiated by the patient's medical record, and that record must be available to payers upon request.

Test Your Knowledge

Code the following diagnostic statements using both the Alphabetic Index and Tabular List of ICD-10-CM.

1. _____ congestive heart failure

2. _____ attention deficit disorder with hyperactivity (combined type)

3. _____ sore throat

4. _____ headache

5. _____ acute bronchitis

6. _____ prostatitis with hematuria

7. _____ hyperlipidemia, unspecified

8. _____ pain in the neck

9. _____ atrial fibrillation

10. _____ acute upper respiratory infection

11. _____ malignant hypertension

12. _____ cervical sprain, initial encounter

13. _____ brain abscess

14. _____ diminished vital capacity

15. _____ pelvic inflammatory disease

16. _____ septic shock due to severe sepsis

17. _____ laceration of right foot with foreign body

18. _____ abnormal weight loss

19. _____ abscess of the prostate due to streptococcus group b

20. _____ acute and chronic respiratory failure

Reference

1. Centers for Medicare & Medicaid Services. ICD-10-CM Official Guidelines for Coding and Reporting. 2011.

Resource

Centers for Medicare & Medicaid Services. ICD-10-CM Official Guidelines for Coding and Reporting. 2011. http://www.cms.hhs.gov/ICD10.

CHAPTER 5

Certain Infectious and Parasitic Diseases

Neoplasms Diseases of the Blood and Blood Forming Organs, Certain Disorders Involving the Immune Mechanism, Endocrine, Nutritional, and Metabolic Diseases (A00-E89.89)

LEARNING OBJECTIVES

- Review specific guidelines for systems and organs in Chapters 1 through 4 of ICD-10-CM

- Understand the complexities of coding multiple procedures

- Review coding examples and scenarios

- Test your skills by completing Checkpoint Exercises

- Test your knowledge by answering additional chapter questions

Chapter 1 of the Tabular List of ICD-10-CM includes certain infectious and parasitic diseases. There are specific guidelines for conditions such as human immunodeficiency virus (HIV), sepsis, infectious agent as the cause of the diseases classified to other chapters, and nosocomial infections.

Chapter 1 in the Tabular List includes the following sections:

- Infectious and parasitic diseases (A00-A09)

- Tuberculosis (A15-A19)

- Certain zoonotic bacterial diseases (A20-A28)

- Other bacterial diseases (A30-A49)

- Infections with a predominately sexual mode of transmission (A50-A64)

- Other spirochetal diseases (A65-A69)

- Other diseases caused by *Chlamydia* (A70-A74)

- Rickettsioses (A75-A79)

- Viral and prion infections of the central nervous system (A80-A89)

- Arthropod-borne viral fevers and viral hemorrhagic fevers (A90-A99)

- Viral infections characterized by skin and mucous membrane lesions (B00-B09)

- Other human herpes viruses (B10)

- Viral hepatitis (B15-B19)

- Human immunodeficiency virus (HIV) disease (B20)

- Other viral diseases (B25-B34)

- Mycoses (B35-B49)

- Protozoal diseases (B50-B64)

- Helminthiases (B65-B83)

- Pediculosis, acriasis, and other infestations (B85-B89)

- Sequelae of infectious and parasitic diseases (B90-B94)

- Bacterial and viral infectious agents (B95-B97)

- Other infectious diseases (B99)

Chapter 1 of ICD-10-CM covers transmissible infections and parasitic diseases, classified according to cause or etiology. Infectious or parasitic conditions can affect different parts of the body. The organism responsible for the condition is classified in several different ways, so use your index carefully so as not to code inappropriately. This chapter does not include acute respiratory infections (J00-J37); certain localized infections and influenza (J11.2 and J12.9), which are found in Chapter 10; and carriers or suspected carriers of infectious organisms (Z22.1-Z22.9) located in Chapter 21. Diseases not considered easily transmissible or communicable are classified in the appropriate organ or system chapter.

Many of the diseases in this chapter are coded by using combination or multiple codes. Although this type of coding was described in chapter 4 chapter of this book, it may be worthwhile to do a quick review of these codes before proceeding with this category.

Following are two examples, one of combination coding and one of multiple coding, with a review of the required steps.

> **EXAMPLE 1:** *A patient visits an ophthalmologist with a complaint of a red and swollen left eye. Upon reviewing the patient's medical history, the ophthalmologist discovers that the patient has a history of herpes zoster and is currently taking medication prescribed by his family physician for the condition. After the examination, the ophthalmologist determines the diagnosis to be conjunctivitis*

of the left eye due to herpes zoster and prescribes an antibiotic ointment for use daily for 7 days. The patient is asked to return in one week for a follow-up examination.

In order to correctly code this encounter, determine the principal diagnosis. In this example, the patient went to the ophthalmologist because of a red and swollen eye. The ophthalmologist made the diagnosis of conjunctivitis due to herpes zoster. How would you code this encounter? Review this example and follow the steps below.

Step 1

Look up conjunctivitis in the ICD-10-CM Alphabetic Index. You will find several options to choose from when you locate this category (see Figure 5.1).

Under the heading Conjunctivitis, there is a subheading "due to." Select the code based on the reason for the condition of conjunctivitis. The reason stated in the ophthalmologist's medical record is "herpes zoster." Review Figure 5.1 and find the code category. If you selected conjunctivitis due to herpes zoster (B02.31), you are correct. However, you are not finished yet. The rule of thumb is to never code from the Alphabetic Index alone; it should be used only as a reference to the Tabular List.

Step 2

Locate the ICD-10-CM code for conjunctivitis due to herpes zoster in the Tabular List. The Alphabetic Index directed you to ICD-10-CM code B02.31.

You will notice that category B02 includes herpes zoster. Find B02.31 in the Tabular List. As you can see, only one code is necessary because the condition is listed with one code. This is a good example of combination coding. As shown in Figure 5.2, the correct code is B02.31, Zoster conjunctivitis. As you see in this example, combination codes are common in coding infectious and parasitic diseases.

FIGURE 5.1 Excerpt from the Alphabetic Index: *Conjunctivitis*

Conjunctivitis
  In (due to)
  herpes (simplex) virus B00.53
    zoster (B02.31)

FIGURE 5.2   Excerpt from the Tabular List: *B02*

B02   Zoster [herpes zoster]
    B02.3   Zoster ocular disease
      B02.30   Zoster ocular disease, unspecified
      B02.31   Zoster conjunctivitis   ⟵
      B02.32   Zoster iridocyclitis
      B02.33   Zoster keratitis
      B02.34   Zoster scleritis
      B02.39   Other herpes zoster eye disease

FIGURE 5.3   Excerpt from the Tabular List: *Urinary Tract Infection*

N39.0   Urinary tract infection, site not specified
Use additional code B95-B97 to identify infectious agent
   EXCLUDES 1   *candidiasis of urinary tract (B37.4-)*
            neonatal urinary tract infection (P39.3)
            urinary tract infection of unspecified site,
            such as
                cystitis (N30.-)
                urethritis (N34.-)

The second type of coding that is common in Chapter 1 of ICD-10-CM is multiple coding. As discussed earlier, multiple coding involves assigning more than one code to provide information about a manifestation and the associated underlying condition.

Review the following example.

> **EXAMPLE 2**: *A five-year-old boy is brought to the emergency department by his parents. He has had an elevated temperature for the past 12 hours; the high was 103°F. He also complains of stomach pains and is vomiting. The parents are very concerned. Past medical history is negative. The patient lives with his parents and is taking no medications.*
>
> *Examination shows a well-developed, well-nourished child who is lethargic and pale. His temperature is 101°F. Pulse is 110/min. Respirations are 28/min. Eyes are normal. There is a minimal amount of inflammation of the tonsils. Ears, nose, and mouth are normal. The neck is supple. Lung sounds are normal. The heart has normal rhythm with no murmurs noted. The abdomen has diffuse tenderness. No masses or organomegaly are noted.*
>
> *Renal x-ray was normal. Lab tests are normal except for urinalysis, which was positive. Urine culture is pending. Lab results indicate that urine culture shows* Escherichia coli, *with a count greater than 100,000. The diagnosis is urinary tract infection. The patient is discharged with Bactrim and will follow up with his physician.*

Pay special attention to the diagnosis—urinary tract infection. Also notice the addendum to the chart note that indicates that the urine culture showed *E coli* bacteria. Because this is documented in the chart note, you must code for both the urinary tract infection (UTI) and the *E coli*. Review Figure 5.3 and follow the next set of steps.

Remember your main term is "infection":

Diagnosis: Urinary tract infection due to *E coli* (*Escherichia*)

Index: Infection, infected, infective, urinary (tract) N39.0

Step 1

Go to the Alphabetic Index and look up the main term, which is "infection" in this example. Under infection, go to "urinary" and note that the Index refers you to N39.0.

Step 2

Go to the Tabular List and look up code N39.0. You will find a note under N39.0 that indicates the need to use an additional code to identify the infectious agent.

Step 3

It is now time to identify the *E coli*. Read the instructions after N39.0, which does not fully describe the condition. The instructions for N39.0 state that you must also code the infectious agent that is causing the urinary tract infection. Go to the Alphabetic Index and look up *E coli*. Note that, for this example, you will need to reference the clinical infection (*Escherichia (E) coli*), not the commonly used term.

Multiple coding is necessary to fully describe the urinary tract infection and the cause (organism). After reviewing the Alphabetic Index, you will find that *Escherichia (E) coli* as cause of disease classified elsewhere is reported as B96.2. Now turn to the Tabular List and look up B96.2 (see Figure 5.4). Make sure to read all the notes in the category before selecting the code.

FIGURE 5.4   Excerpt from the Tabular List: *E. coli*

B96	Other bacterial agents as the cause of diseases classified elsewhere
B96.1	Klebsiella pneumoniae [K. pneumoniae] as the cause of diseases classified elsewhere
B96.2	**Escherichia coli [E. coli] as the cause of diseases classified elsewhere**
B96.3	Hemophilus influenzae [H. influenzae] as the cause of diseases classified elsewhere

The correct codes are N39.0, Urinary tract infection as the first listed diagnosis, and B96.2 to identify *E coli* as the underlying infection (secondary diagnosis).

Now that we have reviewed combination and multiple coding, you are ready to review codes related to specific diseases. The material in this section will focus on the most common infectious and parasitic diseases.

CODING TIP   When referencing the index, remember to find the main term in the diagnosis first, then look up the reference "infection." Refer to Urinary Tract and look up the code in the Tabular List (N39.0). Make sure to read all notes in the code category and follow the instructions.

Tuberculosis (A15-A19)

Tuberculosis is an infectious disease usually caused by the bacterium *Mycobacterium tuberculosis*. Infection may result from inhalation of minute droplets of infected sputum or from drinking infected milk. If the person is not immune, the bacteria grow freely within the body and spread from the lungs to other parts of the body.

SYMPTOMS

Symptoms of tuberculosis occur when the body's immunity does not develop fast enough to prevent the infection from spreading to various parts of the body or when immunity is interrupted by age, certain drugs, or diseases. Many months may go by before symptoms appear. In most cases, the infection involves primarily the top of one of the lungs, although it may spread to other parts of the body.

Initial symptoms may include:

- Weight loss

- Fatigue

- Fever during the evening

- Profuse sweating at night

As the infection progresses, the patient begins to cough up blood-stained sputum, which may be infectious. If a large area of the lung is affected, pleurisy may develop. The most frequently affected areas include the following:

- Meninges (membranes covering the brain and spinal cord)

- Kidneys

- Bones

- Lungs

CODING ISSUES

Tuberculosis is classified A15-A19 in the Tabular List. Be careful when selecting a code that confirms an active condition of tuberculosis from a confirmed positive tuberculin skin test and no diagnosis of active tuberculosis (R76.1, Abnormal reaction to tuberculin test). Code R76.1 classifies a nonspecific reaction to a tuberculin skin test without active tuberculosis and includes:

- Abnormal result of Mantoux test

- PPD **(Purified Protein Derivative)** positive

- Tuberculin (skin test)

- Positive

- Reactor

Within this family of codes, a fourth or fifth is available to indicate the method with which the diagnosis was determined. Review Figure 5.5 for tuberculosis of the bronchus.

FIGURE 5.5   Excerpt from the Tabular List: *Tuberculosis*

A 15	Respiratory tuberculosis
A15.5	Tuberculosis of larynx, trachea and bronchus
	Tuberculosis of bronchus
	Tuberculosis of glottis
	Tuberculosis of larynx
	Tuberculosis of trachea

A symbol next to the code or category is an alert that an additional digit is required. Publishers of ICD-10-CM use different symbols to indicate additional digits are required in the subclassification. For purposes of the examples below, we will use an x to indicate that a fifth digit is required.

EXAMPLE 1: A female patient visits her family physician with complaints of fatigue, a 20-lb weight loss in two weeks, and episodic fevers, particularly at night. After a detailed history and examination in which the physician discovers the patient's lymph nodes are enlarged, he orders a sputum culture and a chest x-ray to rule out tuberculosis. The culture is sent to the lab for confirmation. The physician informs the patient that he will call her when her test results are available. The specimen is examined by microscopy, and the laboratory notifies the physician that tubercle is found in the sputum. The result of the chest x-ray is positive. The patient is notified via telephone, and medication is prescribed to treat the early stages of her condition. The physician documents in the chart a diagnosis of infiltrative tuberculosis of the lung.

Before selecting the appropriate code from the Tabular Listing, locate the condition/disease in the Alphabetic Index. The main term, "tuberculosis," should include the following:

Tuberculosis ➝ Lung—see Tuberculosis, pulmonary

This directs you to the next step—pulmonary.

Under the subcategory, tuberculosis pulmonary, you will find infiltrative.

Return to the Tabular List and look up the diagnosis code A15.0.

The correct diagnosis for this encounter is A15.0, Tuberculosis of lung, infiltrative. If this was your selection, good job!

EXAMPLE 2: A patient visits the emergency department with complaints of excessive sweating, loss of appetite, excessive coughing, and extreme fatigue. After extensive testing and a chest x-ray, the emergency department physician diagnoses tuberculous meningoencephalitis. The patient is placed on oral medications and asked to follow up with his family physician in one week.

In the ICD-10-CM codebook, review the following steps in selecting a diagnosis code for tuberculous meningoencephalitis:

Alphabetic Index:
   Tuberculosis ➝ meningoencephalitis A17.82

Tabular List:
   A17.82 Tuberculous meningoencephalitis

Correct code:
   A17.82

LATE EFFECTS OF TUBERCULOSIS

Late effects of tuberculosis are located in the Alphabetic Index under sequela and are classified in category B90.–. This category is used to indicate conditions classifiable as late effects, which are themselves classified elsewhere. This includes "due to old or inactive tuberculosis" without evidence that the disease is currently active or has recurred. First code the active condition being treated as the primary diagnosis and code the "late effect" as the secondary diagnosis.

Review the following example:

EXAMPLE: A family physician treated a female patient for tuberculosis eight months ago. The patient presents with persistent cough and excessive excretion of mucus. After a detailed history and examination, the physician orders a chest x-ray. The chest x-ray comes back positive, and the physician makes a diagnosis of bronchiectasis with acute exacerbation, a late effect of pulmonary tuberculosis.

Review Figure 5.6

FIGURE 5.6	Excerpt from the Tabular List: *Sequela of Tuberculosis*

B90   Sequelae of tuberculosis
    B90.0   Sequelae of central nervous system tuberculosis
    B90.1   Sequelae of genitourinary system tuberculosis
    B90.2   Sequelae of tuberculosis of bones and joints
    B90.8   Sequelae of tuberculosis of other organs
        EXCLUDES 2   Sequelae of respiratory tuberculosis
    B90.9   Sequelae of respiratory tuberculosis

Review the steps in coding this case.

Alphabetic Index:
   Bronchiectasis ➝ with ➝ exacerbation (acute) J47

Tabular List:
   J47.1 ➝ Bronchiectasis with (acute) exacerbation

Alphabetic Index:
   Sequela ➝ Tuberculosis ➝ B90.–

Tabular List:
   B90 Sequela of tuberculosis ➝ ✓4ᵗʰ ➝ B90.9 Sequela of respiratory tuberculosis

Correct code(s):
   J47.1 Bronchiectasis with (acute) exacerbation

   B90.9 Sequela of respiratory tuberculosis

Correct code sequence:
   J47.1, B90.9

CODING TIP Late effect—residual effect (condition produced) after the acute phase of an illness or injury had terminated or resolved.

CODING TIP All late effects are listed in the Index under the main term "sequela."

CHECKPOINT EXERCISE 5-1

Using your ICD-10-CM codebook, code the following:

1. _____ Tuberculoma of meninges

2. _____ Episcleritis tuberculosis

3. _____ Late effects of respiratory tuberculosis

4. _____ Tuberculosis infection of hip diagnosed by CT scan

5. _____ Renal tuberculosis with pyelonephritis

6. _____ Tuberculosis peritonitis

7. _____ Salmonella meningitis

8. _____ Tuberculosis of the small intestine

9. _____ Gastroenteritis due to rotavirus

10. _____ Staphylococcus enterocolitis

11. _____ Tuberculosis laryngitis that was confirmed histologically but not by bacteriological examination

12. _____ A 45-year-old patient is diagnosed with epididymis tuberculosis

13. _____ Tuberculous mastoiditis

14. _____ A patient was treated in the emergency room after eating bad mayonnaise and was diagnosed with botulism

15. _____ Sixteen patients aboard a cruise ship bound for Alaska had to be returned after the ship's doctor diagnosed the patients with the Norwalk virus

---

Human Immunodeficiency Virus

In the case of HIV, it is extremely important to understand the disease in order to select the correct diagnosis code(s). Following is a brief review of HIV.

TRANSMISSION OF HIV

HIV is spread most commonly by:

- Sexual contact with an infected partner

- Contact with infected blood

- Drug users who share needles or syringes

- Accidental needle sticks from contaminated needles by health care workers

- Accidental bodily fluid exposure

Before the screening of blood for evidence of HIV infection and before the introduction in 1985 of heat-treating techniques to destroy HIV in blood products, HIV was transmitted through transfusions of contaminated blood or blood components.

Almost all HIV-infected children acquire the virus from their mothers before or during birth, a process called perinatal transmission. In the United States, approximately 25% of pregnant HIV-infected women not receiving therapy pass on the virus to their babies.

Other factors that may increase the risk of perinatal transmission are:

- Maternal drug use

- Severe inflammation of fetal membranes

- Prolonged period between membrane rupture and delivery

HIV also may be transmitted from a nursing mother to her infant. Recent studies suggest that breastfeeding introduces an additional risk of HIV transmission among women with chronic HIV infection.

DIAGNOSIS

Because early HIV infection often causes no symptoms, it is primarily detected by testing blood for the presence of antibodies to HIV. Babies born to HIV-positive mothers may or may not be infected with the virus, but all carry their mothers' antibodies to HIV for several months. If these babies lack symptoms, a definitive diagnosis of HIV infection using standard antibody tests cannot be made until after 15 months of age.

By then, babies are unlikely to still carry their mothers' antibodies and will have produced their own if they are infected.

SYMPTOMS

Many people have no symptoms when they first become infected with HIV. Some people, however, have a flu-like illness within a month or two after exposure to the virus. Some signs and/or symptoms you might encounter are:

- Fever
- Headache
- Malaise
- Enlarged lymph nodes in the neck and groin

These symptoms usually disappear within a week to a month and are often mistaken for those of another viral infection. As the immune system deteriorates, a variety of complications begins to surface. One of the first such symptoms experienced by many people infected with HIV is enlarged lymph nodes for a period that may exceed 3 months. Other symptoms often experienced months to years before the onset of AIDS include:

- Lack of energy
- Weight loss
- Frequent fevers and sweats
- Persistent or frequent yeast infections (oral or vaginal)
- Persistent skin rashes or flaky skin
- Pelvic inflammatory disease that does not respond to treatment
- Short-term memory loss
- Delayed development or failure to thrive in children

AIDS

Acquired immunodeficiency syndrome (AIDS) is characterized by the loss of a specific subset of T lymphocytes. Progressive loss of these cells, known as CD4+ lymphocytes, leads to severe immunosuppression, neurologic complications, opportunistic infections, and neoplasms that rarely occur in healthy people with intact immune systems.

Most AIDS-defining conditions are opportunistic infections that rarely cause harm in healthy individuals. In people with AIDS, these infections are often severe and sometimes fatal because the immune system is so ravaged by HIV that the body cannot fight off certain bacteria, viruses, and other microbes. Infections cause a range of symptoms, including:

- Cough
- Dyspnea
- Seizures
- Confusion
- Memory loss
- Vision impairment
- Severe and persistent diarrhea
- Fever
- Severe headaches
- Extreme fatigue
- Nausea
- Vomiting
- Lack of coordination
- Coma

As AIDS further debilitates the immune system, patients become more susceptible to a variety of infections, including:

- Tuberculosis
- Cytomegalovirus infections
- Candidiasis
- Histoplasmosis
- Toxoplasmosis
- Pneumocystis carinii pneumonia (PCP)
- Kaposi sarcoma

CODING ISSUES

HIV disease is an important category in Chapter 1. HIV has become a major health care concern in the past decade, making the collection of accurate data vital to planning for treatment in the future. Diagnosis code B20 is assigned for all types of symptomatic HIV infections. HIV infection is only reported when confirmed by a positive serology report or the physician's diagnostic statement that the patient is HIV-positive or has an HIV-related illness.

Some of the conditions you may find in the documentation related to the patient's diagnosis are:

- Acquired immunodeficiency syndrome
- AIDS
- AIDS-related conditions
- HIV
- Prodromal AIDS
- AIDS-related complex or conditions (ARC)
- AIDS-like syndrome

The code for HIV (B20) is found in Chapter 1 of the Tabular List of ICD-10-CM and is not assigned when the diagnostic statement indicates "suspected," "probable," or "rule out."

Outpatient and/or physician diagnoses are selected based on confirmation of a diagnosis, not on suspicion or probability. However, the physician's documentation of a positive serology for HIV or a statement indicating the patient is HIV-positive or has an HIV-related illness is sufficient.

When coding HIV infection or an HIV-related illness, it is important to understand the codes available and their proper uses.

HIV ICD-10-CM GUIDELINES FOR HUMAN IMMUNODEFICIENCY VIRUS DISEASES

In ICD-10-CM the following codes are used when reporting the HIV virus, exposure, or screenings:

- B20, Human immunodeficiency virus (HIV) disease
- Z21, Asymptomatic human immunodeficiency virus (HIV) infection status
- R75, Inconclusive laboratory evidence of human immunodeficiency virus (HIV)
- Z20.6, Exposure to HIV virus
- Z11.4, Special screening for the human immunodeficiency virus (HIV)
- Z71.7, Human immunodeficiency virus (HIV) counseling
- O98.7, Human immunodeficiency (HIV) disease complicating pregnancy, childbirth and the puerperium

One complication subcategory exists for HIV complicating pregnancy, childbirth, and the puerperium, which is reported with subcategory O98.7–. Special

screening for the HIV virus is reported with code Z11.4, Screening for the human immunodeficiency virus (HIV).

B20 Human immunodeficiency virus (HIV) disease

Category B20 is used for symptomatic HIV patients. The patient will have had any of the opportunistic infections associated with HIV virus. The code for HIV is synonymous with the terms "acquired immune deficiency syndrome (AIDS)" and "AIDS replaced complex (ARC)" and includes acquired immune deficiency syndrome (AIDS) and AIDS-related complex (ARC) HIV infection, symptomatic.

Instructional notes in Category B20 indicate that all manifestations of the disease should be reported in addition to B20.

Use additional code(s) to identify all manifestations of HIV infection. This excludes:

- Asymptomatic human immunodeficiency virus (HIV) infection status (Z21)
- Exposure to HIV virus (Z20.6)
- Inconclusive serologic evidence of HIV (R75)

The appropriate code for a symptomatic HIV patient is B20 (HIV), adding an additional diagnosis code to identify the manifestations of the disease.

Review the following example:

> *EXAMPLE 1: A 42-year-old man arrives at his physician's office for a return visit. After examination, the physician reviews previous data and documents the diagnosis as HIV and Kaposi sarcoma of the lymph nodes.*

The encounter should be coded:

> *Primary Diagnosis:*
> *B20 HIV*
>
> *Secondary Diagnosis:*
> *C46.3 Kaposi sarcoma of lymph nodes*
>
> *Correct code sequencing:*
> *B20, C46.3*

CODING TIP When the patient is treated for an illness that is related to AIDS (HIV), B20 is reported as the first listed diagnosis followed by the condition treated.

CODING TIP When a patient is treated for an illness unrelated to HIV, list the unrelated illness as the first listed diagnosis and any HIV-related condition as secondary.

Sequencing

Patients with HIV-related illness should be assigned a minimum of two codes:

1. Assign B20 to identify the HIV disease.

2. Sequence additional codes to identify the other diagnosis/diagnoses.

If the patient with HIV disease has an unrelated condition, such as an injury (fracture), the code for the unrelated condition should be the first listed diagnosis. Other diagnoses would be B20 (HIV) followed by additional diagnosis codes for all reported HIV-related conditions treated. Review the following example.

> *EXAMPLE 2:* A 42-year-old patient falls off a riding lawn-mower and visits his local emergency room at the hospital, complaining of pain in his left arm. After examining the patient, the emergency room physician calls in the ortho-pedic surgeon who determines that the patient suffered a Galeazzi fracture of the left forearm with an injury to the distal radioulnar joint of the wrist. The patient is taken to surgery for repair of the fracture. The orthopedic surgeon also examines the patient regarding his AIDS condition prior to surgery. The surgeon performs a closed reduction with internal fixation to repair the fracture.

CODING TIP A Galeazzi fracture is a variant of a radius fracture of the forearm. In addition to the fracture of the radius, the patient also has an injury of the distal radial-ulnar joint of the wrist.

CODING TIP At the elbow, the humerus connects with two bones: the radius and the ulna. These bones go from the elbow to the wrist and are regarded as the forearm. The diagnosis indicated fracture of the left arm at the radius and that the patient has AIDS.

Open the ICD-10-CM codebook to the Alphabetic Index. Keep in mind the main term is "fracture." Review Figure 5.7:

FIGURE 5.7   Excerpt from the Alphabetic Index: *Fracture*

Fracture, traumatic
Forearm S52.9.-
  radius—see Fracture, radius
  ulna—see Fracture ulna

Now review the Tabular List S52.9.-, which is an unspecified fracture of the forearm. We know that this is a Galeazzi fracture, which is the lower shaft of

the radius. Return to the Index under the main term "fracture" radius. Now review Figure 5.8.

FIGURE 5.8   Excerpt from the Alphabetic Index: *Fracture*

Fracture, traumatic, radius
  shaft S52.30-
  bent bone S52.38-
  comminuted (displaced) S52.35-
  nondisplaced S52.335-
  Galeazzi's—see Galeazzi's fracture

Galeazzi's fracture S52.37.-

CODING TIP A (–) in the Index indicates additional digits are required and can only be located in the category or sub-classification for the particular code in the Tabular List.

Now turn to the Tabular List in ICD-10-CM and locate subclassification S52.37. Review Figure 5.9.

FIGURE 5.9   Excerpt from the Tabular List: *S52.37–*

S52.37 Galeazzi's fracture
    Fracture of lower shaft of radius with radioulnar joint
      dislocation

    ✓7th S52.371 Galeazzi's fracture of right radius
    ✓7th S52.372 Galeazzi's fracture of left radius
    ✓7th S52.379 Galeazzi's fracture of unspecified radius

In order to complete the code selection, this classifica-tion requires a seventh character, which is found in the Tabular List. Review Figure 5.10 (page 60).

Since this is a closed reduction and the initial encoun-ter, the seventh character is reported as "A."

The encounter should be coded:

> *First listed diagnosis:*
> S52.372A Galeazzi's fracture of left radius (left forearm), initial encounter

> *Secondary diagnosis:*
> B20 AIDS

> *Correct code sequencing:*
> S52.372A, B20

Note: People with HIV can get many infections. These are called opportunistic infections, or OIs.

FIGURE 5.10   Excerpt from the Tabular List: *Seventh character for S52.–*

The appropriate seventh character is to be added to each code from category S52:

A initial encounter for closed fracture

B initial encounter for open fracture type I or II initial encounter for open fracture NOS

C initial encounter for open fracture type IIIA, IIIB, or IIIC

D subsequent encounter for closed fracture with routine healing

E subsequent encounter for open fracture type I or II with routine healing

F subsequent encounter for open fracture type IIIA, IIIB, or IIIC with routine healing

G subsequent encounter for closed fracture with delayed healing

H subsequent encounter for open fracture type I or II with delayed healing

J subsequent encounter for open fracture type IIIA, IIIB, or IIIC with delayed healing

K subsequent encounter for closed fracture with nonunion

M subsequent encounter for open fracture type I or II with nonunion

N subsequent encounter for open fracture type IIIA, IIIB, or IIIC with nonunion

P subsequent encounter for closed fracture with malunion

Q subsequent encounter for open fracture type I or II with malunion

R subsequent encounter for open fracture type IIIA, IIIB, or IIIC with malunion

S sequela

Code Z21 is used for reporting a patient diagnosed with HIV-positive status but no opportunistic infections. One a patient gets his/her first opportunistic infection, the patient is assigned code B20 thereafter. The draft guidelines state: "A patient should never be assigned a Z21 code, even if at a particular encounter no infection or HIV related condition is present. Codes B20 and Z21 should never appear on the same record."

Confirmation of HIV status does not require documentation of positive serology or culture for HIV. Reporting is based on the physician's documentation that the patient has an HIV-related illness or is HIV positive.

Review the following example:

> **EXAMPLE:** *A patient visited an infectious disease specialist in follow-up after a positive HIV test. The physician took a detailed history and completed a comprehensive examination, determining the patient was otherwise healthy but needed routine follow-up to monitor his positive HIV status.*

Open the ICD-10-CM codebook to the Index and locate the main term. In this example, it is "status." Review Figure 5.11.

FIGURE 5.11   Excerpt from the Alphabetic Index: *Status*

Status
Human immunodeficiency virus (HIV), infection, asymptomatic Z21

Now review the Tabular List under Code Z21. Review Figure 5.12.

FIGURE 5.12   Excerpt from the Tabular List: *Z21*

Z21   Asymptomatic human immunodeficiency virus (HIV) infection
HIV positive NOS
Code first human immunodeficiency (HIV) disease complicating pregnancy, childbirth and the puerperium, if applicable (O98.7-)

EXCLUDES 1   acquired immunodeficiency syndrome(B20)
contact with human immunodeficiency virus (HIV) (Z20.6)
exposure to human immunodeficiency virus (HIV) (Z20.6)
human immunodeficiency syndrome (B20)
inconclusive laboratory evidence of human immunodeficiency virus (HIV) (R75)

The patient encounter is coded as Z21, Asymptomatic human immunodeficiency virus (HIV) infection status.

Z20.6 Contact with and exposure to human immunodeficiency virus (HIV)

Code Z20.6 is reported only when a patient believes he or she has been exposed or has come into contact with the HIV virus. In the instructional note there is an Excludes 1 not to exclude coding in this category for a patient who has been potentially exposed to the HIV virus but is not determined as positive.

Review the following example:

> **EXAMPLE:** *A 35-year-old nurse received a needle stick while drawing blood in the physician's office. She was sent to the hospital for an HIV test. The results were negative and the patient was advised to obtain another HIV test in 3 months.*

The encounter is reported as Z20.6, Contact or exposure to HIV virus.

R75 Inconclusive laboratory evidence of human immunodeficiency virus (HIV)

Code R75 is used when a patient has an inconclusive lab finding for HIV. This code is reported for newborns of HIV-positive mothers whose HIV status has not been confirmed. Review Figure 5.13.

FIGURE 5.13   Excerpt from the Tabular List: *R75*

> **R75   Inconclusive laboratory evidence of human immunodeficiency Virus [HIV]**
> nonconclusive HIV-test finding in infants
> **EXCLUDES 1**: asymptomatic human immunodeficiency
> virus [HIV] infection status (Z21) human
> immunodeficiency virus [HIV] disease (B20)

Review the following example:

> **EXAMPLE:** *A single live male was born to a female patient who is HIV positive. The laboratory finding came back inconclusive for the newborn. The pediatrician decided to watch the baby and repeat the blood work in two days.*
>
> **First listed diagnosis code:**
> *R75 Inconclusive laboratory evidence of human immunodeficiency virus (HIV)*

Z11.4 Encounter for screening for the human immunodeficiency virus (HIV)

If the patient is being tested to determine his or her HIV status, the diagnosis code reported is Z11.4. If the patient has other signs and/or symptoms (ie, abdominal pain, fever, cough, etc) in addition to being tested for HIV status report the signs/symptoms codes along with Z11.4. If the patient returns for his or her HIV results or if the practitioner feels it is appropriate, the practitioner may counsel the patient regarding safe practices, etc. If counseling occurs, also report Z71.7 for HIV counseling.

Review the following example:

> **EXAMPLE:** *A 25-year-old patient had unprotected sex with a stranger. The patient went to her family physician for an HIV test. The patient returned the following week for the results of her HIV test, which were negative. The nurse practitioner met with the patient to discuss safe sex practices at the second visit.*

The encounter should be coded:

> **Visit to hospital for HIV test:**
> *Z11.4 Special screening examination for other specified viral diseases*
>
> **Second visit to receive results:**
> *Z71.7 Human immunodeficiency virus (HIV) counseling*

HIV Infection in Pregnancy, Childbirth and the Puerperium (O98.7–)

The last code related to HIV is O98.7 HIV disease complicating pregnancy, childbirth and the puerperium. Notice in the example that the specificity of the subcategory is 6 digits beginning with the letter O. Diagnosis code(s) O98.71– is reported based on the trimester of pregnancy, whereas O98.72– is reported for HIV disease complicating childbirth and O98.73 is reported for complications of the puerperium.

The ICD-10-CM guidelines state: "during pregnancy, childbirth or the puerperium, a patient admitted (or presenting for a health related encounter) because of an HIV-related illness should receive a principal diagnosis code of O98.7– followed by B20 for the HIV-related illness. Codes from Chapter 15 always take sequencing priority. Patients with asymptomatic infection status either admitted or receiving care during pregnancy, childbirth or the puerperium should be coded as O98.7– and Z21 for the HIV positive status."

Review the following example:

> **EXAMPLE:** *A 27-year-old patient who is in her first trimester of pregnancy visited her obstetrician for her routine monthly visit. The patient is HIV positive with no signs of any manifestations. She is doing well. Her obstetrician reports the following: weight 163, pulse 118, BP 124/82'; Gen: Well developed well nourished, slender female; Alert and oriented and appears calm today. Gravid, non-tender to palpation; Skin: No Rash. No edema. Discussed diet, exercise, and vitamin regimen. Counseled patient on HIV status, and risk to fetus. Ultrasound will be performed at next visit.*

How would you find the code category in the Index? The main term necessary to code this encounter is "pregnancy" followed by "complicated by." Review Figure 5.14.

FIGURE 5.14   Excerpt from the Alphabetic Index: *Pregnancy, Complicated by*

> **Pregnancy, complicated by,**
> HIV O98.71-
> Human immunodeficiency [HIV] disease O98.7-

Open the codebook to the Tabular List in category O98.7–. Review Figure 5.15.

FIGURE 5.15   Excerpt from the Tabular List: *O98.7–*

O98.7	**Human immunodeficiency [HIV] disease complicating pregnancy, childbirth and the puerperium** Use additional code to identify the type of HIV disease: Acquired immune deficiency syndrome (AIDS) (B20) Asymptomatic HIV status (Z21) HIV positive NOS (Z21) Symptomatic HIV disease (B20)
O98.71	**Human immunodeficiency [HIV] disease complicating pregnancy**
O98.711	Human immunodeficiency [HIV] disease complicating pregnancy, first trimester
O98.712	Human immunodeficiency [HIV] disease complicating pregnancy, second trimester
O98.713	Human immunodeficiency [HIV] disease complicating pregnancy, third trimester
O98.719	Human immunodeficiency [HIV] disease complicating pregnancy, unspecified trimester
O98.72	**Human immunodeficiency [HIV] disease complicating childbirth**
O98.73	**Human immunodeficiency [HIV] disease complicating the puerperium**

Notice that the code assignment is based on the trimester of the patient. The instructional notes indicate an additional code must be used to report the status of the patient.

The encounter should be coded as follows:

First listed diagnosis:
O98.711 Human immunodeficiency [HIV] disease complicating pregnancy, first trimester

Secondary diagnosis:
Z21 Asymptomatic HIV status

Correct code sequencing:
O98.711, Z21

CODING TIP When a patient has HIV and is pregnant, codes from Chapter 15 of ICD-10-CM, Pregnancy, childbirth and the puerperium are always sequenced first. Code O98.7– should be sequenced second followed by the appropriate HIV code.

HIV Review Code B20 should be sequenced as the first listed diagnosis when the patient is treated for an

HIV-related condition. Any nonrelated conditions may also be sequenced following the related conditions. When an HIV patient is treated for an unrelated condition, the diagnosis code for the unrelated condition is listed first, followed by the HIV-related diagnosis code, which is either B20 for a symptomatic patient or Z21 for an asymptomatic patient.

GUIDELINE TIP: Code B20 should be sequenced as the first listed diagnosis when the patient is treated for an HIV-related condition.

CHECKPOINT EXERCISE 5-2

Using your ICD-10-CM codebook, code the following:

1. _____ Positive HIV blood test

2. _____ Kaposi sarcoma due to AIDS

3. _____ Asymptomatic HIV infection

4. _____ Exposure to HIV

5. _____ A patient with HIV-2 infection

6. _____ Inconclusive HIV serology

7. _____ Testing for HIV and the test results are negative

8. _____ Pregnant patient in her second trimester who has AIDS

9. _____ Patient with known prior diagnosis of an HIV-related illness should be reported with this diagnosis code.

10. _____ Acute salpingitis due to gonococcal infection

11. _____ A patient with known AIDS is admitted to the hospital for treatment of *Pneumocystis carinii* pneumonia.

12. _____ A patient with known hepatitis C seen in the outpatient department for Interferon treatment

13. _____ Typhoid fever

14. _____ Food poisoning due to Staphylococcus organism

15. _____ Pulmonary tuberculosis, bacilli identified with microscopy

Other Bacterial Diseases (A30-A49)

SEPTICEMIA

Septicemia is a serious, rapidly progressing, life-threatening infection that can arise from infections throughout the body, including infections in the lungs, abdomen, and urinary tract. It may precede or coincide with infections of the bone (osteomyelitis), central nervous system (meningitis), or other tissues.

Septicemia can develop quickly. A rash appears under the skin. This starts as a cluster of tiny spots, which look like pinpricks in the skin. If untreated, they get bigger and become multiple areas of obvious bleeding under the skin surface, like fresh bruises. The rash can appear anywhere on the body—even behind the ears or on the soles of the feet. It is more difficult to see the rash in darker-skinned individuals. The spots or bruises do not turn white when pressed.

Septicemia can rapidly lead to septic shock and death. Septicemia associated with some organisms such as meningococci can lead to shock, adrenal collapse, and disseminated intravascular coagulopathy, a condition called Waterhouse-Friderichsen syndrome.

The infection can begin with spiking fevers and chills, rapid breathing and heart rate, the outward appearance of being seriously ill (toxic), and a feeling of impending doom. These symptoms rapidly progress to shock with decreased body temperature (hypothermia), falling blood pressure, confusion or other changes in mental status, and blood-clotting abnormalities evidenced by hemorrhagic lesions in the skin (petechiae and ecchymosis).

Symptoms include:

- Fever (sudden onset, often spiking)
- Chills
- Toxic looking (looks acutely ill)
- Changes in mental state
  - irritable
  - lethargic
  - anxious
  - agitated
  - unresponsive
  - comatose

- Shock
  - cold
  - clammy
  - pale
  - cyanotic (blue)
  - unresponsive
- Skin signs associated with clotting abnormalities
  - petechiae
  - ecchymosis (often large, flat, purplish lesions that do not blanch when pressed)
  - gangrene (early changes in the extremities suggesting decreased or absent blood flow)
- Decreased or no urine output

Physical examination may reveal:

- Low blood pressure
- Low body temperature or fever
- Signs of associated disease (meningitis, epiglottitis, pneumonia, cellulitis, or others)

Tests that can confirm infection include:

- Blood culture, urine culture, colony-stimulating factor (CSF) culture, culture of any suspect skin lesion, complete blood cell count (CBC)
- Platelet count
- Clotting studies
  - prothrombin time (PT)
  - partial thromboplastin time (PTT)
  - fibrinogen levels
- Blood gas

This disorder must be treated in a hospital, usually with admission to an intensive care unit. Intravenous (IV) fluids are given to maintain blood pressure. Strong IV drugs, called sympathomimetics, are often needed to maintain blood pressure. Oxygen therapy is begun to maintain oxygen saturation.

The infection is treated with broad-spectrum antibiotics (those that are effective against a wide range of organisms) before the organism is identified. Once cultures have identified the specific organism that is responsible for the infection, antibiotics specific for that organism are begun. Plasma or other treatment may be needed to correct clotting abnormalities.

Expectations (prognosis)

Septic shock has a high death rate, exceeding 50%, depending on the type of organism involved. The organism involved and the immediacy of hospitalization will determine the outcome. Complications of this disease include:

- Irreversible shock
- Waterhouse-Friderichsen syndrome
- Adult respiratory distress syndrome (ARDS)

Bacteremia and septic shock are closely related conditions. Bacteremia denotes bacteria in the bloodstream. Septic shock is sepsis with hypoperfusion and hypotension refractory to fluid therapy. Sepsis refers to a serious infection, localized or bacteremic, that is accompanied by systemic manifestations of inflammation. Sepsis due to bacteremia is often called septicemia; this term is often imprecisely used and its use is now being discouraged. The more general term, "systemic inflammatory response syndrome (SIRS)," recognizes that several severe conditions (eg, infections, pancreatitis, burns, trauma) can trigger an acute inflammatory reaction, the systemic manifestations of which are associated with release into the bloodstream of a large number of endogenous mediators of inflammation.

SEPTICEMIA, SYSTEMIC INFLAMMATORY RESPONSE SYNDROME, SEPSIS, SEVERE SEPSIS, AND SEPTIC SHOCK CODING GUIDELINES

Sepsis

Sepsis refers to an infection due to any organism that triggers a systemic inflammatory response, that is, systemic inflammatory response syndrome (SIRS). All codes with sepsis in the title include the concept of SIRS. For cases of sepsis that do not result in any associated organ dysfunction, a single code for the type of sepsis should be used.

Review Table 5.1.

For other infections in which SIRS is present but sepsis is not in the code title, code R65.1, Systemic inflammatory response syndrome (SIRS), may also be assigned. For any infection, if associated organ dysfunction is present, a code from subcategory R65.2, Severe sepsis, should be used and the guidelines for coding of severe sepsis should be followed.

TABLE 5.1   Official Guidelines for Sepsis

1. (a) Sepsis	For a diagnosis of sepsis, assign the appropriate code for the underlying systemic infection. If the type of infection or causal organism is not further specified, assign code A41.9, Sepsis, unspecified.
	A code from subcategory R65.2, Severe sepsis, should not be assigned unless severe sepsis or an associated acute organ dysfunction is documented.
(i) Negative or inconclusive blood cultures and sepsis	Negative or inconclusive blood cultures do not preclude a diagnosis of sepsis in patients with clinical evidence of the condition. However, the provider should be queried.
(ii) Urosepsis	The term "urosepsis" is a nonspecific term. It is not to be considered synonymous with sepsis. It has no default code in the Alphabetic Index. If a provider uses this term, he/she must be queried for clarification.
(iii) Sepsis with organ dysfunction	If a patient has sepsis and associated acute organ dysfunction or multiple organ dysfunction (MOD), follow the instructions for coding severe sepsis.
(iv) Acute organ dysfunction that is not clearly associated with sepsis	If a patient has sepsis and an acute organ dysfunction, but the medical record documentation indicates that the acute organ dysfunction is related to a medical condition other than the sepsis, do not assign a code from subcategory R65.2, Severe sepsis.
	An acute organ dysfunction must be associated with the sepsis in order to assign the severe sepsis code. If the documentation is not clear as to whether an acute organ dysfunction is related to the sepsis or another medical condition, query the provider.
(b) Severe sepsis	The coding of severe sepsis requires a minimum of two codes: first a code for the underlying systemic infection, followed by a code from subcategory R65.2, Severe sepsis. If the causal organism is not documented, assign code A41.9, Sepsis, unspecified, for the infection. Additional code(s) for the associated acute organ dysfunction are also required.
	Due to the complex nature of severe sepsis, some cases may require querying the provider prior to assignment of the codes.

(continued)

TABLE 5.1   *(continued)*

2. Septic shock	Septic shock is circulatory failure associated with severe sepsis; therefore, it represents a type of acute organ dysfunction. For all cases of septic shock, the code for the underlying systemic infection should be sequenced first, followed by code R65.21, Severe sepsis with septic shock. Any additional codes for the other acute organ dysfunctions should also be assigned.
	Septic shock indicates the presence of severe sepsis. Code R65.21, Severe sepsis with septic shock, must be assigned if septic shock is documented in the medical record, even if the term "severe sepsis" is not documented.
3. Sequencing of severe sepsis	If severe sepsis is present on admission and meets the definition of principal diagnosis, the underlying systemic infection should be assigned as the principal diagnosis, followed by the appropriate code from subcategory R65.2 as required by the sequencing rules in the Tabular List. A code from subcategory R65.2 can never be assigned as a principal diagnosis.
	When severe sepsis develops during an encounter (it was not present on admission), the underlying systemic infection and the appropriate code from subcategory R65.2 should be assigned as secondary diagnoses.
	Severe sepsis may be present on admission, but the diagnosis may not be confirmed until some time after admission. If the documentation is not clear whether severe sepsis was present on admission, the provider should be queried.
4. Sepsis and severe sepsis with a localized infection	If the reason for admission is both sepsis or severe sepsis and a localized infection, such as pneumonia or cellulitis, a code(s) for the underlying systemic infection should be assigned first and the code for the localized infection should be assigned as a secondary diagnosis. If the patient has severe sepsis, a code from subcategory R65.2 should also be assigned as a secondary diagnosis. If the patient is admitted with a localized infection, such as pneumonia, and sepsis/severe sepsis does not develop until after admission, the localized infection should be assigned first, followed by the appropriate sepsis/severe sepsis codes.
5. Sepsis due to a postprocedural infection	Sepsis resulting from a postprocedural infection is a complication of medical care. For such cases, the postprocedural infection code, such as, T80.2, Infections following infusion, transfusion, and therapeutic injection; T81.4, Infection following a procedure; T88.0, Infection following immunization; or O86.0, Infection of obstetric surgical wound, should be coded first, followed by the code for the specific infection. If the patient has severe sepsis, the appropriate code from subcategory R65.2 should also be assigned with the additional code(s) for any acute organ dysfunction.
6. Sepsis and severe sepsis associated with a noninfectious process (condition)	In some cases, a noninfectious process (condition), such as trauma, may lead to an infection that can result in sepsis or severe sepsis. If sepsis or severe sepsis is documented as associated with a noninfectious condition, such as a burn or serious injury, and this condition meets the definition for principal diagnosis, the code for the noninfectious condition should be sequenced first, followed by the code for the resulting infection. If severe sepsis is present, a code from subcategory R65.2 should also be assigned with any associated organ dysfunction(s) codes. It is not necessary to assign a code from subcategory R65.1, Systemic inflammatory response syndrome (SIRS) of noninfectious origin, for these cases.
	If the infection meets the definition of principal diagnosis, it should be sequenced before the noninfectious condition. When both the associated noninfectious condition and the infection meet the definition of principal diagnosis, either may be assigned as the principal diagnosis.
	Only one code from category R65, Symptoms and signs specifically associated with systemic inflammation and infection, should be assigned. Therefore, when a noninfectious condition leads to an infection resulting in severe sepsis, assign the appropriate code from subcategory R65.2, Severe sepsis. Do not additionally assign a code from subcategory R65.1, Systemic inflammatory response syndrome (SIRS) of noninfectious origin.
7. Sepsis and septic shock complicating abortion, pregnancy, childbirth, and the puerperium	See Section I.C.15, Sepsis and septic shock complicating abortion, pregnancy, childbirth, and the puerperium
8. Newborn sepsis	See Section I.C.16, Newborn sepsis

Codes for sepsis and septic shock associated with abortion, ectopic pregnancy, and molar pregnancy are in Chapter 15. Code R65.1 and a code from R65.2 should not be used together on the same record.

Review the following example:

> **EXAMPLE:** *A 78-year-old male is treated in the hospital for symptoms of nausea, persistent fever, hyperventilation, and prostration. After a comprehensive history and examination, the physician determines the patient has streptococcal septicemia with severe SIRS, which is causing the patient to go into acute renal failure.*

Open the ICD-10-CM codebook to Sepsis and review Figure 5.16.

FIGURE 5.16   Excerpt from the Alphabetic Index: *Sepsis*

```
Sepsis
With
  Streptococcus, streptococcal A40.9
  Agalactiae A40.1
  group
          A A40.0
          B A40.1
          D A41.81
  Neonatal P36.10
```

Alphabetic Index:

Sepsis → with → streptococcal → A40.9

Sepsis (generalized) → with acute organ dysfunction R65.2–

Failure → renal → acute N17.9

Tabular List:

A40.9 Streptococcal sepsis, unspecified

R65.20 Severe sepsis without septic shock

N17.9 Unspecified acute renal failure

The correct code sequence is A40.9, R65.20, N17.9.

> **EXAMPLE:** *This is a 53-year-old male who presented in the emergency room for ground-level fall secondary to weak knees. He complained of epigastric pain for at least a month. In the ER he was initially afebrile but then spiked up to 101.3 with heart rate of 130, respiratory rate of 24. White blood cell count was slightly low at 4, and platelet count was only 22,000. Abdominal ultrasound showed mild-to-moderate ascites. The patient was admitted to the hospital from the ER. Laboratory data as follows: White count is down from 35,000 to 15.5. Hemoglobin is 9.5, hematocrit is 30, and platelets are 269,000. BUN is down to 22, creatinine is within normal limits. The patient was*

diagnosed with sepsis due to urinary Escherichia (E) coli. Urine culture shows E. coli resistant to Levaquin. Medication was changed to doripenem. The patient will be treated with doripenem.

In this example, the diagnosis is sepsis due to a urinary tract infection. Open the ICD-10-CM codebook and look up the main term "sepsis." See if you can find the correct code in the tabular list.

> **Alphabetic List:**
>
> Sepsis → due to → Escherichia coli [E. Coli] A41.5
>
> **Tabular List:**
>
> A41.51 → Sepsis due to Escherichia coli [E. Coli]

In this example, there is a combination code to report the sepsis due to the *E. coli* bacteria.

> **Correct code(s):**
>
> A41.51

REVIEW THE ICD-10-CM EXAMPLE OF SIRS AND SEPSIS CATEGORIES

R65.1 Systemic inflammatory response syndrome (SIRS)

Excludes 1: sepsis, code to infection severe sepsis (R65.2–)

R65.2– Severe sepsis infection with organ dysfunction, code first underlying infection, use additional code to identify specific organ dysfunction, such as acute renal failure.

(N17.–) acute kidney failure

(J96.0) acute respiratory failure

(G72.81) critical illness myopathy

(G62.81) critical illness polyneuropathy encephalopathy (metabolic) (septic) (G93.41) hepatic failure (K72.0–)

R65.20 Severe sepsis without septic shock

Severe sepsis NOS

R65.21 Severe sepsis with septic shock

The terms "bacteremia" and "septicemia NOS" are coded to R78.81. If a patient with a serious infection is documented to have septicemia, the physician should be asked if the patient has sepsis. If any organ dysfunction is documented, the physician should be asked if the patient has severe sepsis. Negative or inconclusive blood cultures do not preclude a diagnosis of sepsis in patients with clinical evidence of the condition.

R78.8 Finding of other specified substances, not normally found in blood

R78.81 Bacteremia Septicemia NOS

Excludes 1: sepsis-code to specified infection (A00-B99)

CODING TIP The term "urosepsis" is a nonspecific term. If a physician uses the term in a medical record, he or she should be asked for which specific condition is the term being used.

Infectious Agents as the Cause of Diseases Classified to Other Chapters

Certain infections are classified in chapters other than Chapter 1 and no organism is identified as part of the infection code. In these instances, it is necessary to use an additional code from Chapter 1 of ICD-10-CM to identify the organism. A code from category B95, Streptococcus, Staphylococcus and Enterococcus as the cause of diseases classified to other chapters; B96, Other bacterial agents as the cause of diseases classified to other chapters; or B97, Viral agents as the cause of diseases classified to other chapters is to be used as an additional code to identify the organism. An instructional note will be found at the infection code advising that an additional organism code is required.

Nosocomial Infections

Nosocomial infections are those that originate or occur in a hospital or hospital-like setting. Nosocomial infections are responsible for approximately 20,000 deaths in the United States per year. Approximately 10% of American hospital patients (about 2 million every year) acquire a clinically significant nosocomial infection.

If a patient contracts an infection while in the hospital, assign code Y95, Nosocomial condition, in addition to the diagnosis code for the infection code to identify the infection as nosocomially acquired. ICD-10-CM code Y95 is a 3-digit classification.

ICD-10-CM Chapter 2 Neoplasms

Chapter 2 in the Tabular List includes the following sections:

- Malignant neoplasms (C00-C96)
- Carcinoma in situ (D00-D09)
- Benign neoplasms (D10-D36)
- Uncertain behavior (D37-D48)
- Unspecified behavior (D49)

MALIGNANT NEOPLASMS

Malignant neoplasms are composed of tumor cells that can invade surrounding structures or distant organs. Their growth is more rapid than that of benign neoplasms. ICD-10-CM classifies malignant neoplasms as:

- Primary
- Secondary
- Carcinoma in situ

Primary identifies the site of origin of the neoplasm. The point of origin is determined through the study of the morphology (form and structure) of the tumor cell. Determination of the point of origin and type of cells is important in establishing the severity of illness and in planning treatment.

> **EXAMPLE:** Primary lung cancer—site where cancer originates.

Secondary identifies the site(s) to which the primary tumor has spread by direct extension to surrounding tissues or metastasized by:

- Lymphatic spread
- Invasion of blood vessels
- Implantation as tumor cells are shed into body cavities

The morphology of a metastatic neoplasm is the same as that of the primary neoplasm.

> **EXAMPLE:** Secondary liver cancer—site where cancer has metastasized to or spread to.

CARCINOMA IN SITU

Carcinoma in situ is composed of tumor cells that are undergoing malignant changes. However, these changes do not extend beyond the point of origin or invade surrounding normal tissue.

Carcinoma in situ is also described as:

- Noninfiltrating carcinoma

- Noninvasive carcinoma

- Preinvasive carcinoma

    EXAMPLE: *Carcinoma in situ of the skin.*

BENIGN NEOPLASMS

Benign neoplasms are tumors that do not invade adjacent structures or spread to distant sites. Their growth may displace or exert pressure on adjacent structures. Some benign neoplasms have no potential for malignancy. However, others, such as adenomatous gastric polyps, have a premalignant potential and removal is indicated. Fortunately, most benign tumors can be completely excised.

    EXAMPLE: *Benign neoplasm of liver.*

Uncertain Behavior

The classification of uncertain behavior includes tumors that show features of both benign and malignant behavior. These tumors may require further study before a definitive diagnosis can be established. The codes in this category should be assigned only when documentation by the pathologist clearly indicates that the behavior of the neoplasm cannot be identified.

If neither the behavior nor the histologic type of tumor is specified in the diagnostic statement, a neoplasm is classified to be of unspecified nature. This situation may be encountered when the patient has been treated elsewhere and now is treated at a different facility without accompanying information to identify the nature or type of neoplasm. This situation also may be encountered when the patient is referred elsewhere for definitive workup or when workup is not performed because of the patient's advanced age or poor condition.

    EXAMPLE: *Neoplasm of skin, uncertain behavior.*

Unspecified Behavior

The category for unspecified behavior is to be used only when a diagnosis (behavior or morphology) cannot be clearly identified in the medical record. Many reasons for coding unspecified behavior exist. One reason could be that the patient has moved to a new location and the physician does not have access to the patient's previous medical record or the patient is sent to another facility for further study to determine the exact nature of the neoplasm.

ICD-10-CM classifies neoplasms by:

- System (eg, respiratory)

- Organ (eg, intrathoracic organs)

- Site (eg, tract, upper)

Exceptions to this are:

- Lymphatic neoplasms

- Hematopoietic neoplasms

- Malignant melanoma of the skin

- Some common tumors of

    • bone

    • uterus

    • ovary

Because of these exceptions, the Alphabetic Index should be checked first to see if there is a specific code assigned to a listed morphologic type, such as:

- Sarcoma

- Adenoma

- Melanoma

Codes for neoplasms are indicated by anatomical site. For each site, there are 6 possible codes indicating whether the neoplasm is malignant, primary, secondary, or carcinoma in situ and whether it is benign, of uncertain behavior, or unspecified. Be careful to code to the highest degree of specificity.

When coding neoplasms, ask the following questions:

- Where did it originate?

- Where is the neoplasm currently?

- What has been its cause?

Neoplasms are located in Chapter 2 of the Tabular List. "Neoplasm" is the medical term for any abnormal growth, commonly referred to as a tumor. Benign and/or malignant lesions are called neoplasms. Physicians must distinguish between malignant (cancerous) and benign (noncancerous) neoplasms. Coding neoplasms requires a good understanding of anatomy and medical terminology.

ICD-10-CM Official Guidelines for Coding Neoplasms

It is important before coding neoplasms that you have a good understanding of the types of neoplasms. As we review the guidelines we will discuss the various types of neoplasms. When coding neoplasms, the Alphabetic Index should be referenced first if the histological term is documented rather than going directly to the neoplasm Table. In some cases the histology may not be listed. If the term in the documentation indicates "adenoma," reference the adenoma first instead of immediately referencing the Neoplasm Table for any additional instructional notes. Also before selecting the code, always verify the code in the Tabular List. In this section, we will review the ICD-10-CM Guidelines for reporting neoplasms. It is important to understand the guidelines when coding neoplasms in order to code them accurately. Each time you code a neoplasm it is recommended that you review the guidelines for the particular situation before submitting the claim to an insurance carrier or government carrier.

Neoplasm Table

ICD-10-CM Chapter 2 contains codes for most benign and malignant neoplasms.

In order to properly code neoplasms, the documentation in the medical record must indicate the neoplasm is benign, in situ, malignant, or of uncertain histologic behavior. If there is a malignancy, the secondary (metastatic) site should also be reported as it is currently done with ICD-9-CM.

As noted, there is a separate Table of Neoplasms. Codes should be selected from this table. The guidelines in ICD-10-CM state, "If the histology (cell type) of the neoplasm is documented, that term should be referenced first, in the main section of the Index, rather than going immediately to the Neoplasm Table, in order to determine which column in the Neoplasm Table is appropriate." Before we review neoplasms, open the ICD-10-CM codebook to the Alphabetic Index and find the Neoplasm Table. See Table 6.3 for an example of this table.

The table is divided into the following categories:

- Malignant
- Primary
- Secondary
- Ca in situ
- Benign
- Uncertain behavior
- Unspecified

Now review the guidelines when treatment is directed at the malignancy.

Guideline C2.a Treatment directed at the malignancy

If the treatment is directed at the malignancy, designate the malignancy as the principal diagnosis.

The only exception to this guideline is if a patient admission/encounter is solely for the administration of chemotherapy, immunotherapy, or radiation therapy. In these instances, assign the appropriate Z51.– code as the first listed or principal diagnosis and the diagnosis or problem for which the service is being performed as a secondary diagnosis.

The malignancy may be the primary site or the secondary site. The primary site is where the cancer originated. The secondary site is the site where the cancer metastasized, or spread, to. For example, if the patient has cancer of the bladder (originating site) and the cancer spreads to the lungs and treatment is directed to the lungs, the secondary site will be the principal or first listed diagnosis.

The only time you would not report where treatment is directed is when a patient's admission/encounter is solely for the administration of chemotherapy, immunotherapy, or radiation therapy. In these instances, assign the appropriate Z51.– code as the first listed or principal diagnosis and the diagnosis or problem for which the service is being performed as a secondary diagnosis.

For example, if the patient is being treated for lung cancer and the patient is undergoing chemotherapy, the chemotherapy code Z51.11 is reported first and the malignancy of the lung is reported as the secondary diagnosis. Review the following example:

EXAMPLE: A 37-year-old female patient with a malignant tumor confirmed by pathology was taken to the operating room for an excision of the tumor. The physician was able to get the entire tumor from the lower-outer quadrant of the left breast. The patient will be scheduled for radiation therapy in the next few days.

FIGURE 5.17 Excerpt from the Tabular List: *C50.5*

C50.5 Malignant neoplasm of lower-outer quadrant
of breast
    C50.51 Malignant neoplasm of lower-outer quadrant of
breast, female
        C50.511 Malignant neoplasm of lower-outer
quadrant of right female breast
        C50.512 Malignant neoplasm of lower-outer
quadrant of left female breast
        C50.519 Malignant neoplasm of lower-outer
quadrant of unspecified female breast

Review Figure 5.17.

Neoplasm Table:
Neoplasm ➔ breast ➔ lower-outer quadrant ➔
C50.5–

Tabular List:
C50.5 ➔ C50.512 ➔ Malignant neoplasm of lower-
outer quadrant of left female breast

Correct code(s):
C50.512

CODING TIP Laterality may be important in the proper
selection of a diagnosis code for neoplasms. Pay careful
attention when coding these conditions.

The guidelines for ICD-10-CM indicate that a confirmed malignancy diagnosis is not reported without a pathology report on the record to confirm the histologic type of neoplasm. If the pathology report is not in the medical record, the attending physician must confirm the diagnosis in the medical record documentation. The pathology report is not required for encounters such as chemotherapy or radiation therapy.

> **EXAMPLE:** A physician diagnosed a 54-year-old female patient with cancer of the epiglottis. The physician's documentation indicated it as the primary site. The Alphabetic Index should be reviewed prior to referencing the Neoplasm Table.

The first step is to reference the Alphabetic Index for the main term:

> **Main term:**
> Carcinoma ➔ see also Neoplasm, malignant by site

The Alphabetic Index identifies adenocarcinoma as a malignancy reported by site. The coder then will reference the Neoplasm Table for selection of the correct code. Review Table 5.2 (Neoplasm Table example) and find the correct code for the malignancy.

TABLE 5.2 Excerpt from Neoplasm Table from the ICD-10-CM Codebook

	MALIGNANT PRIMARY	MALIGNANT SECONDARY	CA IN SITU	BENIGN	UNCERTAIN BEHAVIOR	UNSPECIFIED BEHAVIOR
digestive organs, system, tube, or tract NEC	C26.9	C78.89	D01.9	D13.9	D37.9	D49.0
disc, intervertebral	C41.2	C79.51	–	D16.6–	D48.0	D49.2
disease, generalized	C80.0	–	–	–	–	–
disseminated	C80.0	–	–	–	–	–
Douglas' cul-de-sac or pouch	C48.1	C78.6	–	D20.1	D48.4	D49.0
duodenojejunal junction	C17.8	C78.4	D01.49	D13.39	D37.2	D49.0
duodenum	C17.0	C78.4	D01.49	D13.2	D37.2	D49.0
dura (cranial) (mater)	C70.9	C79.49	–	D32.9	D42.9	D49.7
cerebral	C70.0	C79.32	–	D32.0	D42.0	D49.7
spinal	C70.1	C79.49	–	D32.1	D42.1	D49.7
ear (external)	C44.2–	C79.89	–	–	–	–
auricle or auris	C44.2–	C79.2–	D04.2–	D23.2–	D48.5	D49.2
canal, external	C44.2–	C79.2–	D04.2–	D23.2–	D48.5	D49.2
cartilage	C49.0	C79.89	–	D21.0	D48.1	D49.2
external meatus	C44.2	C79.2–	D04.2–	D23.2–	D48.5	D49.2
inner	C30.1	C78.39	D02.3	D14.0	D38.5	D49.1
lobule	C44.2–	C79.2–	D04.2–	D23.2–	D48.5	D49.2
middle	C30.1	C78.39	D02.3	D14.0	D38.5	D49.1

(continued)

TABLE 5.2 *(continued)*

	MALIGNANT PRIMARY	MALIGNANT SECONDARY	CA IN SITU	BENIGN	UNCERTAIN BEHAVIOR	UNSPECIFIED BEHAVIOR
overlapping lesion with accessory sinuses	C31.8	–	–	–	–	–
skin	C44.2–	C79.2–	D04.2–	D23.2–	D48.5	D49.2
earlobe	C44.2–	C79.2–	D04.2–	D23.2–	D48.5	D49.2
ejaculatory duct	C63.7	C79.82	D07.69	D29.8	D40.8	D49.5
elbow NEC	C76.4–	C79.89	D04.6–	D36.7	D48.7	D49.89
endocardium	C38.0	C79.89	–	D15.1	D48.7	D49.89
endocervix (canal) (gland)	C53.0	C79.82	D06.0	D26.0	D39.0	D49.5
endocrine gland NEC	C75.9	C79.89	D09.3	D35.9	D44.9	D49.7
endometrium (gland) (stroma)	C54.1	C79.82	D07.0	D26.1	D39.0	D49.5
ensiform cartilage	C41.3	C79.51	–	D16.7–	D48.0	D49.2
enteric-see Neoplasm, intestine						
ependyma (brain)	C71.5	C79.31	–	D33.0	D43.0	D49.6
fourth ventricle	C71.7	C79.31	–	D33.1	D43.1	D49.6
epicardium	C38.0	C79.89	–	D15.1	D48.7	D49.89
epididymis	C63.0–	C79.82	D07.69	D29.3–	D40.8	D49.5
epidural	C72.9	C79.49	–	D33.9	D43.9	D49.7
epiglottis	C32.1	C78.39	D02.0	D14.1	D38.0	D49.1
anterior aspect or surface	C10.1	C79.89	D00.08	D10.5	D37.05	D49.0
cartilage	C32.3	C78.39	D02.0	D14.1	D38.0	D49.1
free border (margin)	C10.1	C79.89	D00.08	D10.5	D37.05	D49.0
junctional region	C10.8	C79.89	D00.08	D10.5	D37.05	D49.0
posterior (laryngeal) surface	C32.1	C78.39	D02.0	D14.1	D38.0	D49.1
suprahyoid portion	C32.1	C78.39	D02.0	D14.1	D38.0	D49.1
esophagogastric junction	C16.0	C78.89	D00.2	D13.1	D37.1	D49.0
esophagus	C15.9	C78.89	D00.1	D13.0	D37.8	D49.0
abdominal	C15.5	C78.89	D00.1	D13.0	D37.8	D49.0
cervical	C15.3	C78.89	D00.1	D13.0	D37.8	D49.0

If you selected C32.1 from the Neoplasm Table, you are correct. Since this is a malignant neoplasm and the primary site is the epiglottis, the code is selected from the first column, or "Malignant primary." Don't forget to reference the Tabular List to confirm the correct code. Now find C32.1 in the Tabular List of ICD-10-CM.

Tabular List:
C32.1 Malignant neoplasm of supraglottic →
Malignant neoplasm of epiglottis

NOS

Correct code(s):
C32.1

The Neoplasm Table provides proper coding based on the histology of the neoplasm by site. The Tabular List should be referenced to verify that the correct code has been selected and a more specific code does not exist.

Guideline C2.b Treatment of Secondary Site

When a patient is admitted because of a primary neoplasm with metastasis and treatment is directed toward the secondary site only, the secondary neoplasm is designated as the principal diagnosis even though the primary malignancy is still present. However, in this instance, the primary site or origin of the cancer is reported as the secondary diagnosis. Review the following example. Open your ICD-10-CM codebook and locate the code for this situation.

CODING TIP When an encounter is for primary malignancy with metastasis and treatment is directed at the metastatic site only:

- The secondary site (metastatic site) is designated as the first listed diagnosis

- The primary site is listed with an additional code

    EXAMPLE: A patient was diagnosed with a malignant cancer of the left bronchus with metastasis to the liver and intraheptic bile duct. The patient's treatment is for liver cancer.

    Neoplasm Table:
        Neoplasm ➞ *liver* ➞ *C78.7*

    Tabular List:
        C78.7 ➞ *Secondary malignant neoplasm of liver and intrahepatic bile duct*

Note: The code in the Neoplasm Table is selected from the secondary column because the treatment is directed to the metastasis site.

But you are not finished yet. In order to properly report the patient encounter, the primary site must be coded as the secondary diagnosis even when treatment is not directed to this site. The primary site in this encounter is the malignant neoplasm of the bronchus, which must be coded as follows:

Neoplasm Table:
    Neoplasm ➞ *bronchus* ➞ *C34.9*

Tabular List:
    C34.9 ➞ *Malignant neoplasm of unspecified part of bronchus or lung* ➞ *C34.92 Malignant neoplasm of unspecified part of left bronchus or lung*

Correct code sequencing:
    C78.7, C34.92

Guideline C2.c Coding and Sequencing of Complications

Coding and sequencing of complications associated with malignancies or with the therapy thereof are subject to the following guideline:

1. Anemia associated with malignancy: When admission/encounter is for management of an anemia associated with the malignancy, and the treatment is only for anemia, the appropriate code for the malignancy is sequenced as the principal or first listed diagnosis followed by code D63.0, Anemia in neoplastic disease.

Review the following example:

EXAMPLE: A patient was diagnosed with a primary malignancy of the frontal lobe. The patient was also suffering from anemia due to the tumor.

Alphabetic Index:
    Anemia ➞ *in neoplastic disease D63.0*

Tabular List:
    D63.0 Anemia in neoplastic disease

Coding conventions require that the neoplasm code be sequenced first. Open the ICD-10 codebook to the Neoplasm Table and locate the code for malignant neoplasm of the frontal lobe. Make certain you select the code from the appropriate column and verify the code in the Tabular List.

Here is how the encounter should be coded:

First listed diagnosis:
    C71.1 Malignant neoplasm of frontal lobe

Secondary diagnosis:
    D63.0 Anemia in neoplastic disease

Correct code sequencing:
    C71.1, D63.0

CODING TIP Always follow the guidelines carefully when coding neoplasms because each situation is unique.

2. Anemia associated with chemotherapy, immunotherapy, and radiation therapy: When the admission/encounter is for management of an anemia associated with an adverse effect of chemotherapy or immunotherapy and the only treatment is for the anemia, the appropriate adverse effect code should be sequenced first, followed by the appropriate codes for the anemia and neoplasm.

Review the following example.

EXAMPLE: A patient was experiencing nausea and vomiting following radiation therapy for treatment of a malignant tumor of the parathyroid gland. After examination, the physician determined the patient was suffering from dehydration and ordered IV therapy.

Open the ICD-10-CM codebook and locate the correct codes and sequencing. Because the reason for the encounter is the condition, that is, nausea and vomiting, this is the first listed code. The secondary code will be the anemia, and the third listed code is the reason for the treatment, the malignant neoplasm. Review how the encounter should be coded.

First listed diagnosis:
  R11.0 Nausea with vomiting

Secondary diagnosis:
  D63.0 Anemia in neoplastic disease

Tertiary diagnosis:
  C75.0 Malignant neoplasm of parathyroid gland

Correct code sequencing:
  R11.0, D63.0, C75.0

When the admission/encounter is for management of an anemia associated with an adverse effect of radiotherapy, the anemia code should be sequenced first, followed by the appropriate neoplasm code, and then code Y84.2, Radiological procedure and radiotherapy as the cause of abnormal reaction of the patient, or of later complication, without mention of misadventure at the time of the procedure.

3. Management of dehydration due to the malignancy: When the admission/encounter is for management of dehydration due to the malignancy and only the dehydration is being treated (intravenous rehydration), the dehydration is sequenced first, followed by the code(s) for the malignancy.

Review the following example:

  EXAMPLE: A patient was admitted to the hospital for IV rehydration following chemotherapy for a primary malignancy of the ethmoidal sinus.

Open the ICD-10-CM codebook and locate the correct code(s) and sequencing based on the guidelines. Here is how the encounter should be coded:

First listed diagnosis:
  E86.0 Dehydration

Secondary diagnosis:
  C31.1 Malignant neoplasm of ethmoidal sinus

Correct code sequencing:
  E86.0, C31.1

4. Treatment of a complication resulting from a surgical procedure: When the admission/encounter is for treatment of a complication resulting from a surgical procedure, designate the complication as the principal, or first listed, diagnosis if treatment is directed at resolving the complication.

Review the following example:

  EXAMPLE: A patient was treated for streptococcal sepsis two days after surgery for the removal of a malignant tumor of the lateral wall of the bladder.

The first listed diagnosis for this encounter is the complication "sepsis" followed by the malignancy.

Open the ICD-10-CM codebook and look up the main term "sepsis."

Alphabetic Index:
  Sepsis ➝ streptococcal ➝ A40.9

Tabular List:
  A40.9 ➝ Streptococcal sepsis unspecified

Note: There is an instructional note under the classification A40.9 that directs the user to code the postprocedural streptococcal sepsis (T81.4) first. The next step is to reference T81.4.

Tabular List:
  ✓7th T81.4 ➝ Infection following a procedure

This code category requires a seventh character extension. However, this code has only 4 digits. In order to report the seventh character, we must use dummy placeholders (x) to complete the code. Review Figure 5.18. Because this is the initial encounter, the seventh character reported is "A."

FIGURE 5.18   Excerpt from the Tabular List: *T81.4*

The appropriate seventh character is to be added to each code from category T81

A	initial encounter
D	subsequent Encounter
S	sequela

But you are not finished yet. The malignant neoplasm of the lateral wall of the bladder must be reported as an additional diagnosis. Refer to the Neoplasm Table.

Neoplasm Table:
  Neoplasm ➝ bladder ➝ lateral wall ➝ primary site ➝ C67.2

Tabular List:
  C67.2 ➝ Malignant neoplasm of lateral wall of bladder

First listed diagnosis:
  A40.9 Streptococcal sepsis unspecified

Secondary diagnosis:
  T81.4xxA Infection following a procedure, not elsewhere classified

Tertiary diagnosis:
  C67.2 Malignant neoplasm of lateral wall of bladder

Correct code sequencing:
  A40.9, T81.4xxA, C67.2

C2.d Primary Malignancy Previously Excised

When a primary malignancy has been previously excised or eradicated from its site and there is no further treatment directed to that site and there is no evidence of any existing primary malignancy, a code from category Z85, Personal history of malignant neoplasm, should be used to indicate the former site of the malignancy. Any mention of extension, invasion, or metastasis to another site is coded as a secondary malignant neoplasm to that site.

> **EXAMPLE:** *A 56-year-old male was seen in follow-up after removal of the prostate 3 years ago for a malignancy.*
>
> **First listed diagnosis code:**
> *Z85.46 Personal history of primary malignant neoplasm of prostate*

CODING TIP The secondary site may be the principal or first listed, with the Z85 code used as a secondary code.

C2.e Admission/encounters involving chemotherapy, immunotherapy and radiation therapy

1. Episode of care involves surgical removal of neoplasm.

When an episode of care involves the surgical removal of a neoplasm, primary or secondary site, followed by adjunct chemotherapy or radiation treatment during the same episode of care, the code for the neoplasm should be assigned as principal, or first listed, diagnosis. Review the following example.

> **EXAMPLE:** *A patient was referred to a surgeon with suspected carcinoma of the colon. Laparotomy was carried out, and a significant mass (malignancy) was discovered in the sigmoid colon. The affected part of the colon was resected and closed with an end-to-end anastomosis. The patient received the first course of chemotherapy the same day.*

Open the ICD-10-CM codebook and locate the code(s) for this encounter. When following the guidelines, the first listed diagnosis code is the malignancy followed by the chemotherapy treatment.

> **Neoplasm Table:**
> *Neoplasm ➝ colon ➝ sigmoid ➝ C18.7*
>
> **Tabular List:**
> *C18.7 ➝ Malignant neoplasm of sigmoid colon*
>
> **Alphabetic Index:**
> *Chemotherapy ➝ session (for) ➝ cancer ➝ Z51.11*
>
> **Tabular List:**
> *Z51.11 ➝ Encounter for actineoplastic chemotherapy*
>
> **Correct code sequencing:**
> *C18.7, Z51.11*

2. Patient admission/encounter solely for administration of chemotherapy, immunotherapy, and radiation therapy.

If a patient admission/encounter is solely for the administration of chemotherapy, immunotherapy, or radiation therapy, assign code Z51.0, Encounter for antineoplastic radiation therapy, or Z51.11, Encounter for antineoplastic chemotherapy, or Z51.12, Encounter for antineoplastic immunotherapy as the first listed, or principal, diagnosis. If a patient receives more than one of these therapies during the same admission, more than one of these codes may be assigned, in any sequence.

The malignancy for which the therapy is being administered should be assigned as a secondary diagnosis.

> **EXAMPLE:** *A physician removed a malignant tumor from the descending colon in the outpatient surgery center. The physician recommended that the patient undergo chemotherapy in one week. The patient returned today for his chemotherapy treatment.*
>
> **First listed diagnosis:**
> *Z51.11 Encounter for actineoplastic chemotherapy*
>
> **Secondary diagnosis:**
> *C18.6 Malignant neoplasm of descending colon*
>
> **Correct code sequencing:**
> *Z51.11, C18.6*

3. Patient admitted for radiation therapy, chemotherapy, or immunotherapy and develops complications. When a patient is admitted for the purpose of radiotherapy, immunotherapy, or chemotherapy and develops complications such as uncontrolled nausea and vomiting or dehydration, the principal or first listed diagnosis is Z51.0, Encounter for antineoplastic radiation therapy, or Z51.11, Encounter for antineoplastic chemotherapy, or Z51.12, Encounter for antineoplastic immunotherapy followed by any codes for the complications.

Review the following example:

> **EXAMPLE:** *The patient who was experiencing nausea and vomiting immediately after chemotherapy was admitted for treatment of a primary malignancy of the left lower inner quadrant breast.*

First listed diagnosis:
Z51.11 Encounter for actineoplastic chemotherapy

Secondary diagnosis:
R11.0 Nausea with vomiting

Tertiary diagnosis:
C50.312 Malignant neoplasm of lower-inner quadrant of left female breast

C2.f Admission/encounter to determine extent of malignancy

When the reason for admission/encounter is to determine the extent of the malignancy or for a procedure such as paracentesis or thoracentesis, the primary malignancy or appropriate metastatic site is designated as the principal or first listed diagnosis, even though chemotherapy or radiotherapy is administered.

Review the following example.

EXAMPLE: *A patient is diagnosed with Burkitt's lymphoma of the intrapelvic lymph nodes and is admitted to the hospital by his oncologist . The patient was admitted to determine the extent of the malignancy. A biopsy is scheduled for tomorrow.*

Open the ICD-10-CM codebook and review the index for the main term "Burkitt."

Alphabetic Index:
Burkitt ➡ lymphoma (malignant) ➡ C83.7

Tabular List:
C83.7 ➡ Burkitt lymphoma ➡ C83.76 ➡ Burkitt lymphoma, intra pelvic lymph nodes

Correct code(s):
C83.76 Burkitt lymphoma, intra pelvic lymph nodes

C2.g Symptoms, signs, and abnormal findings listed in Chapter 18 associated with neoplasms

Symptoms, signs, and ill-defined conditions listed in Chapter 18 characteristic of, or associated with, an existing primary or secondary site malignancy cannot be used to replace the malignancy as the principal or first listed diagnosis, regardless of the number of admissions or encounters for treatment and care of the neoplasm.

See section I.C.21. Factors influencing health status and contact with health services, Example:

Encounter for prophylactic organ removal of the ovary for neoplastic management

Alphabetic Index:
Prophylactic ➡ organ removal (for neoplastic management ➡ ovary ➡ Z40.02

Tabular List:
Z40.02 ➡ Encounter for prophylactic removal of ovary

Correct Code:
Z40.02

C2.h Admission/encounter for pain control management

When an encounter is for pain management due to the malignancy, one of the pain codes should be sequenced first followed by the appropriate neoplasm code(s). There is an instructional note to code also the neoplasm.

Review the following example.

EXAMPLE: *A patient with a malignancy of the frontal lobe of the brain was in acute pain during his follow-up visit. The physician prescribed a drug to relieve the patient's pain.*

Alphabetic Index:
Pain ➡ neoplasm related ➡ G89.3

Tabular List:
G89.3 ➡ Neoplasm related pain (acute) (chronic)

First listed diagnosis:
G89.3 Neoplasm related pain (acute) (chronic)

Secondary diagnosis:
C71.1 Malignant neoplasm of frontal lobe

Correct code sequencing:
G89.3, C71.1

C2. i Malignancy in two or more noncontiguous sites

A patient may have more than one malignant tumor in the same organ. These tumors may represent different primaries or metastatic disease, depending on the site. If the documentation is unclear, the provider should be queried as to the status of each tumor so that the correct codes can be assigned.

C2. j Disseminated malignant neoplasm, unspecified

Code C80.0, Disseminated malignant neoplasm, unspecified, is for use only in those cases where the patient has advanced metastatic disease and no known primary or secondary sites are specified. It should not be used in place of codes for the primary site and all known secondary sites.

C2. k Malignant neoplasm without specification of site

Code C80.1, Malignant (primary) neoplasm, unspecified, equates to cancer, unspecified. This code should only be used when no determination can be made as to the primary site of a malignancy. This code should rarely be used in the inpatient setting.

> **EXAMPLE:** *Example from the Tabular List*
>
> *C80 Malignant neoplasm without specification of site*

> **EXCLUDES 1** *Malignant carcinoid tumor of unspecified site – C7a.00*
> *Malignant neoplasm of specified multiple sites – code to each site*

C2. l. Sequencing of neoplasm codes

1. Encounter for treatment of primary malignancy: If the reason for the encounter is for treatment of a primary malignancy, assign the malignancy as the principal or first listed diagnosis. The primary site is to be sequenced first, followed by any metastatic sites.

2. Encounter for treatment of secondary malignancy: When an encounter is for a primary malignancy with metastasis and treatment is directed toward the metastatic (secondary) site(s) only, the metastatic site(s) is designated as the principal or first listed diagnosis. The primary malignancy is coded as an additional code.

3. Malignant neoplasm in a pregnant patient: When a pregnant woman has a malignant neoplasm, a code from subcategory O9a.1–, Malignant neoplasm complicating pregnancy, childbirth, and the puerperium, should be sequenced first, followed by the appropriate code from Chapter 2 to indicate the type of neoplasm.

Review the following example:

> **EXAMPLE:** *A 32-year-old female who is in her second trimester of pregnancy underwent Mohs micrographic surgery for basal cell carcinoma of the lip.*

> **First listed diagnosis:**
> *O9A.112* → *Malignant neoplasm complicating pregnancy, second trimester*

> **Secondary diagnosis:**
> *C44.0 Malignant neoplasm of skin of lip* → *Malignant neoplasm of basal cell carcinoma of lip*

> **Correct code sequencing:**
> *O9a.112, C44.0*

4. Encounter for complication associated with a neoplasm: When an encounter is for management of a complication associated with a neoplasm, such as dehydration, and the treatment is only for the complication, the complication is coded first, followed by the appropriate code(s) for the neoplasm.

The exception to this guideline is anemia. When the admission/encounter is for management of an anemia associated with the malignancy and the treatment is only for anemia, the appropriate code for the malignancy is sequenced as the principal or first listed diagnosis followed by code D63.0, Anemia in neoplastic disease.

5. Complication from surgical procedure for treatment of a neoplasm: When an encounter is for treatment of a complication resulting from a surgical procedure performed for the treatment of the neoplasm, designate the complication as the principal or first listed diagnosis. See guideline regarding the coding of a current malignancy versus personal history to determine if the code for the neoplasm should also be assigned.

6. Pathologic fracture due to a neoplasm: When an encounter is for a pathological fracture due to a neoplasm and if the focus of treatment is the fracture, a code from subcategory M84.5, Pathological fracture in neoplastic disease, should be sequenced first, followed by the code for the neoplasm. Review the following example.

> **EXAMPLE:** *A patient was treated for a pathologic fracture of the right tibia due to the malignant neoplasm of the right lower limb.*

The codes would be reported in the following sequence:

> **First listed diagnosis:**
> *M84.561A Pathologic fracture of bone in neoplastic disease, right tibia, initial encounter*

Secondary diagnosis:
C76.51 Malignant neoplasm of right lower limb

Correct code sequencing:
M84.561A, C76.51

If the focus of treatment is the neoplasm with an associated pathological fracture, the neoplasm code should be sequenced first, followed by a code from M84.5 for the pathological fracture.

Now review how the reverse scenario can change the reporting of the diagnosis code(s).

EXAMPLE: A patient was treated for a malignant neoplasm of the right lower limb. The patient also has a pathologic fracture of the right tibia due to the malignant neoplasm of the right lower limb.

The codes would be reported in the following sequence:

First listed diagnosis:
C76.51 Malignant neoplasm of right lower limb

Secondary diagnosis:
M84.561A Pathologic fracture of bone in neoplastic disease, right tibia, initial encounter

Correct code sequencing:
C76.51, M84.561A

C2.m Current malignancy versus personal history of malignancy

When a primary malignancy has been excised but further treatment, such as an additional surgery for the malignancy or radiation therapy or chemotherapy directed to the site, the primary malignancy code should be used until treatment is completed.

When a primary malignancy has been previously excised or eradicated from its site, there is no further treatment (of the malignancy) directed to that site, and there is no evidence of any existing primary malignancy, a code from category Z85, Personal history of malignant neoplasm, should be used to indicate the former site of the malignancy.

Review the following example:

EXAMPLE: A 56-year-old male was seen in follow-up after removal of the prostate 3 years ago for a malignancy.

Open the ICD-10-CM codebook to the Index and locate the main term. The main term in this encounter is not the malignant neoplasm but "history, personal (of)." When you reference the main term, where does it tell you to go next? Under "history, personal (of)," the next step is to reference cancer. The reference of personal history of cancer directs the user to the phrase "history, personal, malignant neoplasm." Once you have located this information, the site will determine the correct code.

Alphabetic Index:
History → personal (of) → malignant neoplasm → prostate → Z85.46

Now turn to the Tabular List and reference Z85.46.

Tabular List:
Z85.46 → Personal history of malignant neoplasm of prostate

Correct code:
Z85.46

Due to the potentially toxic nature of many chemotherapy agents, certain tests may be performed prior to the administration of chemotherapy as well as during the course of the chemotherapy treatment. The malignancy should be coded as the principal diagnosis for encounters for these tests. The code for long-term (current) use of drug, Z79.8–, should be used as a secondary code if documented in the medical record.

A malignant neoplasm of a transplanted organ should be coded as a transplant complication. First assign the appropriate code from category T86.–, Complications of transplanted organs and tissue, followed by code C80.2, Malignant neoplasm associated with transplanted organ. Use an additional code for the specific malignancy.

Endocrine therapy, such a tamoxifen, may be given prophylactically, for women at high risk of developing breast cancer. It may also be given during cancer treatment as well as following treatment to help prevent recurrence. The use of endocrine therapy does not affect the guidelines for coding of neoplasms.

CHECKPOINT EXERCISE 5-3

Use the current edition of ICD-10-CM and answer the following:

1. _____ Primary pancreatic cancer

2. _____ Secondary tumor found in the bronchus in the middle lobe of the lung

3. _____ Bronchial adenoma in a 70-year-old woman

4. _____ Carcinoma in situ of the right eyeball

5. _____ Tumor of the hilus of lung, unspecified

6. _____ Lymphoid leukemia in remission in a 40-year-old man

7. _____ Malignant lymphosarcoma

8. _____ Carcinoma in situ of the vermilion border of the lip

9. _____ Cancer in situ of the right ovary

10. _____ Metastatic cancer to the lung from the breast in a male patient

11. _____ Severe dysplasia of the cervix in a 50-year-old female

12. _____ A 52-year-old patient is treated for prophylactic chemotherapy treatment. The patient has acute monoblastic leukemia.

13. _____ A patient is diagnosed with chronic myelogenous leukemia with blastic exacerbation.

14. _____ A patient with myeloblastic leukemia in the remission stage underwent a bone marrow transplant on 7/1/20xx.

15. _____ A patient diagnosed by the physician with Hodgkin's lymphoma is scheduled for a follow-up visit.

Chapter 3, Diseases of the Blood and Blood-Forming Organs and Certain Disorders Involving the Immune Mechanism (D50-D89)

In this chapter of ICD-10-CM there are no chapter-specific guidelines other than the general guidelines and conventions.

Chapter 3 of ICD-10-CM contains the following classifications:

- Nutritional anemias (D50-D53)

- Hemolytic anemias (D55-D59)

- Aplastic and other anemias and other bone marrow failure syndromes (D60-D64)

- Coagulation defects, purpura, and other hemorrhagic conditions (D65-D69)

- Other disorders of the blood and blood-forming organs (D70-D77)

- Intraoperative and postprocedural complications of the spleen (D78)

- Certain disorders involving the immune mechanism (D80-D89)

The conditions in Chapter 3 include:

- Anemia

- Bone marrow

- Lymphatic tissue

- Platelets

- Coagulation factors

The most common conditions will be reviewed in this chapter.

ANEMIA

Anemia is a reduction in hemoglobin or in the volume of packed red blood cells. Anemia is attributed to a number of causes. They include:

- Bleeding

- Aging

- Cell destruction

Accuracy is important when coding anemia. You may need to refer to a laboratory or pathology report for a more precise diagnosis. However, make sure the documentation in the medical record supports your code selection. When the diagnosis is unclear or unspecified, check with the physician for the most accurate diagnosis.

"Anemia" is the main term, under which you will find many subterms that relate to anemia. Many of the subterms for anemia have lengthy additional subterms listed under them. Anemia complicating pregnancy or the puerperium is excluded from this category and is coded as O99.0.

Iron deficiency anemias (D50)

The conditions in category D50 may be due to a chronic blood loss from such conditions as:

- Blood loss
- Menorrhagia
- Iron deficiency

When the specific type of iron deficiency anemia is unknown, code D50.9 is assigned.

Secondary Anemia

Secondary anemia often results from chronic conditions such as infection or blood loss. Anemia should be coded to the specific type of anemia, when the information is available. Use "anemia unspecified" only when the type of anemia cannot be identified. There are two types of anemia that are often confusing, "anemia of chronic disease" and "chronic anemia." These two diagnostic statements are not the same. In "anemia of chronic disease," chronic describes the name of the disease that is the cause of the anemia. Review the following:

> **EXAMPLE:** *A 46-year-old male patient is admitted by his internist with a diagnosis of chronic kidney disease. After the lab results are received, the physician documents in the patient's chart anemia due to chronic renal failure.*

Review the steps in coding this encounter, Anemia due to chronic kidney disease.

Turn to the Alphabetic Index and look up the main term "failure."

> **Find the subcategory: kidney.**
> *Under the subcategory kidney, find chronic.*
>
> *You should have found failure* ➝ *kidney* ➝ *chronic N18.9.*
>
> *Go to the Tabular List under category N18.– and review the codes in this category (chronic kidney disease).*

Since we do not know the stage of the kidney disease, the only code in the category that can be used is N18.9 for the chronic kidney disease unspecified, which includes chronic renal failure.

Now we will code the anemia. Again, turn to the Alphabetic Index and look up the main term "anemia."

> *Under anemia you will locate anemia* ➝ *due to* ➝ *chronic kidney disease. This information directs the user to D63.1.*

Return to the Tabular List and find D63.1. You will find the description as "Anemia in chronic kidney disease." There is an instructional note to "code first the underlying chronic kidney disease (CKD)" (N18.–).

In this example, chronic renal failure is the disease causing the anemia. Code the chronic renal failure as the primary diagnosis and the anemia as the secondary diagnosis.

> **Correct code(s):**
> **Primary diagnosis:**
> *N18.9 Chronic renal failure*
>
> **Secondary diagnosis:**
> *D63.1 Anemia in chronic kidney disease*
>
> **Correct code sequencing:**
> *N18.9, D63.1*

Now, review this example:

> **EXAMPLE:** *A patient is diagnosed with chronic anemia.*
>
> **Alphabetic Index:**
> *Anemia* ➝ *chronic simple D53.9*

In this example, the Alphabetic Index indicates a subterm "chronic simple" that directs you to D53.9. Now review the Tabular List under the subcategory D53.9.

> **Tabular List:**
> *D53.9* ➝ *Nutritional anemia unspecified* ➝ *chronic simple anemia*
>
> *Notice that "simple chronic" is listed under the subcategory D53.9.*
>
> **Correct code:**
> *D53.9 Nutritional anemia, unspecified*

Sickle-cell Anemia (D57)

Category D57 contains hereditary conditions characterized by escalated erythrocyte (red blood cell) destruction. Sickle-cell anemia is a common disorder within this category of diagnosis codes. When coding sickle-cell disorders, it is important to understand the difference between the sickle-cell trait and sickle-cell anemia. Sickle-cell anemia is a hereditary disease of the red blood cells passed to a child when both parents carry the genetic trait. It is present in up to 1% of the black population. The cells contain an abnormal type of hemoglobin that, when deoxygenated, precipitates into long crystals, deforming the cells and damaging the membrane. Organ damage and death may result from this very serious condition.

Clinical manifestations of sickle-cell disease include anemia, susceptibility to infection, impaired growth and development, hepatosplenomegaly, cardiomegaly, and episodes of pain. Many are a result of increased blood viscosity. The disruption of blood flow causes hemorrhage, infarction, vascular occlusions, and ischemic necrosis in tissues and organs.

Some complications of sickle-cell disease that are not all inclusive are:

- Skin ulcers
- Anemia
- Nocturia
- Cardiomegaly
- Chest syndrome
- Renal failure
- Sepsis
- Cholelithiasis
- Aplastic crisis
- Hemolysis
- Infections
- Chronic pain

Sickle-cell trait is also hereditary. It is passed to a child from only one parent who carries the genetic trait. Persons who carry the sickle-cell trait do not necessarily develop the disease; they are carriers. This condition is coded as D57.3, HB-S trait or heterozygous hemoglobin S.

Diagnosis code D57.0 is reported when Hb-SS disease is present with crisis. The documentation must indicate a vasoocclusive crisis. If crisis is not mentioned, code with D57.1 (without mention of crisis). Review Figure 5.19.

FIGURE 5.19   Excerpt from the Tabular List: *D57.–*

D57	Sickle Cell Disorders
	D57.0 HB-SS disease with crisis
	Sickle-cell disease NOS with crisis
	HB-SS disease with vasoocclusive pain
	D57.00 HB-SS disease with crisis, unspecified
	D57.01 HB-SS disease with acute chest syndrome
	D57.02 HB-SS disease with splenic sequestration
	D57.1 Sickle-cell disease without crisis
	HB-SS disease without crisis
	Sickle-cell anemia, NOS
	Sickle-cell disease NOS
	Sickle-cell disorder-NOS

CHECKPOINT EXERCISE 5-4

Using your ICD-10-CM, code the following:

1. _____ Addison's anemia
2. _____ Imerslund syndrome
3. _____ Physical retardation due to malnutrition
4. _____ Acquired sideroblastic anemia
5. _____ Scorbutic anemia
6. _____ Chlorotic anemia
7. _____ Pseudocholinesterase deficiency
8. _____ Stomatocytosis
9. _____ Anemia due to acute blood loss
10. _____ Christmas disease
11. _____ Von Willebrand disease
12. _____ A 10-year-old sickle-cell patient presents with severe chest pain, dyspnea, cough, fever, and pain. The physician documents sickle-cell Hb-SS disease and administers a transfusion and oxygen.
13. _____ A patient with polyuria, muscle weakness, chronic fatigue, and failure to grow is diagnosed with primary aldosteronism.
14. _____ A patient who is morbidly obese is diagnosed with dysmetabolic syndrome X.
15. _____ A patient presents with symptoms of severe lethargy, pain in the joints, and feelings of overall illness. Blood levels reveal decreased potassium. He is diagnosed with hypopotassemia.

Review the following example:

EXAMPLE: *A five-year-old male patient with sickle-cell disease is admitted to the hospital with severe abdominal pain, abdominal wall rigidity, distension, and diffuse tenderness. The physician examines him noting an enlarged spleen and diagnosis sickle-cell thalassemia.*

Analyze the coding steps:

Alphabetic Index:
Disease → sickle cell → thalassemia → with splenic sequestration → with crisis → D57.412

Tabular List:
D57.412 → Sickle-cell thalassemia with splenic sequestration with crisis

Correct code:
D57.412

Splenic sequestration (D57.412) identifies when sickle cells occlude the vessels leading from the spleen and blood is entrapped in the spleen, resulting in a sharp drop in hemoglobin and decreased hematocrit.

Chapter 4, Endocrine, Nutritional, and Metabolic Diseases

Chapter 4 in the Tabular List includes the following sections:

- Disorders of the thyroid gland E00-E07

- Diabetes mellitus E08-E13

- Other disorders of glucose regulation and pancreatic internal secretion (E15-E16)

- Disorders of other endocrine glands (E20-E35)

- Intraoperative complications of endocrine system (E36)

- Malnutrition (E40-E46)

- Other nutritional deficiencies (E50-E64)

- Overweight, obesity, and other hyperalimentation (E65-E68)

- Metabolic disorders (E70-E88)

- Postprocedural endocrine and metabolic complications and disorders, not elsewhere classified (E89)

Chapter 4 in the Tabular List describes diseases or conditions that affect the endocrine system. The endocrine system involves the glands that are located throughout the body. The function of these glands is to secrete hormones into the bloodstream. The thyroid, an important endocrine gland, varies greatly in size. This gland secretes hormones governing the body's metabolic rate. Two common disorders of the thyroid are hyperthyroidism and hypothyroidism. Also included in this section are diseases and conditions that affect nutritional and metabolic conditions and disorders of the immune system.

Some of the common disorders that are identified in Chapter 4 of the Tabular List are:

- Disorders of the thyroid gland

- Disorders of the pituitary gland

- Disorders of the adrenal gland

- Diabetes mellitus

- Disorders of the parathyroid gland

- Disorders relating to metabolism

Following is a review of some of the common conditions in these categories.

DISORDERS OF THE THYROID GLAND

Hyperthyroidism is a condition in which excessive levels of hormones are secreted, resulting in abnormal enlargement of the gland (goiter) in numerous forms. Some of the symptoms and characteristics of this disease are:

- Nervousness

- Weight loss

- Diarrhea

- Heat intolerance

- Palpitations

- Insomnia

- Weakness

- Bulging eyes

- Lymph system swelling

- Blurred or double vision

- Skin problems

Thyroid storm or (thyrotoxic crisis) is uncontrolled hyperthyroidism, a life-threatening condition caused by underproduction of follicle-stimulating hormone (FSH). Open the ICD-10-CM codebook to the Tabular List and review Figure 5.20. There are several choices in this category. It is very important to document what is affected (nodule, goiter, etc.) and whether the patient is in crisis or storm.

FIGURE 5.20   Excerpt from the Tabular List: *E05.–*

E05 **EXCLUDES 1**	**Thyrotoxicosis [hyperthyroidism]** chronic thyroiditis with transient thyrotoxicosis (E06.2) neonatal thyrotoxicosis (P72.1)
E05.0	**Thyrotoxicosis with diffuse goiter** Exophthalmic or toxic goiter NOS Graves' disease Toxic diffuse goiter
E05.00	Thyrotoxicosis with diffuse goiter without thyrotoxic crisis or storm
E05.01	Thyrotoxicosis with diffuse goiter with thyrotoxic crisis or storm
E05.1	Thyrotoxicosis with toxic single thyroid nodule
E05.10	Thyrotoxicosis with toxic single thyroid nodule without thyrotoxic crisis or storm
E05.11	Thyrotoxicosis with toxic single thyroid nodule with thyrotoxic crisis or storm
E05.2	Thyrotoxicosis with toxic multinodular
E05.20	Thyrotoxicosis with toxic multinodular goiter without thyrotoxic crisis or storm
E05.21	Thyrotoxicosis with toxic multinodular goiter with thyrotoxic crisis or storm
E05.3	Thyrotoxicosis from ectopic thyroid tissue
E05.30	Thyrotoxicosis from ectopic thyroid tissue without thyrotoxic crisis or storm
E05.31	Thyrotoxicosis from ectopic thyroid tissue with thyrotoxic crisis or storm
E05.4	Thyrotoxicosis factitia
E05.40	Thyrotoxicosis factitia without thyrotoxic crisis or storm
E05.41	Thyrotoxicosis factitia with thyrotoxic crisis or storm
E05.8	Other thyrotoxicosis
E05.80	Other thyrotoxicosis without thyrotoxic crisis or storm
E05.81	Other thyrotoxicosis with thyrotoxic crisis or storm
E05.9	Thyrotoxicosis, unspecified
E05.90	Thyrotoxicosis, unspecified without thyrotoxic crisis or storm
E05.91	Thyrotoxicosis, unspecified with thyrotoxic crisis or storm

Review the following example:

> **EXAMPLE:** *A patient was diagnosed with thyroidtoxicosis factitia in crisis.*

Open the ICD-10-CM codebook, start with the Alphabetic Index and then locate the correct diagnosis code in the Tabular List.

> **Alphabetic Index:**
> *Thyrotoxicosis* ➝ *due to* ➝ *factitia* ➝ *with thyroid storm* ➝ *E50.41*

> **Tabular List:**
> *E05.41* ➝ *Thyrotoxicosis factitia with thyrotoxic crisis or storm*

> **Correct code:**
> *E50.41*

DIABETES MELLITUS

Diabetes mellitus is one of the most frequently used categories in Chapter 4 of the ICD-10-CM codebook. Diabetes mellitus is a chronic metabolic disease of the pancreatic islet cells. Millions of people have this serious, lifelong condition, and more than 650 000 people are newly diagnosed with diabetes each year. Although it occurs most often in older adults, diabetes is also one of the most common chronic childhood diseases in the United States today.

Types of Diabetes

In order to code diabetes mellitus correctly, it is critical that the coder understand the types of diabetes and underlying conditions related to diabetes mellitus.

The 3 main types of diabetes are:

- Type 1, insulin dependent
- Type 2, non-insulin dependent
- Gestational diabetes, which occurs during pregnancy

Many patients with diabetes mellitus also have manifestations associated with diabetes. In ICD-10-CM there are combination codes to identify the type of diabetes along with any associated manifestations.

CODING TIP   Be careful when coding diabetes mellitus. Make sure the documentation in the medical record indicates controlled or uncontrolled. Also be sure the documentation indicates whether the patient is IDDM (insulin dependent) or NIDDM (non-insulin dependent).

IDDM, or type 1 diabetes, usually results from damage or destruction of the pancreatic islets, leading to reduction or absence of insulin secretion. Diabetes sometimes follows a viral infection, which suggests that the virus may have induced the disease by injuring or destroying the islets. Many patients with this type of diabetes have antibodies directed against their own islet cells, indicating that an abnormal immune response may also play a part in causing the disease. IDDM most often develops in children and young adults. For this reason, IDDM used to be known as "juvenile" diabetes. It is one of the most common chronic disorders in American children.

A patient with type 1, insulin-dependent diabetes mellitus requires insulin to live. The patient must be monitored to identify complications of the disease, monitor insulin levels, and control diet. Type 1 diabetes mellitus indicates that:

- Insulin is not produced by the body or
- Production of insulin is decreased.

NIDDM, or type 2 diabetes, is the most common type of diabetes. It accounts for 90% to 95% of diagnosed diabetes. NIDDM usually develops in adults over age 40 and is most common in overweight people. People with NIDDM usually produce some insulin, but the body's cells cannot use it efficiently because the cells are insulin resistant. The result is hyperglycemia and inability of the body to use its main source of fuel.

Gestational diabetes is demonstrated by abnormal glucose tolerance test results during pregnancy. It usually ends after delivery, but women with gestational diabetes may develop NIDDM later in life.

Gestational diabetes results from the body's resistance to the action of insulin. Hormones produced by the placenta cause this resistance. Women with gestational diabetes require treatment for blood glucose control during pregnancy to prevent adverse effects to the fetus. However, they return to normal glucose tolerance after pregnancy.

Gestational diabetes is usually treated with dietary adjustments, although some women may need insulin. Gestational diabetes cannot be treated with oral hypoglycemic medications because these medicines can harm the fetus.

Now that you have a good understanding of the disease, look at this subcategory in the Tabular List, Diabetes mellitus (E08-E13).

Diabetes mellitus codes in ICD-10-CM are combination codes that include:

- Type of diabetes mellitus
- Body system affected, and;
- The complications affecting that body system.

In order to code diabetes mellitus in ICD-10-CM, the following are necessary:

- Type of diabetes
- Body system affected
- Use of insulin
- Complication(s)
- Manifestation(s)

There are 5 diabetes mellitus categories in the ICD-10-CM. They are:

- E08   Diabetes mellitus due to an underlying condition
- E09   Drug- or chemical-induced diabetes mellitus
- E10   Type 1 diabetes mellitus
- E11   Type 2 diabetes mellitus
- E13   Other specified diabetes mellitus

Documentation requirements for coding diabetes mellitus include:

- Type of diabetes
- Body system affected
- Complication or manifestation
- If type 2 diabetes mellitus, whether use of insulin is long term

All of the above categories with the exception of E10 include a note directing users to use an additional code to identify any insulin use; the code is Z79.4. The concept of requiring insulin and not requiring insulin is not a component of the diabetes mellitus categories in ICD-10-CM. Code Z79.4, Long-term current use of insulin, is added to identify the use of insulin for diabetic management even if the patient is not insulin dependent in code categories E08-E09 and E11-E14.

The character under these categories refers to underlying conditions with specified complications, whereas the fifth character defines the specific manifestation such as neuropathy and angiopathy.

Definitions for the types of diabetes mellitus are included in the Includes Notes under each diabetes mellitus category. Sequencing of diabetes codes from categories E08-E09 have a "Code first" note indicating that diabetes is to be sequenced after the underlying condition, drug, or chemical that is responsible for the diabetes. Codes from categories E-10-E14, Diabetes mellitus, are sequenced first, followed by codes for any additional complications outside of these categories, if applicable.

With the exception of category E10, all ICD-10-CM categories for diabetes mellitus include a note that directs the coder to use an additional code to identify insulin usage (Z79.4). Fourth characters under these categories refer to underlying conditions with specified complications. Fifth characters define the specific manifestation (eg, ketoacidosis, nephropathy, neuropathy, peripheral angiopathy). Sixth characters define the manifestations further.

CODING TIP Use an additional code to identify insulin usage (Z79.4) if applicable when coding diabetes mellitus.

Review the guidelines for Diabetes Mellitus

C4. a. Diabetes mellitus The diabetes mellitus codes are combination codes that include the type of diabetes mellitus, the body system affected, and the complications affecting that body system. As many codes within a particular category as are necessary to describe all of the complications of the disease may be used. They should be sequenced based on the reason for a particular encounter. Assign as many codes from categories E08-E13 as needed to identify all of the associated conditions that the patient has.

1. Type of diabetes

The age of a patient is not the sole determining factor, although most patients with type 1 diabetes develop the condition before reaching puberty. For this reason type 1 diabetes mellitus is also referred to as juvenile diabetes.

Review the following example:

> **EXAMPLE:** *A 60-year-old patient presents with type 1 diabetes. The patient has a **chronic left foot ulcer** with **muscle necrosis** due to the **diabetes**.*

Review Figures 5.21 and 5.22 from the Alphabetic Index and Tabular List.

FIGURE 5.21   Excerpt from the Alphabetic Index: *Diabetes, diabetic*

Diabetes, diabetic
    Type 1
    With
    foot ulcer NEC E10.621

FIGURE 5.22   Excerpt from the Tabular List: *E10.621*

E10.621   **Type 1 diabetes mellitus with foot ulcer**
           Use additional code to identify site of ulcer
           (L97.4-, L97.5-)

There is an instructional note that instructs the user to "use additional code to identify site of ulcer." Open the ICD-10-CM codebook to L97.4- to L97.5- and select the appropriate secondary diagnosis. You will also notice that laterality is important to identify left or right foot.

> **Alphabetic Index:**
> *Diabetes, diabetic → type 1 → with → foot ulcer → E10.621*

> **Tabular List:**
> *E10.621 → E10.621 Type 1 diabetes mellitus with foot ulcer*

Don't forget to assign the secondary diagnosis to identify the ulcer of the foot.

> **First listed diagnosis:**
> *E10.621 Type 1 diabetes mellitus with foot ulcer*

> **Secondary diagnosis:**
> *L97.523 Nonpressure chronic ulcer of left foot with necrosis of muscle*

> **Correct code sequencing:**
> *E10.621, L97.523*

CODING TIP Type 1 diabetes mellitus is only assigned when the physician's documentation indicates insulin dependent.

2. Type of diabetes mellitus not documented

If the type of diabetes mellitus is not documented in the medical record, the default is E11.–, Type 2 diabetes mellitus.

Review the following example:

> **EXAMPLE:** *A patient is treated in the internist's office for diabetes mellitus. The patient is doing well and will follow up in 4 weeks.*

In this example, the type of diabetes is unknown. It is important to code as specifically as possible so that when the information is not complete, it is recommended to query the physician. However, if this is not possible, the default of E11.– is the only recourse the user may have. This type of code selection should be used rarely; always query the provider for more details in order to select to the highest level of specificity.

The default is type 2 when no more information is available.

This is how this patient encounter is coded:

Alphabetic Index:
Diabetes, diabetic ➞ type 2 ➞ E11.9

Tabular List:
E11.9 ➞ Type 2 diabetes mellitus without complications

Correct code:
E11.9

3. Diabetes mellitus and the use of insulin

If the documentation in a medical record does not indicate the type of diabetes but does indicate that the patient uses insulin, code E11, Type 2 diabetes mellitus, should be assigned. Code Z79.4, Long-term (current) use of insulin, should also be assigned to indicate that the patient uses insulin. Code Z79.4 should not be assigned if insulin is given temporarily to bring a type 2 patient's blood sugar under control during an encounter.

Review the following example:

EXAMPLE: A 45-year-old type 2 patient returns to his physician's office for a 3-month follow-up visit. The patient has been on insulin for the past 8 months because the diabetes was not well controlled. The patient is also suffering from diabetic gastroparesis. After an expanded problem-focused history and physical examination, the physician documents in the medical record, "Type 2 diabetes mellitus currently maintaining good control with insulin, diet, and exercise. Patient will continue with same medication dosage, monitor glucose levels with home monitoring system, and return in 3 months for recheck. We may consider discontinuing insulin if patient remains in good control."

Open the ICD-10-CM codebook and code this encounter.

Alphabetic Index:
Diabetes, diabetic ➞ type 2 ➞ with ➞ gastroparesis ➞ E11.43

Tabular List:
E11.43 ➞ Type 2 diabetes mellitus with diabetic gastroparesis

The Tabular List instructs to use Z79.4 for long-term insulin use, which would be reported in this situation.

Correct Code Sequencing:
E11.43, Z79.4

4. Diabetes mellitus in pregnant patient

Codes for pregnancy, childbirth, and the puerperium, which are located in Chapter 15 of ICD-10-CM, are always sequenced first on the medical record. A patient who has a preexisting diabetes mellitus (DM) and becomes pregnant should be assigned a code from category O24, Diabetes mellitus in pregnancy, childbirth, and the puerperium, followed by the diabetes code from Chapter 4 of ICD-10-CM. These codes have been expanded in ICD-10-CM. The fourth character subcategory codes identify the type of diabetes as preexisting type 1 or type 2, unspecified, or gestational.

The fifth character indicates whether the diabetes is treated during pregnancy, childbirth, or the puerperium. The sixth character indicates the trimester during which treatment is sought. With gestational diabetes, the sixth character identifies whether the gestational diabetes is diet controlled, insulin controlled, or unspecified control.

Review the following example:

EXAMPLE: A 25-year-old patient with diabetes mellitus type 1 with diabetic neuralgia in her second trimester visited her OB/GYN for her routine follow-up visit. The patient's blood sugar was well controlled and the patient indicated she was doing well with her diet and exercise regimen. The physician scheduled the patient for follow-up in one month.

Open the ICD-10-CM codebook and begin with the Tabular List to locate the correct code. In this instance, the main term is not "diabetes," but "pregnancy, complicated by."

Alphabetic Index:
Pregnancy ➞ complicated by ➞ diabetes mellitus ➞ type 1 ➞ O24.01-

Tabular List:
O24.012 ➞ Pre-existing diabetes mellitus, type 1, in pregnancy, second trimester

You are not finished yet. There is an instructional note in code category O24.01– that instructs the use of an additional code in category E10 to identify any manifestations.

Alphabetic Index:
Diabetes, diabetic ➞ with ➞ neuralgia ➞ E10.42

Tabular List:
E10.42 ➞ Type 1 diabetes mellitus with diabetic polyneuropathy

Correct code sequencing:
O24.012, E10.42

In this patient encounter two codes are need to fully describe the patient's condition.

Review the following example:

> **EXAMPLE:** *A 27-year-old patient developed gestational diabetes in her third trimester. The patient's condition is controlled with diet and exercise.*

Review Figure 5.23 from the Tabular List for category O24.41.

FIGURE 5.23   Excerpt from the Tabular List: *O24.41–*

O24.41	Gestational diabetes mellitus in pregnancy
O24.410	**Gestational diabetes mellitus in pregnancy, diet controlled**
O24.414	Gestational diabetes mellitus in pregnancy, insulin controlled
O24.419	Gestational diabetes mellitus in pregnancy, unspecified control
O24.420	Gestational diabetes mellitus in childbirth, diet controlled
O24.424	Gestational diabetes mellitus in childbirth, insulin controlled
O24.429	Gestational diabetes mellitus in childbirth, unspecified control
O24.430	Gestational diabetes mellitus in the puerperium, diet controlled
O24.434	Gestational diabetes mellitus in the puerperium, insulin controlled
O24.439	Gestational diabetes mellitus in the puerperium, unspecified control

---

Now open the ICD-10-CM codebook to the Alphabetic Index to locate the appropriate code.

Alphabetic Index:
Pregnancy → complicated by → diabetes mellitus → gestational → see diabetes gestational → diabetes, diabetic → gestational (in pregnancy) → diet controlled → O24.410

Tabular List:
O24.410 → Gestational diabetes mellitus in pregnancy, diet controlled

In this example only one code is reported.

Correct code:
O24.410

5. Complications due to insulin pump malfunction

(a) Underdose of insulin due to insulin pump failure An underdose of insulin due to an insulin pump failure should be assigned to a code from subcategory T85.6–, Mechanical complication of other specified internal and external prosthetic devices, implants and grafts, that specifies the type of pump malfunction, as the principal or first listed code, followed by code T38.3x6–, Underdosing of insulin and oral hypoglycemic [antidiabetic] drugs. Additional codes for the type of diabetes mellitus and any associated complications due to the underdosing should also be assigned.

Review the following example:

> **EXAMPLE:** *A 46-year-old woman with type 1 IDDM is seen in the emergency department while on vacation. She presents with complaints of fatigue, excessive thirst, and sudden weight loss. The physician performs a detailed history and examination and runs blood tests to determine the patient's blood glucose level. The physician reviews the lab results. The patient has a blood glucose level of 350 mg/dL, and the physician documents that the insulin level is uncontrolled and the patient is hyperglycemic. The patient is on an insulin pump. The pump was tested and the physician determined that the pump was not working. The physician adjusts her insulin regimen, gives the patient a new pump, and advises her to see her physician when she returns from vacation.*

Open the ICD-10-CM codebook and locate the correct codes for this encounter. Review the following steps:

Step 1: The guidelines instruct the user to report the first listed code from category T85.6–. Turn to the Tabular List and review the codes in this category.

First listed diagnosis:
T85.614 → Breakdown (mechanical of insulin pump), initial encounter

Step 2: The guidelines instruct the secondary code selected is T38.3x6, which is the code to report for the underdosing of insulin. Go to the Tabular List and reference T38.3x6. Notice that in this classification a seventh character is required for the initial, subsequent, or sequela encounter. Because we can assume this is the first encounter, the seventh character will be "A."

Secondary diagnosis:
T38.3x6A → Underdosing of insulin and oral hypoglycemic [anti-diabetic] drugs, initial encounter

Step 3: You are not finished yet. The type of diabetes mellitus must be reported in addition to the insulin pump failure and the underdosing. Review the Alphabetic Index for type 1 diabetes with hyperglycemia and verify the correct code in the Tabular List.

Tertiary diagnosis:
E10.65 ➔ *Type 1 diabetes mellitus with mention of hyperglycemia*

Correct code sequencing:
T85.614A, T38.3x6A, E10.65

(b) Overdose of insulin due to insulin pump
failure The principal or first listed code for an encounter due to an insulin pump malfunction resulting in an overdose of insulin should also be T85.6–, Mechanical complication of other specified internal and external prosthetic devices, implants and grafts, followed by code T38.3x1–, Poisoning by insulin and oral hypoglycemic [antidiabetic] drugs, accidental (unintentional).

An insulin overdose can be extremely dangerous. Insulin can be a difficult medication to properly dose, and it is actually quite easy to accidentally overdose on this medication.

Review the following example:

EXAMPLE: An 85-year-old woman with type 1 IDDM is seen in the emergency department with very low blood sugar. She presents with complaints of sweating, dizziness, and cold sweats. The physician performs a detailed history and examination and runs blood tests to determine the patient's blood glucose level. The physician reviews the lab results, documents that the insulin level is very low, and admits the patient to the medicine unit. The patient is on an insulin pump; the pump was tested and the physician determined that the pump was not working properly, causing too much insulin to be administered (overdosing). This is the second time the pump has malfunctioned in the past two months. The patient was treated two months ago for the same symptoms and was hypoglycemic during the previous encounter, but was not hospitalized. The physician orders a new pump, adjusts her insulin regimen, and contacts the endocrinologist on call to take over management of the patient.

Review the steps in the previous example and locate the correct codes and sequencing.

First listed diagnosis:
T85.6 ➔ *T85.614D* ➔ *Breakdown (mechanical) of insulin pump*

Secondary diagnosis:
T38.3x1D ➔ *Poisoning by insulin and oral hypoglycemic [antidiabetic] drugs, accidental (unintentional)* ➔ *subsequent encounter*

Tertiary diagnosis:
E10.649 ➔ *Type 1 diabetes mellitus with hypoglycemia without coma*

6. Secondary diabetes mellitus

Secondary diabetes is a form of the disease that develops as a result of, or secondary to, another disease or condition.

Secondary diabetes can be caused by a wide range of health problems that damage, injure, interfere with, or destroy the pancreas. For example, secondary diabetes may develop from inflammation of the pancreas (pancreatitis), cystic fibrosis, or conditions related to the overproduction of growth hormone or cortisol. Some medicines may also affect how the body uses insulin or prevent the pancreas from producing enough insulin.

Codes under categories E08, Diabetes mellitus due to underlying condition, and E09, Drug or chemical induced diabetes mellitus, identify complications/manifestations associated with secondary diabetes mellitus. Secondary diabetes is always caused by another condition or event (eg, cystic fibrosis, malignant neoplasm of the pancreas, pancreatectomy, adverse effect of drug, or poisoning).

(a) Secondary diabetes mellitus and the use of insulin
For patients who routinely use insulin, code Z79.4, Long-term (current) use of insulin, should also be assigned. Code Z79.4 should not be assigned if insulin is given temporarily to bring a patient's blood sugar under control during an encounter.

Review the following example:

EXAMPLE: A 52-year-old patient was diagnosed with diabetes mellitus type 2 with diabetic neuropathy due to acute pancreatitis. The patient is not insulin dependent but is currently on insulin to control blood sugar.

When coding this encounter, it is important to read all the instructional notes. This patient encounter is coded in category E08. Review Figure 5.24. Open the ICD-10-CM codebook and code this patient encounter.

FIGURE 5.24 Excerpt from the Alphabetic Index: *Diabetes*

Diabetes, diabetic
 With
  Neuropathy E08.40

Alphabetic Index:
Diabetes, diabetic ➔ with neuropathy ➔ E08.40

Tabular List:
E08.40 ➔ *Diabetes mellitus due to underlying condition with diabetic neuropathy, unspecified*

After reading the instructional notes, the user is required to code first the underlying condition. In this example, the underlying condition is acute pancreatitis.

>   **Alphabetic Index:**
>   *Pancreatitis* ➔ *K85.9*
>
>   **Tabular List:**
>   *K85.9* ➔ *pancreatitis*

In addition, because this patient is not a type 1 patient but is using insulin, code Z79.4 should be assigned also.

>   **Correct code sequencing:**
>   *K85.9 (per instructional notes), E08.40, Z79.4*

(b) Assigning and sequencing secondary diabetes codes and their causes   The sequencing of the secondary diabetes codes in relationship to codes for the cause of the diabetes is based on the Tabular List instructions for categories E08 and E09. For example, for category E08, Diabetes mellitus due to underlying condition, code first the underlying condition; for category E09, Drug or chemical induced diabetes mellitus, code first the drug or chemical (T36-T65).

(i) Secondary diabetes mellitus due to pancreatectomy

For postpancreatectomy diabetes mellitus (lack of insulin due to the surgical removal of all or part of the pancreas), assign code E89.1, Postprocedural hypo-insulinemia. Assign a code from category E13 and a code from subcategory Z90.41–, Acquired absence of pancreas, as additional codes.

(ii) Secondary diabetes due to drugs

Secondary diabetes may be caused by an adverse effect of correctly administered medications, poisoning, or late effect of poisoning.

Manifestations and Complications of Diabetes Mellitus

Patients with diabetes mellitus are susceptible to other chronic conditions as a result of this disease.

Some body systems that can be affected are:

- Renal system
- Nervous system
- Peripheral vascular system
- Eyes and feet (most commonly affected)

Use your medical dictionary to identify clinical terms for infectious diseases.

When coding chronic complications, the code for diabetes mellitus, in most cases, is a combination code that is available to describe both the diabetes and the manifestation of the diabetes.

The manifestation is the complication or condition caused by diabetes mellitus.

Review the following example:

>   **EXAMPLE:** *A patient with IDDM develops mild nonproliferative diabetic retinopathy.*

Now open the ICD-10-CM codebook and code diabetic retinopathy.

CODING TIP   The acronym IDDM stands for insulin-dependent diabetes mellitus. The term "NIDDM" is non–insulin-dependent diabetes mellitus.

>   **Alphabetic Index:**
>   *Retinopathy* ➔ *see diabetes, retinopathy* ➔ *diabetes, diabetic* ➔ *type 1* ➔ *retinopathy* ➔ *nonproliferative* ➔ *E10.329*
>
>   **Tabular List:**
>   *E10.329* ➔ *Type 1 diabetes mellitus with mild nonproliferative diabetic retinopathy without macular edema*
>
>   **Correct code:**
>   *E10.329*

Review the following example. Open the ICD-10-CM codebook and try to find the correct code.

>   **EXAMPLE:** *A type 1 diabetic patient with Kimmelstiel-Wilson disease visited his endocrinologist in follow-up.*
>
>   **Alphabetic Index:**
>   *Diabetes, diabetic* ➔ *with* ➔ *Kimmelstiel-Wilson disease* ➔ *E10.21*
>
>   **Tabular List:**
>   *E10.21* ➔ *Type 1 diabetes mellitus with diabetic nephropathy Type 1 diabetes mellitus with Kimmelstiel-Wilson disease*

Diabetic patients who receive a new pancreas for treatment of diabetes mellitus may no longer require insulin or other care for their diabetes mellitus. However, preexisting complications from the diabetes may still exist after transplant. Codes from the diabetes mellitus categories are still applicable to describe the complication is these cases. A transplant status code should be used with the diabetes code in this circumstance.

Review the following example:

EXAMPLE: *A type 2 diabetic patient visited the physician in follow-up 6 months postsurgical transplant of a pancreas. The patient is doing well, medication is adjusted, and the patient will be seen in two weeks. The patient has no complications.*

Alphabetic Index:
Status ➞ Transplant ➞ Pancreas

Tabular List:
Z94.83 ➞ Pancreas transplant status

Correct code:
Z94.83

Because there are no further complications documented for the diabetes, it is only necessary to code the pancreas transplant status with this patient encounter. If there were still complications or residual effects of the diabetes, a diabetes code would be required.

Hypoglycemia

Very low blood sugar is called hypoglycemia and is sometimes referred to as an "insulin reaction." This condition can be caused by too much insulin, too little or delayed food intake, exercise, alcohol, or any combination of these factors. The patient with IDDM must constantly adjust the insulin dose to match exercise and eating patterns. If there is too much insulin, blood sugar drops and hypoglycemia results.

Because the nervous system requires glucose to function properly, neurologic symptoms occur if the blood sugar continues to fall. The patient becomes confused, may lose consciousness or experience convulsions, and, if left untreated, will lapse into a coma.

You will find these conditions in several classifications, and the code category will depend on whether the condition is due to: diabetes, non-diabetes (E15) drug-induced, or pregnancy.

Before selecting a code, make sure to read all notes carefully within the code selection.

Review the following example:

EXAMPLE: *A 37-year-old patient was having difficulty maintaining the diet and exercise program prescribed by her doctor. She was not eating properly and on many occasions went without food because of her busy schedule at work. She became ill at home and was rushed to the emergency department by her husband. Upon arrival at the emergency department, the patient was unconscious. After reviewing the patient's history with her husband, the doctor discovered that the patient had never been diagnosed with diabetes mellitus. The emergency department physician examines her and diagnoses hypoglycemic coma.*

To code, first refer to the Alphabetic Index and find "hypoglycemia." See excerpt below. Then refer to the excerpt from the Tabular List.

Alphabetic Index:
Non-diabetic hypoglycemia (spontaneous) ➞
E16.2 ➞ Coma E15

Tabular List:
E15

Correct code:
E15 Hypoglycemic coma

Resources

Clinical reference: Merck Manual on line Published by Merck Sharp & Dohme Corp., a subsidiary of Merck & Co., Inc., Whitehouse Station, N.J., U.S.A.

National Institute of Allergy and Infectious Disease; HIV/AIDS; April 2009

Medline Plus; Medical Encyclopedia; Sepsis and Septicemia; http://www.nlm.nih.gov/medlineplus/ency/article/001355.htm

Stedman's Electronic Medical Dictionary, 26th edition, Williams and Wilkins, 1999.

ICD-10-CM Official Guidelines for Coding and Reporting, Centers for Medicare and Medicaid Services, 2008; ICD-10-CM January 2011 release; http://www.cms.hhs.gov/ICD10.

ICD-10-CM; Ingenix, 2011

Test Your Knowledge

Provide the ICD-10-CM code(s) for the following diagnostic statements:

1. _____ A 45-year-old man with HIV infection

2. _____ Type 1 diabetic patient is brought to the ER by ambulance in a coma. The patient is pale, has rapid heart beat, and his face is covered in sweat. The physician finds that the insulin pump is not delivering insulin. After reviewing the lab results, the patient is diagnosed with diabetic coma.

3. _____ Vitamin K deficiency

4. _____ Graves' disease with thyrotoxic crisis

5. _____ Addison's disease

6. _____ Morbid obesity

7. _____ Gout

8. _____ Alders' syndrome

9. _____ A patient with type 1 diabetes is seen for an eye checkup. After a thorough examination, the ophthalmologist determines the patient has retinal edema.

10. _____ A patient diagnosed with ovarian cancer

11. _____ Subcutaneous lipoma of the face

12. _____ A 12-year-old male patient diagnosed with acute poliomyelitis

13. _____ A 28-year-old female patient in her first trimester of pregnancy developed gestational diabetes. The patient was monitored with diet and exercise during pregnancy. She delivered a healthy female infant at week 40 without complications. Her postpartum examination revealed the diabetes mellitus was gestational. No further indication of the condition was present. She will be monitored twice in the next year at 6-month intervals.

14. _____ Wiskott-Aldrich syndrome

15. _____ A patient is diagnosed with a benign neoplasm of the occipital bone.

True or False

16. _____ A benign neoplasm is a noncancerous tumor that does not worsen over time.

17. _____ A patient who has non–insulin-dependent diabetes mellitus that is out of control is coded using category E-10.–.

18. _____ Chronic hepatitis C with hepatic coma is located in Chapter 2 of the Tabular List.

19. _____ Late effects of tuberculosis are never coded.

20. _____ Diabetic complications of pregnancy are coded using only category O24.–.

Mental and Behavioral Disorders, Diseases of the Nervous System, Diseases of the Eye, and Diseases of the Ear (F01-H95)

LEARNING OBJECTIVES

- Understand the guidelines for mental health coding
- Review and understand guidelines for nervous system coding
- Review and understand guidelines for diagnosis coding of the eye and ear
- Review coding and coding scenarios
- Test your skill by completing checkpoint exercises
- Test your knowledge by answering additional questions

Chapter 6 in the Tabular List includes the following sections:

- Mental disorders due to known physiological conditions (F01-F09)
- Mental and behavioral disorders due to psychoactive substance use (F10-F19)
- Schizophrenia, schizotypal and delusional, and other nonmood psychotic disorders (F20-F29)
- Mood [affective] disorders (F30-F39)
- Anxiety, dissociative, stress-related, somatoform, and other nonpsychotic mental disorders (F40-F48)
- Behavioral syndromes associated with physiological disturbances and physical factors (F50-F59)
- Disorders of adult personality and behavior (F60-F69)
- Mental retardation (F70-F79)
- Pervasive and specific developmental disorders (F80-F89)
- Behavioral and emotional disorders with onset usually occurring in childhood and adolescence (F90-F98)
- Unspecified mental disorders (F99)

The psychiatric terms that appear in Chapter 6 are based on material furnished by the American

Psychiatric Association's Task Force on Nomenclature and Statistics and from the Psychiatric Glossary, as indicated in the *Diagnosis and Statistical Manual of Mental Disorders, Fourth Edition* (DSM-IV), which can be obtained by most health care publishers. The Psychiatric Glossary is part of the DSM-IV manual. Understanding the terminology of mental conditions is critical for coding the conditions. The publication to refer to when assigning codes in this category is the DSM-IV, published by the American Psychiatric Association. Most of the diagnosis codes found in DSM-IV are also found in the *International Classification of Diseases, 10th Revision, Clinical Modification* (ICD-10-CM) manual; however, the terminology may be different. It is important to become familiar with DSM-IV, even though the diagnosis code selection will be taken from the ICD-10-CM manual.

Mental health (psychiatric) disorders involve disturbances in thinking, emotion, and behavior. These disorders are caused by complex interactions including the following:

- Physical factors
- Psychological factors
- Social factors
- Cultural influences
- Hereditary influences

Classification and Diagnosis of Mental Illness

In the field of medicine, the classification of diseases is constantly changing as knowledge changes. In psychiatry, the knowledge of how the brain functions and is influenced by the environment and other factors is constantly becoming more sophisticated. Despite advances, knowledge of the intricate mechanisms involved in brain functioning is still in its infancy. However, because many research studies have shown that mental illnesses can be distinguished from one another with a high degree of reliability, a standardized approach to diagnosis is becoming more and more refined.

PSYCHOTHERAPY

In recent years, significant advances have been made in the field of psychotherapy. *Psychotherapy* is the treatment of a patient by a therapist using psychological techniques and making systematic use of the patient-therapist relationship. Psychiatrists are not the only mental health professionals trained to practice psychotherapy. Others include clinical psychologists, social workers, nurses, some pastoral counselors, and many paraprofessionals; however, psychiatrists are the only mental health professionals licensed to prescribe drugs.

MENTAL DISORDERS DUE TO KNOWN PHYSIOLOGICAL CONDITIONS (F01-F09)

This category includes mental disorders grouped together based on etiology in cerebral disease, brain injury, and other conditions leading to cerebral dysfunction. Conditions in this category include the following:

- Delirium
- Dementia
- Mood disorder due to know physiological conditions
- Personality and behavioral disorders due to known physiological conditions

Psychosis is defined as a personality derangement and loss of contact with reality and is frequently associated with the following:

- Delusions
- Hallucinations
- Illusions

Delirium

Delirium is defined as an acute state of confusion and is characterized by fluctuating disturbances in the following:

- Cognition
- Mood
- Attention
- Arousal
- Self-awareness

These disturbances arise acutely without prior intellectual impairment or are superimposed on chronic intellectual impairment.

A person who is less alert and has difficulty paying attention will have difficulty accurately perceiving and interpreting data from the environment, may misinterpret factual information or have illusions, and will have difficulty acquiring or remembering new information. With difficulty receiving, perceiving, interpreting, and remembering things, the person will not reason logically, will have difficulty manipulating symbolic data (eg, performing arithmetic or explaining proverbs), will become very anxious and agitated or withdraw from the environment, will become less active and involved, and may think in paranoid and delusional ways (see Figure 6.1).

Etiology of Delirium Many conditions can cause delirium. Initially, the causes can be classified as primary brain diseases (organic brain disease) or diseases that occur primarily elsewhere in the body but affect the brain, usually through associated toxic or metabolic changes.

The causes of delirium can be further categorized as metabolic, toxic, structural, or infectious.

FIGURE 6.1   Criteria for Diagnosis of Delirium

Reduced ability to maintain attention to external stimuli

Need to repeat questions because patient's attention wanders and to appropriately shift attention to new external stimuli

Persistence in answering previous question

Disorganized thinking, indicated by rambling, irrelevant, or incoherent speech

---

For a patient with delirium, at least two of the following signs/symptoms are present:

1. Reduced level of consciousness (eg, difficulty staying awake during examination)

2. Perceptual disturbances, misinterpretations, illusions, or hallucinations

3. Disturbance of sleep-wake cycle, with insomnia or daytime sleepiness

4. Increased or decreased psychomotor activity

5. Disorientation to time, place, or person

6. Memory impairment (eg, inability to learn new material, such as memorizing the names of several unrelated objects to be repeated after 5 minutes or to remember past events, such as history of current episode of illness)

Metabolic or Toxic Causes of Delirium Virtually any metabolic disorder can cause delirium in elderly people. Some of the more important metabolic and toxic causes of delirium include:

- Electrolyte imbalances
- Hyperkalemia
- Hypokalemia

- Metabolic acidosis nutritional deficiencies
- Chronic endocrine abnormalities
  - hypothyroidism
  - hyperthyroidism
  - hyperparathyroidism; confusion brought on by hyperparathyroidism
- Transient ischemia
- Hypoglycemia

Confusion can often occur in a patient with poorly managed diabetes. It may also occur without evidence of intracranial bleeding.

Delirium and Dementia

The most common syndromes that affect cognitive, physical, or behavioral functions and are associated with an acute or chronic central nervous system (CNS) disorder are dementia and delirium. Other forms of cognitive decline in elderly people include the amnestic syndromes, which are rare. All of these terms refer to dysfunction or loss of cognitive functions, the processes by which knowledge is acquired, retained, and used.

Traditionally, cognitive change in elderly people has been classified as delirium or dementia. Although delirium and dementia have separate and distinct characteristics, distinguishing between them can be difficult. Because no laboratory test can reliably establish a definitive cause of cognitive failure, evaluation is usually based on patient history and physical examination. Knowledge of baseline function is essential for determining the extent of change and the rate at which it has occurred. Table 6.1 lists the differences between delirium and dementia.

TABLE 6.1   Differences Between Delirium and Dementia

DELIRIUM	DEMENTIA
Rapid onset	Develops slowly
Fluctuating course	Slow, progressive course
Potentially reversible	Not reversible
Profoundly affects attention	Profoundly affects memory
Focal cognitive deficits	Global cognitive deficits
Usually caused by systemic medical drugs	Usually caused by Alzheimer illness or disease
Requires immediate evaluation and treatment	Does not require immediate treatment

For example, traumatic brain injury occurs suddenly but may result in severe, permanent dementia; hypothyroidism may produce the slowly progressive picture of dementia but be completely reversible with treatment.

Alzheimer's Disease

Alzheimer's disease is one of several disorders that cause the gradual loss of brain cells. The disease was first described in 1906 by German physician, Dr Alois Alzheimer. Although the disease was once considered rare, research has shown that it is the leading cause of dementia. "Dementia" is an umbrella term for several symptoms related to a decline in thinking skills. Common symptoms include a gradual loss of memory, problems with reasoning or judgment, disorientation, difficulty in learning, loss of language skills, and decline in the ability to perform routine tasks.

People with dementia also experience changes in their personalities and behavioral problems, such as agitation, anxiety, delusions (believing in a reality that does not exist), and hallucinations (seeing things that do not exist).

Alzheimer's disease advances at widely different rates. The duration of the illness may vary from 3 to 20 years. The areas of the brain that control memory and thinking skills are affected first, but as the disease progresses, cells die in other regions of the brain. Eventually, the person with Alzheimer's disease will need complete care. If the person has no other serious illness, the loss of brain function itself will cause death.

Alzheimer's disease is coded to F02, Dementia in other diseases classified elsewhere. Alzheimer's disease typically has an associated physiological condition associated with the dementia, and the condition is coded as the first listed diagnosis followed by a code in category F02.–.

CODING ISSUES

When coding mental disorders, it is extremely important to read the Includes and Excludes notes. These notes guide coders to the most accurate code category. When assigning codes from this category, it is essential to:

- Code only the diagnoses documented in the medical record

- Use caution to select the appropriate ICD-10-CM code

- Verify the diagnosis with the physician when in doubt

Review the following examples using the Index to Diseases and the Tabular List for coding dementia (see Figure 6.2).

> **EXAMPLE:** *A patient is diagnosed with senile dementia with paranoia.*

FIGURE 6.2 Excerpt from the Alphabetic Index: *Dementia*

Dementia (degenerative) (primary) (old age) (persisting) F03
    Alzheimer's type—see Disease, Alzheimer's Disease
      Alzheimer's G30.9 [F02.80]
      with behavioral disturbance G30.9 [F02.81]

1. First look in the Alphabetic Index: Dementia.

2. Locate "senile" under the category "Dementia."

3. The next step is to find "with paranoia."

4. The most accurate selection is "paranoid type F03."

Refer to Figure 6.3 to code the diagnosis accurately.

FIGURE 6.3 Excerpt from the Tabular List: *Senile dementia (F03)*

F03   Unspecified dementia
      Presenile dementia NOS
      Presenile psychosis NOS
      Primary degenerative dementia NOS
      Senile dementia NOS
      Senile dementia depressed or paranoid type
      Senile psychosis NOS
      EXCLUDES 1 *senility NOS (R41.81)*
      EXCLUDES 2 *senile dementia with delirium or acute confusional state (F05)*

Tabular List:
   F03 Senile dementia depressed or paranoid type

EXAMPLE: *A 76-year-old man has been in a nursing home for 6 months and is evaluated monthly. He has a history of* **left-sided cerebrovascular accident with right-sided paralysis**. *He has had* **dementia** *since his stroke and has been seen by a psychiatrist who diagnosed* **cerebral atherosclerosis with arteriosclerotic dementia**. *He is acutely delusional and does not answer any questions. He has swallowing problems but has not had signs of choking. General physical examination shows a blood pressure of 125/78 mm Hg, pulse of 78 beats per minute, and weight of 108 lb with a loss of 5 lb since last month. Examination of head, eyes, ears, nose, and throat shows laxity of the lower jaw and cataracts bilaterally. Lungs are clear to auscultation and percussion. Heart shows normal sinus rhythm. There is a 2/6 heart murmur. On CNS examination, the patient responds to name only, is delusional, and has right-sided paralysis due to an old cerebrovascular accident.* **Cerebral atherosclerosis** *along with arteriosclerotic dementia and* **acute confusional state** *are present, with acute cerebrovascular insufficiency. Current medications and dosage will be continued, and he will be seen again in 1 month.*

Figure 6.4 shows the appropriate part of the Alphabetic Index for vascular dementia and Figure 6.5 of the Tabular List.

FIGURE 6.4   Excerpt from the Alphabetic Index:
              Vascular Dementia

Dementia
    Vascular (acute onset) (mixed) (multi-infarct)
    subcortical F01.50
    with behavioral disturbance F01.51

FIGURE 6.5   Excerpt from the Tabular List: *F01.–*

F01   Vascular dementia
    F01.5   Vascular dementia
    F01.50 Vascular dementia without behavioral disturbances
    F01.51 Vascular dementia with behavioral disturbances
             Vascular dementia with aggressive behavior
             Vascular dementia with combative behavior
             Vascular dementia with violent behavior
             Vascular dementia with wandering off

Alphabetic Index:
  Dementia ➞ *vascular F01* ➞ *without behavioral disturbances* ➞ *F01.50*

Tabular List:
  F01.50 Vascular dementia without behavioral disturbances

The instructional notes under category F01 indicate that the user must "Code first the underlying physiological condition or sequelae of cerebrovascular disease." In this example the underlying condition is the "acute delusional state."

Open the ICD-10-CM codebook to the Alphabetic Index and look up "delusion." You will notice that there is an instructional note to "see disorder." Review Figure 6.6.

FIGURE 6.6   Excerpt from the Alphabetic Index:
              Disorder, Delusional

Disorder
    Delusional (persistent) (systematized) F22
    Induced F24

Now review both categories F22 and F24 and select the appropriate principal diagnosis. The correct diagnosis code for this encounter is F22.

An additional code is required to identify cerebral atherosclerosis. The physician identified cerebral atherosclerosis as a diagnosis. The cerebral atherosclerosis is coded as a secondary diagnosis to the arteriosclerotic dementia, with delirium. When reviewing the index under atherosclerosis, it refers the user to "arteriosclerosis." Under arteriosclerosis you will need to locate "cerebral." Cerebral arteriosclerosis is classified to I67.2.

Tabular List:
  I67.2 ➞ *Cerebral atherosclerosis*

The correct ICD-10-CM codes for this patient encounter are as follows:

First listed diagnosis:
  F22 Delusional disorder

Secondary diagnosis:
  F01.50 Vascular dementia without behavioral disturbances

Tertiary diagnosis:
  I67.2 Cerebral atherosclerosis

Correct coding sequencing:
  F22, F01.50, I67.2

ALCOHOL-INDUCED MENTAL DISORDERS

Alcoholic hallucinosis follows abrupt abstinence from prolonged, excessive use of alcohol. Symptoms include auditory illusions and hallucinations, frequent accusatory and threatening behavior, apprehension, terror caused by the hallucinations, and vivid, frightening dreams.

Delirium tremens usually begins soon after alcohol withdrawal, with the following:

- Anxiety attacks

- Increasing confusion

- Poor sleep (with frightening dreams or nocturnal illusions)

- Marked sweating

- Profound depression

Coding Issues

Alcoholism is coded with category F10, Alcohol related disorders. An additional code is required to identify blood alcohol levels if applicable and is coded in sub-classification Y90.–.

An associated condition related to the alcohol abuse or dependence should be coded as an additional diagnosis such as the following:

- Alcoholic psychoses

- Drug dependence

- Other related conditions

Some physical complications of alcohol include the following:

- Cerebral degeneration

- Alcoholic cirrhosis of liver

- Epilepsy

- Alcoholic gastritis

- Acute alcoholic hepatitis

- Liver damage

Conditions of alcoholic psychoses include the following:

- Withdrawal delirium

- Alcoholic dementia

- Hallucinosis

- Psychosis with hallucinosis

- Alcohol intoxication

- Alcohol withdrawal syndrome

- Alcoholic mania

- Chronic alcoholism with psychosis

Open the ICD-10-CM codebook, start with the Alphabetic Index and verify the code in the Tabular List.

Review the following example:

EXAMPLE: *A 42-year-old woman enters an alcohol treatment facility in the hospital to withdraw from alcohol. She is alcohol dependent. Twenty-four hours after her arrival, she experiences acute hallucinations, profuse sweating, increased confusion, and anxiety. The physician overseeing her care diagnoses the patient with hallucinosis alcohol withdrawal.*

Alphabetic Index:
Psychosis, psychotic → *F29* → *with* → *hallucinosis* → *F10.251* → *dependence* → *F10.250*

Tabular List:
F10.251 → *Alcohol dependence with alcohol-induced psychotic disorder with hallucinations*

Notice that when reviewing the Tabular List that F10.250 is with delusions and F10.251 is with hallucinations, which is what this patient is experiencing.

Correct diagnosis code:
F10.251

ICD-10-CM OFFICIAL GUIDELINES FOR MENTAL HEALTH DISORDERS: CHAPTER 5: MENTAL AND BEHAVIORAL DISORDERS (F01-F99)

C5 a. Pain Disorders Related to Psychological Factors

Assign code F45.41 for pain that is exclusively psychological. Code F45.41, Pain disorder exclusively related to psychological factors, should be used following the appropriate code from category G89, Pain, not elsewhere classified, if there is documentation of a psychological component for a patient with acute or chronic pain. See Section I.C.6, Pain.

C5 b. Mental and Behavioral Disorders due to Psychoactive Substance Use

1. In remission

   Selection of codes for "in remission" for categories F10-F19, Mental and behavioral disorders due to psychoactive substance use (categories F10-F19) requires the provider's clinical judgment. The appropriate codes for "in remission" are assigned only on the basis of provider documentation (as defined in the Official Guidelines for Coding and Reporting).

2. Psychoactive substance use, abuse, and dependence

   When the provider documentation refers to use, abuse, and dependence of the same substance (eg, alcohol, opioids, cannabis), only one code should be assigned to identify the pattern of use based on the following hierarchy:

- If both use and abuse are documented, assign only the code for abuse

- If both abuse and dependence are documented, assign only the code for dependence

- If use, abuse, and dependence are all documented, assign only the code for dependence

- If both use and dependence are documented, assign only the code for dependence.

C3 Psychoactive Substance Use

As with all other diagnoses, the codes for psychoactive substance use (F10.9–, F11.9–, F12.9–, F13.9–, F14.9–, F15.9–, F16.9–) should only be assigned based on provider documentation and when they meet the definition of a reportable diagnosis (see Section III, Reporting Additional Diagnoses). The codes are to be used only when the psychoactive substance use is associated with a mental or behavioral disorder and such a relationship is documented by the provider.

ALCOHOL DEPENDENCE F10.2–

Alcohol dependence is a state resulting from drinking alcohol on a continuous or periodic basis to experience its psychic effects and sometimes to avoid discomfort of its absence.

Alcoholism

Alcoholism is associated with deviant behaviors with prolonged consumption of excessive amounts of alcohol. Alcoholism is considered a chronic illness of undetermined etiology, with recognizable signs and symptoms. Consumption of large amounts of alcohol usually causes the following:

- Significant clinical toxicity and tissue damage

- Significant physical dependence

- A dangerous withdrawal syndrome

A person with alcoholism is identified by severe dependence or addiction and a cumulative pattern of characteristic behaviors. Frequent intoxication is obvious and destructive; it interferes with the ability to socialize and to work. Eventually, drunkenness may lead to failed relationships and to job loss due to work absenteeism. People with alcoholism may incur physical injury, be apprehended for driving while intoxicated, or be arrested for drunkenness.

People with alcoholism may seek medical treatment for their drinking. Eventually, they may be hospitalized for delirium tremens or cirrhosis. The earlier in life these behaviors are evident, the more crippling the disorder. Women alcoholics are, in general, more likely to drink alone and are less likely to experience some of the social stigmas.

Alcohol Dependence

Category F10.2– is used to identify the following:

- Alcohol dependence in uncomplicated (F10.20)

- Alcohol dependence in remission (F10.21)

- Alcohol dependence with intoxication (F10.22–)

- Alcohol dependence with withdrawal (F10.23)

- Alcohol dependence with alcohol-induced mood disorder (F10.24)

- Alcohol dependence with alcohol-induced psychotic disorder (F10.25–)

- Alcohol dependence with alcohol-induced amnestic disorder (F10.26)

- Alcohol dependence with alcohol-induced persistent dementia (F10.27)

- Alcohol dependence with other alcohol-induced disorders (F10.28–)

- Alcohol dependence with unspecified alcohol-induced disorder (F10.29)

A sixth digit subclassification is required in many of these categories to identify the associated disorder associated with the alcohol dependence (see Figure 6.7).

FIGURE 6.7   Excerpt from the Tabular List: *F10.23–*

✓6ᵗʰ F10.23 Alcohol dependence with withdrawal
EXCLUDES 1 *Alcohol dependence with intoxication (F10.22)*
F10.230 Alcohol dependence with withdrawal, uncomplicated
F10.231 Alcohol dependence with withdrawal delirium
F10.232 Alcohol dependence with withdrawal with perceptual disturbance
F10.239 Alcohol dependence with withdrawal, unspecified

It is important to understand the following terms when selecting the appropriate category for alcoholism and drug usage:

Continuous: Daily intake of large amounts of alcohol or drugs or regular, heavy drinking on weekends or days off work. For drugs, daily or almost daily use.

Episodic: Alcoholic binges that last weeks or months, with sobriety for long periods afterward or use of drugs on weekends or short periods between drug use.

In remission: Complete cessation of alcohol or drug intake for a length of time or a gradual trend toward cessation.

When a patient is admitted for withdrawal or when alcohol withdrawal develops after admission, the code for alcoholism is reported as the first listed diagnosis, and the blood alcohol level (if known) is selected as the secondary diagnosis.

Open the ICD-10-CM codebook to the Alphabetic Index and refer to the Tabular List to select the appropriate code.

Review the following examples:

> **EXAMPLE:** *A 27-year-old woman is admitted to an alcohol treatment facility to help withdraw from alcohol. The patient has had alcoholism since age 20 years and is now experiencing hallucinations. The patient has chronic alcoholism and has been drinking on a daily basis for 7 years. She has not had a drink for 24 hours and believes this is the reason she is having acute hallucinations. The patient was recently fired from her job for drinking while at work.*

Open the ICD-10-CM codebook to the Alphabetic index and reference the main term "alcohol." Review the following:

> **Alphabetic Index:**
> *Alcohol, alcoholic, alcohol-induced → hallucinosis (acute) → in dependence → F10.251*

> **Tabular List:**
> *F10.251 → Alcohol dependence with alcohol-induced psychotic disorder with hallucinations*

> **Correct coding:**
> *F10.251*

> **EXAMPLE:** *A 45-year-old man is admitted to a hospital-based alcohol treatment facility. The patient's history includes a previous 5-day stay in the alcohol treatment facility and alcohol binges that sometimes lasted for several weeks. The patient's medical history is unremarkable. The patient denies hallucinations, psychosis, and delirium. He does admit to becoming angry and explosive to his family while drinking and admits to hitting his wife. He has been drinking for 3 days continuously and has decided to again seek help for chronic episodic alcohol dependence. His blood alcohol level is 22mg/100ml upon admission.*

Open the ICD-10-CM codebook to the Alphabetic Index and identify the main term. The main term in this patient encounter is "dependence" followed by the term "alcohol."

The medical record documentation indicates chronic episodic alcohol dependence.

> **Alphabetic Index:**
> *Alcohol → dependence → with → mood disorder → F10.24*

> **Tabular List:**
> *F10.24 → Alcohol dependence with alcohol-induced mood disorder*

The instructional note in this classification requires an additional code to identify the blood alcohol level if known. In this case the blood alcohol level is 22.

> **Tabular List:**
> *Y90.1 → Blood alcohol level of 20-39 mg/100 mL*

> **Correct code sequencing:**
> *F10.24, Y90.1*

NONDEPENDENT ABUSE OF ALCOHOL (F10.1.–)

This category is used for alcohol abuse. For alcohol, it is used with the following diagnoses:

- Drunkenness
- Excessive drinking
- Inebriety
- Alcohol hangover

However, there is no indication in this category that the patient is dependent on alcohol. Review the following example.

> **EXAMPLE:** *A 21-year-old female college student is sent to the emergency department after excessive drinking at a fraternity party and was observed as being intoxicated. The patient states that she does not drink very often, but at the party she drank several glasses of wine along with several mixed drinks. The patient complains of headache, excessive vomiting, nausea, and fatigue. The patient was given intravenous fluids, counseled on excessive drinking by the physician, and released the next morning.*

This encounter does not indicate that the patient is an alcoholic. The documentation, however, states that the patient drank excessively at a party and indicates alcohol abuse. Open the ICD-10-CM codebook and review the main term "abuse" in the Alphabetic Index.

Alphabetic Index:
Abuse ➞ alcohol (non dependent) ➞ with intoxication ➞ F10.129

Tabular List:
F10.12 ➞ Alcohol abuse with intoxication ➞ F10.129 unspecified

In this example the correct code to report is F10.129. Because the blood alcohol level is not documented, only the alcohol abuse is reported. The signs/symptoms are the result of the alcohol abuse and would not be reported. However, you are not finished yet. Counseling of the patient should also be reported.

Review the Alphabetic Index under the main term "counseling."

Alphabetic Index:
Counseling ➞ alcohol abuser ➞ Z71.41

Tabular List:
Z71.41 ➞ Alcohol abuse counseling and surveillance of alcoholic

Correct code sequencing:
F10.129, Z71.41

Substance Abuse

Drug addiction and substance abuse are chronic mental and physical conditions related to the patient's pattern of drug use. Codes in this classification are defined by type of drug or substance along with whether the encounter is abuse or dependence. In addition, a sixth character may be required in many instances to identify the condition related to the abuse or dependence.

The following subclassifications identify specific drugs:

- Opioid-related disorders F11.–
- Cannabis-related disorders F12.–
- Sedative-, hypnotic-, or anxiolytic-related disorders F13.–
- Cocaine-related disorders F14.–
- Other stimulant-related disorders F15.–
- Hallucinogen-related disorders F16.–
- Nicotine dependence F17.–
- Inhalant-related disorders F18.–
- Other psychoactive substance-related disorders F19.–

EXAMPLE: A 16-year-old boy is admitted to a drug treatment facility by his father. The patient has a history of cocaine abuse, with continuous use for the past year. The patient indicates that he uses cocaine daily. The parents tried to manage their son as an outpatient, but the patient would sneak out of the house to buy cocaine when the parents were sleeping. The patient does not sleep more than a couple hours a day and paces in his room all night, which has kept the entire family awake. This has been ongoing for the past 6 months. The psychiatrist on call performs a comprehensive examination as well as mental health status evaluation and counsels the patient and parents as to treatment, outcomes, and length of stay. The diagnosis the physician documents is continuous cocaine dependence and abuse.

Alphabetic Index:
Dependence ➞ drug ➞ cocaine ➞ with ➞ sleep disorder ➞ F14.282

Tabular List:
F14.282 ➞ Cocaine dependence with cocaine-induced sleep disorder

Correct code:
F14.282

Principal Diagnosis Selection for Substance Abuse or Dependence

The following guidelines should be reviewed when the principal diagnosis is substance abuse or substance dependence:

- When a patient is admitted for the purpose of detoxification or rehabilitation or both and when withdrawal or other psychotic symptoms are indicated, sequence the substance abuse or dependence as the principal diagnosis.

- When the patient is treated for alcohol abuse or dependence and the blood alcohol level is known use an additional code to identify the blood alcohol level from category Y90.–.

- When a patient is treated for both drug and alcohol abuse or dependence and is admitted for detoxification or rehabilitation, either condition may be designated the principal diagnosis.

- When a patient is diagnosed with substance abuse or dependence and is admitted for treatment or evaluation of a medical or physical condition related to the substance abuse or dependence, follow the directions in the Alphabetic Index for conditions described as alcoholic or due to drugs. Sequence the physical condition as the principal diagnosis, followed by the abuse or drug dependence.

- When a patient with a diagnosis of substance abuse, alcohol or drugs, is admitted for an unrelated condition, follow ICD-10-CM coding guidelines when selecting the principal diagnosis.

SCHIZOPHRENIA, SCHIZOTYPAL, DELUSIONAL, AND OTHER NONMOOD PSYCHOTIC DISORDERS (F20-F29)

Several disorders are listed in this category of codes. Some of the most common disorders are the following:

- Schizophrenia (F20.–)
- Schizotypal disorders (F21)
- Delusional disorders (F22)
- Schizoaffective disorders (F25.–)

Schizophrenia

Schizophrenia is a common and serious mental disorder characterized by loss of contact with reality (psychosis), hallucinations (false perceptions), delusions (false beliefs), abnormal thinking, flattened affect (restricted range of emotions), diminished motivation, and disturbed work and social functioning.

Although its specific cause is unknown, schizophrenia has a biologic basis. A vulnerability-stress model, in which schizophrenia is viewed as occurring in persons with neurologically based vulnerabilities, is the most widely accepted explanation. Onset, remission, and recurrence of symptoms are seen as products of interaction between these vulnerabilities and environmental stressors.

No definitive test for schizophrenia exists. Diagnosis is based on a comprehensive assessment of clinical history, signs, and symptoms. Information from ancillary sources, such as family, friends, and teachers, is often important in establishing the chronology of illness onset. According to DSM-IV, two or more characteristic symptoms (delusions, hallucinations, disorganized speech, disorganized behavior, negative symptoms) for a significant portion of a one-month period are required for the diagnosis, as well as prodromal or attenuated signs of illness with social, occupational, or self-care impairments. The condition must be evident for a 6-month period that includes one month of active symptoms.

Psychotic disorders due to physical disorders or associated with substance abuse, as well as primary mood disorders with psychotic features, must be ruled out by clinical examination and history. In addition, laboratory tests can rule out underlying medical, neurologic, and endocrine disorders that can manifest as psychosis, such as the following:

- Vitamin deficiencies
- Uremia
- Thyrotoxicosis
- Electrolyte imbalance

The types of schizophrenia include the following:

- Paranoid
- Catatonic
- Undifferentiated
- Residual
- Disorganized

Coding Issues

Schizophrenic disorders are classified in category F20.–. The fifth character in this category identifies the type of schizophrenia. For example, if the diagnostic statement indicates the patient is suffering from schizophrenic catalepsy, the correct code would be F20.3, Catatonic schizophrenia, which includes schizophrenic catalepsy.

> **EXAMPLE:** *A patient is diagnosed with chronic residual schizophrenia.*

Open the ICD-10-CM codebook to the Index and reference the main term "schizophrenia."

> ***Alphabetic Index:***
> *Schizophrenia* → *residual (state) (type)* → *F20.5*

> ***Tabular List:***
> *F20.5* → *Residual schizophrenia*

> ***Correct code:***
> *F20.5*

MOOD AFFECTIVE DISORDERS (F30-F39)

Affective psychoses include major depressive, manic, and bipolar disorders. These are common mental conditions characterized by mood disturbances. The major affective disorders are classified according to symptoms. Other nonpsychotic depressive disorders are subclassification F32.- depression. These disorders can be diagnosed and documented in the medical record as:

- Recurrent
- Mild
- Moderate
- Mixed
- Severe, without mention of psychotic behavior
- Severe, specified as with psychotic behavior

- In partial or unspecified remission

- In full remission

Depressive Disorders

Depressive disorders are mental disorders typically without an organic basis. Behavior may be affected, although it usually remains within acceptable social limits. A person diagnosed with a depressive disorder usually manifests the following:

- Sadness

- Despair

- Discouragement

- Low self-esteem

- Guilt

- Self-reproach

- Withdrawal

- Eating and sleeping disturbances

Review the following example:

> **EXAMPLE:** *A patient diagnosed with major depressive disorder returns to her psychiatrist with a complaint that her depression has not subsided even though the physician has prescribed fluoxetine (Prozac). The physician spends 45 minutes counseling the patient, updating her history, and changing the medication dosage. She is to return in one week for a follow-up evaluation. The assessment and plan indicate she has a moderate recurrent major depressive disorder.*

A diagnosis of major depressive disorder indicates that the diagnosis code is selected from category 296. Because the patient has had recurrent episodes, the disease should be coded as recurrent.

> **Alphabetic Index:**
> *Disorder → depressive → recurrent → moderate → F33.1*

> **Tabular List:**
> *F33.1 → Major depressive disorder, recurrent, moderate*

> **Correct code:**
> *F33.1*

MANIC AND BIPOLAR DISORDERS (F30-F31)

Manic disorders are conditions in which a patient exhibits the following symptoms:

- Grandiosity

- Poor judgment

- Rapid speech

- Flight of ideas

- Major depression

Bipolar disorders are classified in category F31.–. Bipolar disorder is a manic depressive psychosis that appears in the manic and depressive forms, alternating or separated by an interval of normality. Many patients experience recurrent mood changes that result in severe depression followed by extreme elation, which are beyond the normal mood swings.

The codes in this category are as follows:

F31	Bipolar disorder	
	F31.0	Bipolar disorder, current episode hypomanic
		F31.10 Bipolar disorder, current episode manic without psychotic features, unspecified
		F31.11 Bipolar disorder, current episode manic without psychotic features, mild
		F31.12 Bipolar disorder, current episode manic without psychotic features, moderate
		F31.13 Bipolar disorder, current episode manic without psychotic features, severe
	F31.2	Bipolar disorder, current episode manic severe with psychotic feature
	F31.3	Major depressive disorder, recurrent
		F31.30 Bipolar disorder, current episode depressed, mild or moderate severity, unspecified
		F31.31 Bipolar disorder, current episode depressed, mild
		F31.32 Bipolar disorder, current episode depressed, moderate
	F31.4	Bipolar disorder, current episode depressed, severe, without psychotic feature
	F31.5	Bipolar disorder, current episode depressed, severe, with psychotic feature
	F31.6	Bipolar disorder, current episode, mixed
		F31.60 Bipolar disorder, current episode mixed, unspecified
		F31.61 Bipolar disorder, current episode mixed, mild
		F31.62 Bipolar disorder, current episode mixed, moderate
		F31.63 Bipolar disorder, current episode mixed, severe, without psychotic feature
		F31.64 Bipolar disorder, current episode mixed, severe, with psychotic features
	F31.7	Bipolar disorder, currently in remission
		F31.70 Bipolar disorder, currently in remission, most recent episode unspecified
		F31.71 Bipolar disorder, in partial remission, most recent episode hypomania
		F31.72 Bipolar disorder, in full remission, most recent episode hypomania
		F31.73 Bipolar disorder, in partial remission, most recent episode mania
		F31.74 Bipolar disorder, in full remission, most recent episode mania

F31.75   Bipolar disorder, in partial remission, most recent episode depressed

F31.76   Bipolar disorder, in full remission, most recent episode depressed

F31.77   Bipolar disorder, in partial remission, most recent episode mixed

F31.78   Bipolar disorder, in full remission, most recent episode mixed

F31.81   Bipolar II disorder

F31.89   Other bipolar disorder

F31.9   Bipolar disorder, unspecified

Review the following example:

EXAMPLE: *A patient was referred to a psychiatrist for treatment. After a comprehensive history and mental status examination, the psychiatrist diagnoses the patient with mild hypomania. The physician spends 30 minutes counseling the patient and prescribing medications. The patient is scheduled to return for a follow-up appointment in two weeks.*

Alphabetic Index:
Hypomania, hypomanic reaction F30.8

Tabular List:
F30.8 ➡ Other manic episodes ➡ hypomania

Correct code:
F30.8

EXAMPLE: *A woman visits her psychiatrist for a follow-up visit. After a mental status evaluation along with a psychotherapy session, the psychiatrist determines the patient is exhibiting signs of manic and depressive behavior. The documentation in the medical record states, "severe bipolar disorder, mixed."*

Alphabetic Index:
Disorder ➡ bipolar ➡ mixed ➡ severe ➡ F31.63

Tabular List:
F31.63 Bipolar disorder, current episode mixed, severe, without psychotic features

Because there is no mention of a psychotic condition with the bipolar disorder, the code selection is based on the statement "without psychotic features."

Correct code:
F31.63

ANXIETY, DISSOCIATIVE, STRESS-RELATED, SOMATOFORM, AND OTHER NONPSYCHOTIC MENTAL DISORDERS (F40-F48)

These types of disorders are mental disorders without demonstrable organic basis in which the person may have considerable insight but impaired reality perception. The person usually does not confuse morbid subjective experiences and fantasies with external reality.

These disorders include the following:

- Excessive anxiety
- Hysterical symptoms
- Phobias
- Obsessive symptoms
- Compulsive symptoms
- Depression

Some of the ICD-10-CM codes in this category include the following:

- Obsessive compulsive disorder (F42)
- Posttraumatic stress disorder (F43.1–)
- Agoraphobia with panic disorder (F40.01)
- Somatoform disorders (F45.–)
- Fear of flying (F40.243)
- Psychogenic deafness (F44.6)
- Psychogenic pruritus (F45.8)

Review the following example:

EXAMPLE: *Patient: Mary Jones   Date: 06/30/20xx*

Time spent with patient: 45 minutes

Session focus: To cope with lifestyle changes, which are causing her panic.

The patient stated, "I have had a bad week, I am still having crying spells and tension." Patient states crying spells have decreased in frequency. Patient states panic attacks are worsening and occurring every time she leaves the house. Patient discussed her anger, need for distraction, and anger at loss of a travel opportunity. She reports a solid block of sleep at night and adds that she has been spending a lot of time in bed. She is afraid to leave the house. Every time she leaves the house, she cannot breathe and is dizzy and fearful.

Assessment: Four of 12 planned counseling sessions completed, patient still experiencing panic attacks frequently.

Plan: Will continue therapy as planned, next session in two weeks, continue current medications.

Alphabetic Index:
Panic (attack) (state) ➡ F41.0

Tabular List:
F41.0 ➡ Panic disorder [episodic paroxysmal anxiety] without agoraphobia

Correct code(s):
F41.0

STRESS AND ADJUSTMENT REACTIONS (F43.-)

The ICD-10-CM manual provides a category to classify transient mental disorders that are reactions to physical or mental stress. Acute stress reactions are the result of an acute stressor (eg, being mugged) and include disorders of any severity and nature (eg, depression, anxiety, panic). These reactions usually subside in a matter of hours or days.

Adjustment reactions (F43.2–) are the result of chronic stressors (eg, bereavement, divorce) and last usually no longer than a few months. Conditions classified to these categories are considered situational and reversible and, therefore, need to be differentiated from other mental disorders.

Review the following example:

> **EXAMPLE**: *A 30-year-old woman who was trapped under debris from a tornado for 12 hours was having a difficult time one year after the incident. She went to a psychiatrist with symptoms of nightmares reliving the experience, fear of storms, and difficulty concentrating. The physician diagnosed chronic posttraumatic stress disorder.*
>
> **Alphabetic Index:**
> *Disorder* ➞ *posttraumatic stress* ➞ *chronic F43.12*
>
> **Tabular List:**
> *F43.12* ➞ *Posttraumatic stress disorder, chronic*
>
> **Correct code:**
> *F43.12*

BEHAVIORAL SYNDROMES ASSOCIATED WITH PHYSIOLOGICAL DISTURBANCES AND PHYSICAL FACTORS (F50-F59)

Codes F50-F59 are intended to be used if the psychopathology is manifested by a single, specific symptom (or group of symptoms) that is not part of an organic illness or other mental disorder classifiable elsewhere.

Some common conditions listed in this category include the following:

- Eating disorders
- Sleep disorders
- Anorexia nervosa
- Tic disorders
- Speech disorders
- Bulimia
- Psychogenic pain
- Sexual disorders

- Nail biting
- Thumb sucking

Figure 6.8 shows several exclusions noted for anorexia nervosa. Caution must be used when selecting a code in this category.

FIGURE 6.8   Excerpt from the Tabular List: *Anorexia Nervosa*

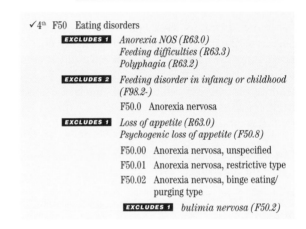

The following are some of the codes in this category:

- Sleepwalking (F51.3)
- Sexual aversion disorder (F52.1)
- Orgasmic disorder (F52.3)
- Abuse of laxatives (F55.2)

PERSONALITY [ADULT] DISORDERS (F60-F69)

Personality disorders include pervasive, inflexible, and stable personality traits that deviate from cultural norms and cause distress or functional impairment.

Personality traits are patterns of thinking, perceiving, reacting, and relating that are relatively stable over time and in various situations. Personality disorders occur when these traits are so rigid and maladaptive that they impair interpersonal or vocational functioning. These traits and their potential maladaptive significance are usually evident from early adulthood and persist throughout much of life. Without environmental frustration, persons with personality disorders may or may not be dissatisfied with themselves.

They may seek help because of symptoms such as the following:

- Anxiety
- Depression
- Maladaptive behavior
- Substance abuse
- Vengefulness that results from the personality disorder

Often they do not see a need for therapy, and their peers, their families, or a social agency refer them because their maladaptive behavior causes difficulties for others. Because these patients usually view their difficulties as discrete and outside of themselves, mental health professionals have difficulty getting them to see that the problem is really based on their personality.

Persons with severe personality disorders are at high risk of the following:

- Hypochondriasis
- Alcoholism
- Drug abuse
- Violent behavior
- Self-destructive behavior

Coding Issues

The following are examples of coding personality disorders. Open the ICD-10-CM codebook to the Alphabetic Index and confirm the correct diagnosis code in the Tabular List for the following examples:

EXAMPLE: Chronic obsessional personality disorder

Alphabetic Index:
Personality → obsessional → F60.5

Tabular List:
F60.5 → Obsessive-compulsive personality disorder

Correct code:
F60.5

EXAMPLE: A 56-year-old established patient visits her internist complaining of fatigue, constant crying, feelings of aggressiveness, and constant fighting with her coworkers and her family. She indicates this has been going on for 6 months. She also has had a 20-pound weight gain in the past 3 months. The physician performs a detailed history and examination and diagnosis the patient with explosive personality disorder.

Alphabetic Index:
Personality → explosive → F60.3

Tabular List:
F60.3 → Borderline personality disorder → explosive personality (disorder)

Correct code:
F60.3

PERVASIVE DEVELOPMENTAL DISORDERS (F80-F89)

Codes F80 to F89 are reported for conditions that relate to childhood. These disorders include reading disorders, Asperger's syndrome, speech and language developmental delay, and autism.

Review the following example:

EXAMPLE: An 8-year-old child in the third grade is having difficulty reading. He appears to read backwards and does not appear to understand what he is reading. The teacher counseled the parents. The mom took the child to the pediatrician who diagnosed the patient with developmental dyslexia. No other problems were identified during the visit.

Alphabetic Index:
Dyslexia → developmental → F81.0

Tabular List:
F81.0 → Specific reading disorder → developmental dyslexia

Correct code:
F81.0

BEHAVIORAL SYNDROMES ASSOCIATED WITH PHYSIOLOGICAL DISTURBANCES AND PHYSICAL FACTORS (F50-F59)

The ICD-10-CM code book differentiates between physiological malfunctions arising from mental disorders and psychic conditions associated with underlying physical disorders. The distinction between the two categories is the nature of the physical condition. Physical conditions that manifest as functional disorders (eg, vomiting) are classified to category F45.-. Physical conditions that manifest as structural disturbances or tissue damage (eg, ulcerative colitis) are classified to category F50-F54. The underlying physical condition is coded and is sequenced as a secondary diagnosis.

Review the following examples:

> **EXAMPLE:** *A 32-year-old patient experiences nervous gastritis when under stress and anxiety. The patient's symptoms include belching, excessive swallowing of air, and a distended abdomen. The physician diagnoses the patient with an acute gastric ulcer due to the nervous gastritis.*
>
> **Alphabetic Index:**
> *Gastritis → nervous → F54*
>
> **Tabular List:**
> *F54 → Psychological and behavioral factors associated with disorder or diseases classified elsewhere*

There is an instructional note to code first the associated physical disorder. The patient's condition in this example is nervous gastritis. The final diagnosis in this example is the acute gastric ulcer that was caused by the stress and anxiety.

> **Alphabetic Index:**
> *Ulcer → gastric → K25.–*
>
> **Tabular List:**
> *K25.3 → Acute gastric ulcer without hemorrhage or perforation*
>
> **Correct code sequencing:**
> *K25.3, F54*

CODING TIP Always follow the instructional notes in the Tabular List to identify the first listed or additional diagnoses associated with the condition.

> **EXAMPLE:** *A 40-year-old woman is treated by her internist for chronic eczema due to anxiety. Every time she gets anxious or agitated, the eczema reoccurs. This is the fifth time in a year she has had this condition. The physician prescribed medication for the eczema and the anxiety.*
>
> **Alphabetic Index:**
> *Psychogenic—see also condition factors associated with physical conditions F54*
>
> **Tabular List:**
> *F54 → Psychological and behavioral factors associated with disorders or diseases classified elsewhere*

Note: There are instructions to use an additional code to identify the associated psychological factors associated with the physical condition → eczema → see dermatitis contact.

> **Tabular List:**
> *L25.9 Contact dermatitis and other eczema → unspecified cause*
>
> **Correct code sequencing:**
> *L25.9, F54*

CHECKPOINT EXERCISE 6-1

Using the ICD-10-CM manual, code the following:

1. _____ Anorexia nervosa

2. _____ Attention deficit disorder

3. _____ Moderate pyromania

4. _____ Narcissistic personality

5. _____ Chronic alcoholism in remission

6. _____ Oppositional defiant disorder

7. _____ Phonological disorder

8. _____ Acute stress disorder

9. _____ Psychogenic pain

10. _____ Night terrors

True or False

11. _____ The term "abuse" means the same as dependence when coding with ICD-10-CM.

12. _____ ICD-10-CM code F20.1 requires a fifth character.

13. _____ Use code category F20 when coding childhood-type schizophrenic disorders.

14. _____ Alcohol withdrawal hallucinosis excludes alcohol withdrawal with delirium.

15. _____ Bulimia Nervosa is classified as F50.9.

Diseases of the Nervous System and Sense Organs (G00-G99)

Chapter 6 in the Tabular List includes the following sections:

- Inflammatory diseases of the central nervous system (G00-G09)

- Systemic atrophies primarily affecting the central nervous system (G10-G14)

- Extrapyramidal and movement disorders (G20-G26)

- Other degenerative diseases of the nervous system (G30-G32)

- Demyelinating diseases of the central nervous system (G35-G37)

- Episodic and paroxysmal disorders (G40-G47)

- Nerve, nerve root, and plexis disorders (G50-G59)

- Polyneuropathies and other disorders of the peripheral nervous system (G60-G64)

- Diseases of the myoneural junction and muscle (G70-G73)

- Cerebral palsy and other paralytic syndromes (G80-G83)

- Other disorders of the nervous system (G89-G99)

The brain, the spinal cord, and the nerves throughout the body make up the nervous system. The nervous system, which is vulnerable to disease and injury, contains 100 billion or more nerve cells that run throughout the body, making connections with the brain, the body, and each other. Nerve cells called *neurons* are largely responsible for sending messages. The brain and nerves compose a communication system able to send and receive information simultaneously. It is divided into two main parts:

- Central nervous system

- Peripheral nervous system

Central Nervous System

The central nervous system (CNS) is composed of the brain and the spinal cord.

THE BRAIN

The brain is the site of thinking and the control center for the rest of the body. It coordinates the ability to move, touch, smell, hear, and see. It allows people to form words, understand and manipulate numbers, compose and appreciate music, see and understand geometric shapes, and communicate with others. It even has the capacity to plan ahead and fantasize. The brain is protected by cerebrospinal fluid and has 3 major anatomic components: the cerebrum, the brain stem, and the cerebellum.

The brain is divided into 4 major sections:

- Cerebrum/cerebral cortex—the main portion of brain tissue

- Brain stem—below the cerebrum, the stem of tissue that connects into the spinal cord

- Midbrain, pons, medulla oblongata—make up the brain stem diencephalon (interbrain)

- Cerebellum—behind the brain stem and below the cerebrum; consists of the median lobe and two lateral lobes

SPINAL CORD

The spinal cord is the main pathway of communication between the brain and the rest of the body. The spinal cord is protected by the spinal column, which consists of 33 vertebrae. The spinal cord consists of nerve tissue that extends down from the brain through the vertebrae in the spinal column to the first and second lumbar vertebrae. Its purpose is to conduct nerve impulses to and from the brain. These nerve branches provide communication with all parts of the body.

Peripheral Nervous System

The peripheral nervous system consists of the following:

- 12 pairs of cranial nerves

- 31 pairs of spinal nerves

- Autonomic nervous system

It is a network of nerves that connects the brain and spinal cord to the rest of the body. The peripheral nervous system includes all the nerves outside the CNS (brain and spinal cord). Cranial nerves connect the head and face directly to the brain, and the nerves connect the eyes and nose to the brain. All nerves connecting the spinal cord to the body are part of the peripheral nervous system.

INFLAMMATORY DISEASES OF THE CENTRAL NERVOUS SYSTEM (G00-G09)

Diseases in this category include the following:

- Meningitis

- Encephalitis

- Abscesses

- Phlebitis

- Late effects

Meningitis

Meningitis is classified in categories G00 to G03. It is an inflammation of the meninges, the covering of the brain and spinal cord. It is most common in children between the ages of 1 month and 2 years; however, it can afflict adults as well, particularly adults with risk factors such as head trauma.

Aseptic meningitis is caused by a virus or an autoimmune reaction, as sometimes occurs in multiple sclerosis. Bacterial meningitis is an inflammation of the meninges caused by bacteria. The most common bacteria responsible for this condition are *Neisseria meningitidis*, *Haemophilus influenzae*, and *Streptococcus pneumoniae*.

Chronic meningitis is a brain infection that produces inflammation in the meninges lasting a month or longer. This condition usually affects persons who have immune system disorders such as acquired immunodeficiency syndrome (AIDS), cancer, and other severe diseases or have needed long-term use of prednisone or anticancer drugs.

ICD-10-CM code G01, Meningitis in other bacterial diseases classified elsewhere, requires close attention. The note that follows this code indicates that the underlying disease must be coded first, with G01 as the secondary diagnosis. There is an Excludes1 note that excludes meningitis in other conditions/diseases; if that condition exists, it is coded elsewhere. The conditions listed are excluded from this category (see Figure 6.9)

FIGURE 6.9   Excerpt from the Tabular List: *G01*

```
Meningitis (in)
  EXCLUDES 1  gonococcal (A54.81)
              leptospirosis (A27.81)
              listeriosis (A32.11)
              Lyme disease (A69.21)
              meningococcal (A39.0)
              neurosyphilis (A52.13)
              tuberculosis (A17.0)
              meningoencephalitis and meningomyelitis in
              bacterial diseases classified elsewhere (G05)
```

CODING TIP Use caution when coding classification G01 and G02. The underlying condition must be coded first. Make sure the Excludes 1 conditions are not coded in the classification.

Bacterial meningitis is caused by a specific organism and is coded as G00.–. A fourth character is required in the category. There is an instructional note in this section that an additional code should be used to further identify the organism.

Meningitis due to other unspecified causes are coded in G03.–. This subclassification includes the following:

- Arachnoiditis
- Leptomeningitis

- Meningitis NOS
- Pachymeningitis NOS

A fourth character is required when coding in this subclassification. Meningitis, unspecified, is classified as G03.9. This classification includes nonpryogenic meningitis (G03.0), chronic meningitis (G03.1), and meningitis, unspecified (G03.9). Because meningitis, unspecified, is a nonspecific code, all codes in this subclassification should be reviewed in order to code meningitis as specifically as possible. The documentation in the medical record must support the ICD-10-CM code selected. The following is an example:

> **EXAMPLE:** *A patient is admitted by his family physician with headache, nausea, vomiting, and stiffness. The patient indicates that he has been experiencing this condition for several weeks. The physician performs a comprehensive history and physical examination and orders laboratory tests. The laboratory results indicate that the patient has a staphylococcal infection. The family physician calls a neurologist for consultation. A computed tomographic (CT) scan is ordered and shows that the patient's condition is meningitis, staphylococcal.*

Open the ICD-10-CM codebook to the Alphabetic Index and locate the main term "meningitis." The documentation in the patient encounter indicates the patient has staphylococcal meningitis.

Alphabetic Index:
  Meningitis ➝ *staphylococcal G00.3*

Tabular List:
  G00.3 Staphylococcal meningitis

In addition, a code from category B95.0-B95.5 must be listed as an additional diagnosis. Because the information is not specified, the only choice in this category is B95.8 for the unspecified staphylococcal infection.

Tabular List:
  B95.8 Unspecified staphylococcus as the cause of the disease classified elsewhere

Correct code sequencing:
  G00.3, B95.8

Code G00.3 includes the manifestation of meningitis and also the etiology, the staphylococcal organism. Throughout this chapter, there are conditions that are manifestations of other diseases. These categories are given in italics in the Tabular List, which provides instructions to code the underlying disease first.

Review the following example:

> **EXAMPLE:** *A patient who had recent brain surgery arrives at her neurosurgeon's office for a follow-up visit. The patient complains of neck stiffness, headache, nausea, and vomiting of 3 days' duration. The physician suspects the symptoms could be related to meningitis and orders a CT scan. The scan indicates that the patient's condition is a **cerebrospinal fever.***

Open the ICD-10-CM codebook to the main term "fever" and locate Cerebrospinal Fever. Review Figures 6.10 and 6.11.

FIGURE 6.10   Excerpt from the Alphabetic Index: *Fever*

Fever,
    Cerebrospinal meningococcal (A39.0)

Notice that this encounter is coded in the Tabular List located in Chapter 1, Infectious and Parasitic Diseases, instead of Diseases of the Nervous System. Remember to always use the Alphabetic Index as your guide. You would not select a code in category G00.– because the diagnosis in the medical record indicates the patient's condition is cerebrospinal fever. The Alphabetic Index refers you to A39.0.

FIGURE 6.11   Excerpt from the Tabular List: *A39.0*

A39   Meningococcal infection
    A39.0   Meningococcal meningitis
    A 39.1   Waterhouse-Friderichsen syndrome
    A39.2   Acute meningococcemia
    A39.3   Chronic meningococcemia
    A39.4   Meningococcemia, unspecified
    A39.5   Meningococcal carditis
    A39.50   Meningococcal carditis, unspecified

Encephalitis, Myelitis, and Encephalomyelitis (G04-G05)

Encephalitis is inflammation of the brain and is usually caused by a viral infection but may also be caused by an autoimmune reaction. This condition is known as viral encephalitis.

Another condition, encephalomyelitis, is an inflammation of the brain and spinal cord caused by a virus.

Encephalitis disrupts normal brain function, which may cause the following:

- Personality changes
- Weakness
- Confusion
- Sleepiness
- Seizures

Symptoms associated with encephalitis include the following:

- Fever
- Headache
- Vomiting
- Weakness
- Stiff neck
- General feeling of illness

In this category, many of the codes direct coders to code first the underlying condition as the primary diagnosis, with encephalitis as the secondary diagnosis.

Review the following example:

> **EXAMPLE:** *A patient who had been on a camping trip two weeks ago was suffering from nausea, diarrhea, vomiting, and abdominal pain for the past week. He admitted to eating raw hamburger and pork during the trip. The physician ordered blood work and diagnostic tests. The results came back positive for trichinellosis. The physician reviewed all the test results and diagnosed the patient with trichinellosis encephalitis.*

Open the ICD-10-CM codebook to the main term "encephalitis." Review both the Alphabetic Index and the Tabular List. Review Figure 6.12.

FIGURE 6.12   Excerpt from the Alphabetic Index: *Encephalitis*

Encephalitis
    in (due to)
        trichinosis B75 [G05.3]

After reviewing Figure 6.12, you notice that code G05.3 is in brackets. When a code is in brackets in the Alphabetic Index, that code is never used as the first listed or principal diagnosis for the condition. It is always a secondary diagnosis. Now review the Tabular List and find the correct coding and sequencing.

Note there is also an instructional note in the Tabular List that indicates that trichinosis is reported as the first listed or principal diagnosis.

CODING TIP When a code located in the Alphabetic Index is in brackets [ ], the code is never listed as the principal or first listed diagnosis when coding that condition.

OTHER DEGENERATIVE DISEASES OF THE NERVOUS SYSTEM (G30-G32)

Dementia is classified in "Other cerebral degenerations" in the ICD-10-CM code book Dementia is a slowly progressing decline in mental ability in which memory, judgment, thinking, the ability to pay attention, and learning are impaired. With some conditions, personality may deteriorate. Dementia usually affects persons older than 60 years. However, it can develop suddenly in younger people when brain cells are destroyed by trauma, injury, disease, or toxic substances. Dementia is not a normal process of aging, although as people age they often experience short-term memory loss and a decline in learning ability. Dementia is also possible after brain injury or cardiac arrest when the oxygen supply to the brain has been jeopardized.

Symptoms of dementia include the following:

- Loss of memory, specifically recent events

- Wandering attention

- Difficulty finding the right words

- Impaired orientation to surroundings

- Possibly diminished awareness to present time

Alzheimer's disease is a progressive degenerative disease of the brain of unknown cause with diffuse atrophy throughout the cerebral cortex. It initially presents with slight memory disturbance or personality changes that progressively deteriorate to profound memory loss and dementia.

Alzheimer's disease is the most common form of dementia and is classified as G0.30–. The cause of Alzheimer's disease is unknown, but scientists believe the condition may be hereditary. Recent studies have shown that Alzheimer disease tends to run in families and is caused by specific gene abnormalities. Parts of the brain degenerate, destroying cells in patients with Alzheimer's disease. Physicians have recognized abnormal tissue and abnormal proteins in Alzheimer's disease.

Another type of dementia is multi-infarct dementia, in which patients have small successive strokes, leaving none of the immediate weakness or paralysis that often results from larger strokes. The small strokes with this type of dementia destroy brain tissue gradually as the result of blocked blood supply (infarcts). Many people who have this type of dementia have high blood pressure or diabetes, which damages blood vessels in the brain.

Open the ICD-10-CM codebook and locate the correct code(s) for this patient encounter.

Review the following example:

> **EXAMPLE:** *A family practitioner examines a 68-year-old female patient. The patient's daughter, who is with her, tells the physician that her mother is experiencing episodes of memory loss and loss of time and place and sometimes does not know her. The patient has been experiencing these episodes gradually during the past year. In the past two months, her condition has worsened. The reason for the visit to the office is that the patient got lost in the neighborhood she has lived in for more than 30 years. After the physician performs an expanded problem-focused history and examination, the physician explains to the daughter that the patient is experiencing signs of dementia due to Alzheimer's disease and will require constant care because her condition is worsening. The diagnosis documented in the medical record is early onset Alzheimer's disease with dementia.*

Review Figure 6.13 from the Alphabetic Index. The main term in this encounter is "disease." You will also notice that a code from the Mental Disorders category is reported as the secondary diagnosis to identify the dementia. Because there is no mention of a behavioral disturbance it is coded without behavioral disturbance.

FIGURE 6.13 Excerpt from the Alphabetic Index to Diseases: *Alzheimer's*

Disease
    Alzheimer's G30.9 [F02.80]
    with behavioral disturbance G30.9 [F02.81]
    early onset G30.0 [F02.80]
    with behavioral disturbance G30.0 [F02.81]
    late onset G30.1 [F02.80]
    with behavioral disturbance G30.1 [F02.81]
    specified NEC G30.8 [F02.80]
    with behavioral disturbance G30.8 [F02.81]

Alphabetic Index:
Disease → Alzheimer's → early onset → G30.0 [F02.80]

Tabular List:
G30.0 → Alzheimer's disease with early onset

F02.80 → Dementia in other diseases classified elsewhere, without behavioral disturbance

Correct coding sequence:
G30.0, F02.80

The Alphabetic Index directs coders to code the Alzheimer's disease as the first listed diagnosis (underlying condition) and the dementia as the secondary diagnosis. Because the encounter was documented with Alzheimer's disease and dementia, both diagnosis codes would be selected.

Hydrocephalus results when an excess of cerebrospinal fluid, which normally surrounds the brain, fails to be properly reabsorbed and causes decreased mental function and incontinence. These diseases are coded with category G91.–.

Demyelinating Diseases of the Central Nervous System (D35-D37)

Diseases classified in this category include the following:

- Multiple sclerosis

- Diffuse sclerosis

- Acute transverse myelitis

The most common condition in this category is multiple sclerosis. Multiple sclerosis is a disorder in which the nerves of the eye, brain, and spinal cord lose patches of myelin. The term comes from the multiple areas of scarring (sclerosis) that represent many patches of demyelination in the nervous system. Although the disease often worsens slowly over time, affected people usually have periods of relatively good health (remissions) alternating with debilitating flare-ups (exacerbations). This disease occurs mostly in young adults. The cause of multiple sclerosis is unknown, but a virus or an unknown antigen affecting the autoimmune system is suspected.

Common symptoms are as follows:

- Numbness

- Tingling

- Peculiar feeling in the:

  - Arms

  - Trunk

  - Legs

  - Face

- Loss of strength or dexterity in a leg or a hand

- Double vision in some patients

- Partial blindness

- Eye pain, dim or blurred vision

- Optic neuritis

Open the ICD-10-CM codebook and look up the main term "sclerosis" and reference the Tabular List to select the correct code.

Review the following example:

EXAMPLE: *A patient is diagnosed with generalized multiple sclerosis.*

Alphabetic Index:
Sclerosis, sclerotic → brain → multiple (brain stem) G35

Tabular List:
G35 Multiple sclerosis → Multiple sclerosis of brain stem

Correct code:
G35

CODING TIP A fourth or fifth character is not available when coding multiple sclerosis.

Episodic and Paroxysmal Disorders (G40-G47)

Diseases classified in this category include the following:

- Epilepsy

- Epileptic syndromes

- Migraines

- Headache syndrome

- Posttraumatic headaches

- Sleep disorders

Epilepsy is a recurrent disorder of cerebral function characterized by the following:

- Migraine

- Other conditions of the brain

- Other paralytic syndromes

  - Sudden attacks of altered consciousness

  - Altered motor activity

  - Inappropriate behavior caused by excessive discharge of cerebral neurons

There are several types of seizures associated with epilepsy:

- Generalized loss of consciousness and motor functions along with infantile spasms and absence of seizure

- Atonic: brief, generalized seizures in children characterized by complete loss of muscle tone and consciousness

- Petit mal (absence seizures): brief, generalized attacks of 10 to 30 seconds of loss of consciousness without convulsions and without knowledge that an attack has occurred

- Myoclonic: brief, lightning-like jerks of limb(s) or trunk without loss of consciousness

- Tonic-clonic: loss of consciousness followed by tonic, then clonic, contractions of the muscles of the extremities, trunk, and head with seizures usually lasting 1 to 2 minutes

The term "intractable" can be referenced in the medical record under many names including:

- Pharmacoresistant

- Pharmacologically resistant

- Refractory (medically)

- Treatment resistant

- Poorly controlled

Diagnosis coding depends on the type of epilepsy being treated, onset, and other mitigating factors.

Open the ICD-10-CM codebook and locate the main term in each example and reference the Tabular List for the correct code(s).

Review the following examples:

EXAMPLE: A previously diagnosed patient with epilepsy is experiencing tonic-clonic seizures on a daily basis. A neurologist who has been treating the patient for this condition for 3 years prescribed phenytoin (Dilantin) one month ago, which provided little relief to the patient. After a problem-focused history and examination, the neurologist decides to prescribe carbamazepine (Tegretol) in addition to the phenytoin and asks the patient to return to the office in two weeks to monitor the patient's progress.

Alphabetic Index:
Epilepsy, epileptic → tonic-clonic → see Epilepsy generalized idiopathic

Epilepsy → generalized → idiopathic → G40.309

Tabular List:
G40.309 → Generalized idiopathic epilepsy and epileptic syndromes, not intractable, without status epilepticus

Correct code:
G40.309

Note: Epilepticus is a life-threatening condition in which the brain is in a state of persistent seizure. Traditionally it is defined as one continuous unremitting seizure lasting longer than 30 minutes or as recurrent seizures without regaining consciousness between seizures for longer than 30 minutes (or shorter with medical intervention).

EXAMPLE: A 45-year-old female patient has been treated by her neurologist for epilepsy for the past year. The epilepsy was caused by a previous traumatic brain injury, which required a craniotomy with debridement. This resulted in the loss of her right frontal lobe. The patient has focal seizures but does not typically lose consciousness. She has not had a seizure for two days but has been having seizures every couple of day over the past month. The patient was last seen in the office 3 months ago and was doing well with her medication. A detailed history and detailed neurologic examination are performed. The patient is asked to return in one week for follow-up and an EEG. The physician adjusted her medication to hopefully avoid another seizure.

Alphabetic Index:
Epilepsy, epileptic, epilepsia → focal → see localization related symptomatic, with simple partial seizures generalized → without status epilepticus → G40.119

Tabular List:
G40.119 → Localization related (focal) (partial) symptomatic epilepsy and epileptic syndromes with simple partial seizures, intractable, without status epilepticus

In addition, it is recommended that the history of the brain injury is also reported.

Alphabetic Index:
History (personal) → brain injury (traumatic) → Z87.820

Tabular List:
Z87.820 → Personal history of traumatic brain injury

Correct code sequencing:
G40.119, Z87.820

If the episode was for seizure disorder or convulsions other than epilepsy, the code assigned would be R56.9.

CODING TIP In category G40.-, the physician must specifically indicate "epilepsy" in the diagnosis before the code can be assigned.

Migraine

Headaches are classified in category G44.– based on the type of headache. A headache without a specific type is coded as R51 (headache, unspecified), which is located in the Signs and Symptoms chapter in ICD-10-CM. Most generalized headaches involve symptoms of the head and neck.

A migraine headache is a recurring, throbbing, intense pain that usually affects one side or both sides of the head. It begins suddenly and may be preceded or accompanied by the following symptoms:

- Blurred vision

- Photophobia (discomfort in bright lights)

- Nausea

- Vomiting

- Other gastrointestinal symptoms

- Neurologic symptoms

Nausea and blurred vision are very common symptoms. Migraine headaches usually begin in patients between 10 and 30 years of age but can occur at any age. More women than men experience migraine headaches. Migraine headaches are generally more severe than other headaches, and many treatment options are available for relief.

Migraines can last from several hours to several days when untreated. The level of intensity of the migraine varies with the individual. Some are mild and can be relieved with analgesics, whereas others are more severe and can be temporarily disabling.

Migraine with aura is a migraine that's preceded or accompanied by a variety of sensory warning signs or symptoms, such as flashes of light, blind spots, or tingling in the hand or face. Both a migraine with aura and one without are managed by the practitioner in the same manner. Documentation must identify the aura or the symptoms related to a migraine with aura when reporting the diagnosis code.

Status migrainosus is a migraine that has progressed beyond 72 hours. Certain neurochemical changes occur within the brain during a migraine. The longer

a migraine (or any pain for that matter) progresses, the worse it may become and the more difficult to treat.

An intractable migraine is a migraine that typically lasts for more than 3 days.

Figure 6.14 shows the Tabular List for migraine without aura.

FIGURE 6.14   Excerpt from the Tabular List: *G43.–*

G43   Migraine
    G43.0   Migraine without aura
            common Migraine
      EXCLUDES 1 Chronic migraine with aura 643.7
                    headache NOS (R51)
                    headache syndrome (G44.-)
                    lower half migraine (G44.00)
        G43.00   Migraine without aura, not intractable
      EXCLUDES 1 chronic migraine without aura (G43.7)
        G43.01   Migraine without aura, not intractable, with status migrainosus
        G43.001   Migraine without aura, not intractable, with status migrainosus
        G43.009   Migraine without aura, not intractable without status migrainosus
                  Migraine without aura NOS

Open the ICD-10-CM codebook and begin with the Alphabetic Index and reference the correct code in the Tabular List.

Review the following example:

> **EXAMPLE:** *An established patient contacts her physician for an appointment because she had been having painful headaches for the past month. They last for about a day; during that period she has to lay down with cold rags on her head in a dark room. An appointment is scheduled for the following day. After her family physician takes a comprehensive history, along with performing a detailed examination, he diagnoses common migraine headaches and prescribes an oral medication to help relieve the pain. The patient is asked to follow up in 3 weeks to monitor her progress.*

As shown in Figure 6.13, a common migraine is coded to G43.0 and a sixth character is required to code to the highest level of specificity. The difference between code category G43.0– and G43.1– is that G43.0– is a migraine without aura and G43.1– includes migraine with aura. When coding migraines it is important to know what the term aura means. What does the term "aura" mean? The term aura means that a patient who is getting a migraine will start experiencing symptoms shortly before the headaches begin. These symptoms may be called a prodrome in the medical record. However if the physician does not clarify whether an aura is or was present, it is a good idea to query the physician.

Alphabetic Index:
Migraine ➜ common ➜ without aura ➜ G43.009

Tabular List:
G43.009 ➜ Migraine without aura, not intractable, without status migrainosus

Correct code:
G43.009

SLEEP DISORDERS (G47)

Narcolepsy is a serious medical disorder and a key to understanding other sleep disorders. Narcolepsy is a disabling illness affecting more than 1 in 2,000 Americans. Most people with the disorder are not diagnosed and, thus, are not treated. The disease is principally characterized by a permanent and overwhelming feeling of sleepiness and fatigue. Other symptoms involve abnormalities of dreaming sleep, such as dreamlike hallucinations and finding oneself physically weak or paralyzed for a few seconds.

It is the second leading cause of excessive daytime sleepiness diagnosed by sleep centers, after obstructive sleep apnea. In many cases, the diagnosis is not made until many years after the onset of symptoms, often because patients consult a physician after many years of excessive sleepiness, assuming that sleepiness is not indicative of a disease.

The effects of narcolepsy are devastating. Studies have shown that even treated narcoleptic patients are often markedly psychosocially impaired in the areas of work, leisure, and interpersonal relations and are more prone to accidents.

Symptoms

The main symptoms of narcolepsy are as follows:

- Excessive daytime sleepiness
- Abnormal rapid eye movement (REM) sleep

Narcolepsy not only is a serious and common medical problem but it also offers basic sleep researchers a unique opportunity to gather new information on the central mechanisms regulating REM sleep and alertness. Since the 1960s, it has been known that several of the disabling symptoms of narcolepsy, such as sleep paralysis, cataplexy, and hypnagogic hallucinations, are pathological equivalents of REM sleep. In sleep paralysis, a frightening symptom considered to be an abnormal episode of REM sleep atonia, the patient suddenly is unable to move for a few minutes, most often upon falling asleep or waking up. During hypnagogic hallucinations, patients experience dreamlike auditory or visual hallucinations while dozing or falling asleep.

Cataplexy, a pathological equivalent of REM sleep atonia unique to narcolepsy, is a striking, sudden episode of muscle weakness triggered by emotions. Typically, the patient's knees buckle and may give way on laughing, elation, surprise, or anger. In other typical cataplectic attacks, the head may drop or the jaw may become slack. In severe cases, the patient might fall down and become completely paralyzed for a few seconds to several minutes. Reflexes are abolished during the attack.

Diagnosis

Narcolepsy can be diagnosed by using specific medical procedures; the diagnosis of narcolepsy is usually easy if all symptoms of the illness are present. More often, however, the symptoms of dissociated REM sleep, such as cataplexy, are mild and a nocturnal polysomnogram followed by the multiple sleep latency test (MSLT) are suggested. This test, performed at a sleep disorder clinic, will confirm the daytime sleepiness by showing a short sleep latency of usually less than 5 minutes, as well as an abnormally short latency prior to the first REM period. Other causes of daytime sleepiness, such as sleep apnea or periodic leg movements, are also excluded by the nocturnal recordings.

Coding Issues

Narcolepsy is coded in category G47. This category includes a sixth character subclassification to identify narcolepsy with and/or without cataplexy. Code G47.429 is only to be used when narcolepsy is classified elsewhere.

Review the following example:

EXAMPLE: *An elderly man with a previously confirmed diagnosis of narcolepsy and no other significant sleep disorders recently started stimulant treatment. The patient undergoes polysomnography with recording for 7 to 8 hours of one- to four-lead electroencephalography, submental electromyography and electro-olfactography for sleep staging, and electrocardiography, while attended by a technologist. The testing is performed on the night before a repeated MSLT for evaluation of control of somnolence. The physician confirms a diagnosis of narcolepsy with cataplexy in the medical record.*

Alphabetic Index:
Narcolepsy ➜ with cataplexy G47.411

Tabular List:
G47.411 ➜ Narcolepsy with cataplexy

Correct code:
G47.411

NERVE, NERVE ROOT, AND PLEXUS DISORDERS (G50-G59)

One of the most common conditions in this category is carpal tunnel syndrome. Carpal tunnel syndrome is pressure on the median nerve, that is, the nerve in the wrist that supplies feeling and movement to parts of the hand. It can lead to numbness, tingling, weakness, or muscle damage in the hand and finger and is typically treated surgically.

Common symptoms include:

- Numbness or tingling in the thumb and next two or three fingers of one or both hands
- Numbness or tingling in the palm of the hand
- Pain extending to the elbow
- Pain in wrist or hand, in one or both hands
- Problems with fine finger movements (coordination) in one or both hands
- Wasting away of the muscle under the thumb (in advanced or long-term cases)
- Weak grip or difficulty carrying bags
- Weakness in one or both hands

Coding Issues

This condition is coded in category G56, Mononeuropathies of upper limb. The code selection is based on laterality, right versus left. There is a code for unspecified limb (G56.00), but use caution when selecting an unspecified code when the documentation in the medical record should indicate which side of the body is affected.

Open the ICD-10-CM codebook to the Alphabetic Index and reference the Tabular List when selecting the correct code.

Review the following example:

> **EXAMPLE:** *A right-handed female patient who types all day at work was diagnosed with carpal tunnel syndrome of the right hand. The patient had recurring pain and discomfort in the wrist and tendon attachments of the hand, with pain in the elbow and shoulder. The patient is going to undergo a carpal tunnel release to correct the problem.*
>
> **Alphabetic Index:**
> *Syndrome* ➝ *Carpal tunnel* ➝ *C56.0-*
>
> **Tabular List:**
> *C56.01* ➝ *Carpal tunnel syndrome of right upper limb*
>
> **Correct code:**
> *C56.01*

Review the ICD-10-CM Official Guidelines for the Nervous System. After reviewing the guidelines, open the ICD-10-CM codebook and review the examples referencing the Alphabetic Index and Tabular List to locate the appropriate diagnosis code(s).

Dominant/Nondominant Side

Codes from category G81, Hemiplegia and hemiparesis, and subcategories G83.1, Monoplegia of lower limb, G83.2, Monoplegia of upper limb, and G83.3, Monoplegia, unspecified, identify whether the dominant or nondominant side is affected. This category is to be used only when hemiplegia (complete) (incomplete) is reported without further specification or is stated to be old or longstanding but of unspecified cause. The category is also for use in multiple coding to identify these types of hemiplegia resulting from any cause.

Should the affected side be documented but not specified as dominant or nondominant, and the classification system does not indicate a default, code selection is as follows:

- For ambidextrous patients, the default should be dominant.
- If the left side is affected, the default is nondominant.
- If the right side is affected, the default is dominant.

PAIN (G89)

General Coding Information

Codes in category G89, Pain, not elsewhere classified, may be used in conjunction with codes from other categories and chapters to provide more detail about acute or chronic pain and neoplasm-related pain, unless otherwise indicated below.

If the pain is not specified as acute or chronic, postthoracotomy, postprocedural, or neoplasm related, do not assign codes from category G89.

A code from category G89 should not be assigned if the underlying (definitive) diagnosis is known, unless the reason for the encounter is pain control/management and not management of the underlying condition.

When an admission or encounter is for a procedure aimed at treating the underlying condition (eg spinal fusion, kyphoplasty), a code for the underlying condition (eg vertebral fracture, spinal stenosis) should be assigned as the principal diagnosis. No code from category G89 should be assigned.

CATEGORY G89 CODES AS PRINCIPAL OR FIRST LISTED DIAGNOSIS

Category G89 codes are acceptable as principal diagnosis or the first listed code as follows:

- When pain control or pain management is the reason for the admission/encounter (eg a patient with displaced intervertebral disc, nerve impingement, and severe back pain presents for injection of steroid into the spinal canal). The underlying cause of the pain should be reported as an additional diagnosis, if known.

- When a patient is admitted for the insertion of a neurostimulator for pain control, assign the appropriate pain code as the principal or first listed diagnosis. When an admission or encounter is for a procedure aimed at treating the underlying condition and a neurostimulator is inserted for pain control during the same admission/encounter, a code for the underlying condition should be assigned as the principal diagnosis and the appropriate pain code should be assigned as a secondary diagnosis.

Use of Category G89 Codes in Conjunction with Site-Specific Pain Codes

Assigning Category G89 and Site-Specific Pain Codes   Codes from category G89 may be used in conjunction with codes that identify the site of pain (including codes from Chapter 18) if the category G89 code provides additional information. For example, if the code describes the site of the pain but does not fully describe whether the pain is acute or chronic, then both codes should be assigned.

SEQUENCING OF CATEGORY G89 CODES WITH SITE-SPECIFIC PAIN CODES

The sequencing of category G89 codes with site-specific pain codes (including Chapter 18 codes) is dependent on the circumstances of the encounter/admission as follows:

- If the encounter is for pain control or pain management, assign the code from category G89 followed by the code identifying the specific site of pain (eg encounter for pain management for acute neck pain from trauma is assigned code G89.11, Acute pain due to trauma, followed by code M54.2, Cervicalgia, to identify the site of pain).

- If the encounter is for any other reason except pain control or pain management and a related definitive diagnosis has not been established (confirmed) by the provider, assign the code for the specific site of pain first, followed by the appropriate code from category G89.

Postoperative Pain

The provider's documentation should be used to guide the coding of postoperative pain, as well as Section III, Reporting Additional Diagnoses, and Section IV, Diagnostic Coding and Reporting in the Outpatient Setting.

The default for postthoracotomy and other postoperative pain not specified as acute or chronic is the code for the acute form. Routine or expected postoperative pain immediately after surgery should not be coded.

Postoperative Pain not Associated with Specific Postoperative Complication

Postoperative pain not associated with a specific postoperative complication is assigned to the appropriate postoperative pain code in category G89.

Postoperative Pain Associated with Specific Postoperative Complication

Postoperative pain associated with a specific postoperative complication (such as painful wire sutures) is assigned to the appropriate code(s) found in Chapter 19, Injury, poisoning, and certain other consequences of external causes. If appropriate, use additional code(s) from category G89 to identify acute or chronic pain (G89.18 or G89.28).

Chronic Pain

Chronic pain is classified to subcategory G89.2. There is no time frame defining when pain becomes chronic pain. The provider's documentation should be used to guide use of these codes.

Neoplasm-Related Pain

Code G89.3 is assigned to pain documented as being related, associated, or due to cancer, primary or secondary malignancy, or tumor. This code is assigned regardless of whether the pain is acute or chronic.

This code may be assigned as the principal or first listed code when the stated reason for the admission/encounter is documented as pain control/pain management. The underlying neoplasm should be reported as an additional diagnosis.

When the reason for the admission/encounter is management of the neoplasm and the pain associated with the neoplasm is also documented, code G89.3 may be assigned as an additional diagnosis. It is not necessary to assign an additional code for the site of the pain.

See Section I.C.2 for instructions on the sequencing of neoplasms for all other stated reasons for the admission/encounter (except for pain control/pain management).

Chronic Pain Syndrome

Central pain syndrome (G89.0) and chronic pain syndrome (G89.4) are different from chronic pain. Therefore, codes should only be used when the provider has specifically documented this condition. See Section I.C.5, Pain disorders related to psychological factors.

> **EXAMPLE:** *A 60-year-old patient underwent laminectomy 4 weeks ago and visits the pain specialist because of ongoing acute back pain following surgery. The physician prescribed medication to relieve the pain and asked that the patient return to the office in one month for reevaluation.*

> **Alphabetic Index:**
> *Pain* → *postoperative* → *G89.18*

> **Tabular List:**
> *G89.18* → *Other acute postprocedural pain*

> **Correct code:**
> *G89.18*

> **EXAMPLE:** *A 15-year-old girl undergoing treatment for acute lymphoblastic leukemia is referred to the pain specialist for chronic pain related to the leukemia. She has had repeated lumbar punctures and intrathecal chemotherapy treatments during the past 3 months to fight the disease.*

CODING TIP When coding for pain management related to a neoplasm or cancer, related pain, the pain is coded to G89.3 regardless of whether the pain is acute or chronic. When the reason for the encounter is pain management, it is reported as the first listed diagnosis, with the underlying neoplasm or cancer coded as an additional diagnosis.

> **Alphabetic Index:**
> *Pain(s)* → *cancer associated (acute) (chronic) G89.3*

> **Tabular List:**
> *G89.3* → *Neoplasm related pain (acute) (chronic)*

The lymphoblastic leukemia also needs to be coded as the secondary diagnosis because this is the reason for pain management.

> **Alphabetic Index:**
> *Leukemia* → *acute lymphoblastic* → *C91.0–*

> **Tabular List:**
> *C91.00* → *Acute lymphoblastic leukemia not having achieved remission*

> **Correct code(s) and sequencing:**
> *G89.3, C91.00*

CHECKPOINT EXERCISE 6-2

Using the ICD-10-CM codebook, code the following:

1. _____ Parkinson's disease

2. _____ Candidal meningitis

3. _____ Cerebral degeneration in neoplastic disease

4. _____ Infectious mononucleosis

5. _____ Krabbe disease

6. _____ Whooping cough with meningitis

7. _____ Cerebral palsy

8. _____ Horton's neuralgia

9. _____ Temporal lobe epilepsy

10. _____ Paralysis of right lower limb (dominant side)

11. _____ Decubitus ulcer due to autonomic dysreflexia

12. _____ Stiff-man syndrome

13. _____ An elderly patient exhibited Parkinsonian motor features, unexplained repeated falls, decreased ability to reason and carry out simple actions, impaired memory and language skills, and confusion. After a comprehensive physical examination, the physician diagnosed the patient with Lewy body disease.

14. _____ A 56-year-old man saw his physician because of muscle fatigue after exercising. After performing diagnostic tests, the physician documented that the patient's eye muscle displayed diminished muscle response after repeated eye stimulation. The diagnosis recorded in the medical record is myasthenia gravis.

15. _____ Meningitis due to *Proteus morganii*

Chapter 7, Disorders of the Eye and Adnexa (H00–H59)

Chapter 7 in the Tabular List includes the following sections:

- Disorders of the eyelid, lacrimal system, and orbit (H00–H05)

- Disorders of the conjunctiva (H10–H11)

- Disorders of the sclera cornea, iris, and ciliary body (H15-H22)

- Disorders of the lens (H25-H28)

- Disorders of the choroid and retina (H30-H36)

- Glaucoma (H40-H42)

- Disorders of the vitreous body and glob (H43-H44)

- Disorders of the optic nerve and visual pathways (H46-H47)

- Disorders of ocular muscles, binocular movement, accommodation and refraction (H49-H52)

- Visual disturbances and blindness (H53-H54)

- Other disorders of eye and adnexa (H55-H57)

- Intraoperative and postprocedural complications and disorder of eye and adnexa, not elsewhere classified (H59)

The structure and function of the eye are complex and fascinating. The eye constantly adjusts the amount of light it lets in, focuses on objects near and far, and produces continuous images that are instantly transmitted to the brain. Following is a review of some common disorders in this category along with coding issues.

Coding Issues

For most of the categories in Chapter 7 designate codes based on laterality. Most codes in this chapter are selected for right eye, left eye, and bilateral (both eyes). In cases where a code does not provide a designation for which eye is involved, that condition is always bilateral. In cases where a bilateral code is not provided the condition is always unilateral.

This category of codes excludes injuries of the eye and adnexa which are coded in categories S01.1- S05.

Disorders of the Conjunctiva (H10-H11)

Conjunctivitis is an inflammation of the conjunctiva, usually caused by viruses, bacteria, or an allergy. Conjunctivitis can sometimes last for months or years. This type of conjunctivitis may be caused by conditions in which an eyelid is turned outward (ectropion)

or inward (entropion), problems with the tear ducts, sensitivity to chemicals, exposure to irritants, and infection by particular bacteria—typically *Chlamydia*. Conjunctivitis is coded with category H10.-. The diagnosis is coded to the highest level of specificity. Selections are based on etiology and manifestation in some conditions. The following is an example:

> **EXAMPLE:** *A patient has acute toxic conjunctivitis in both eyes.*
>
> **Alphabetic Index:**
> *Conjunctivitis* ➡ *toxic* ➡ *acute* ➡ *H10.21-*
>
> **Tabular List:**
> *H10.213* ➡ *Toxic conjunctivitis, bilateral*
>
> **Correct code:**
> *H10.213*

Note the sixth character "3" identifies the condition affects both eyes.

Disorders of Lens (H26-H28)

CATARACTS

A cataract is a cloudiness (opacity) in the eye's lens that impairs vision. Over time, cataracts produce a progressive loss of vision. Cataracts are most common in older adults but can be congenital or traumatic (due to trauma to the eye). Diabetes can also be the cause of cataracts.

A cataract can be seen while examining the eye with an ophthalmoscope (an instrument used to view the inside of the eye). The exact location of the cataract and the extent of its opacity can be viewed by an instrument called a slit lamp. Surgery is the choice for most patients with this condition, when vision hampers driving, daily tasks, etc. Eyeglasses and contact lenses may improve vision without surgery.

Cataract surgery, which can be performed on a person of any age, usually does not require general anesthesia or an overnight hospital stay. During the operation, the human lens is removed and usually an intraocular lens (lens implant) is inserted. Usually, a patient's vision can be restored without the use of contact lenses or glasses, but these aids may be necessary to sharpen vision after cataract surgery. Review Figure 6.15 which is an example in the Alphabetic Index of a traumatic cataract.

FIGURE 6.15   Excerpt from the Alphabetic Index:
Traumatic Cataract

Cataract
    traumatic H26.10-
        localized H26.11-
        partially resolved H26.12-
        total H26.13-

Now review the following example. Open the codebook and locate the correct code beginning with the Alphabetic Index and reference the Tabular List.

> **EXAMPLE:** *A 30-year-old male patient who suffered an eye injury in an accident is referred to an ophthalmologist for evaluation. The patient complains that since his accident, he is experiencing a complete loss of vision in the left eye. After taking a comprehensive history and performing an ophthalmologic examination, the physician diagnoses a total traumatic cataract of the left eye. The physician discusses options with the patient, and the patient will follow up in one month for a recheck.*

> **Alphabetic Index:**
>   *Cataract → traumatic → total → H26.13-*

> **Tabular List:**
>   *H26.13 → left eye → H25.132*

Note: Laterality is critical when selecting the appropriate sixth character which identifies right, left, or unspecified eye.

> **Correct code:**
>   *H26.132*

Now review the next example and locate the correct code(s).

> **EXAMPLE:** *A 68-year-old male patient is examined by an ophthalmologist. The patient complains of reduced vision that makes it impossible to see traffic lights or signs clearly when driving. The physician examines the patient with a slit lamp and diagnoses a mature senile cataract of the right eye. Cataract extraction with an intraocular lens implant is scheduled for the next week.*

> **Alphabetic Index:**
>   *Cataract → senile → H25.9*

> **Tabular List:**
>   *H25.9 → Unspecified age-related cataract*

CODING TIP When no more information is available, use the unspecified code

CODING TIP When the note states to code the underlying condition first, the underlying condition is the first listed diagnosis.

DISORDERS OF THE CHOROID AND RETINA (H30-H36)

The retina is the light-sensitive membrane on the inner surface of the back of the eye. The optic nerve extends from the brain to about the center of the retina and then branches out. The central area of the retina, called the macula, contains the highest density of light-sensing nerves and, thus, produces the sharpest visual resolution. The retinal vein and artery reach the retina near the optic nerve and then branch out, following the paths of the nerves. Like the optic nerve and its branches, the retina itself has a rich supply of vessels that carry blood and oxygen. The cornea and lens near the front of the eye focus light onto the retina. Then, the branches of the optic nerve sense the light and the optic nerve transmits it to the brain, where it is interpreted as visual images.

Retinal Detachment

Retinal detachment is the separation of the retina from its underlying support. Detachment may begin in a small area, but if it is not treated, the entire retina can detach.

Retinal detachment is painless, and some common symptoms are as follows:

- Images of irregular floating shapes
- Flashes of light
- Blurred vision
- Vision loss

Vision loss begins in one part of the visual field, and, as the detachment progresses, the vision loss spreads. If the macular area of the retina becomes detached, vision rapidly deteriorates and everything becomes blurred. An ophthalmologist will diagnose this condition by examining the retina through an instrument used to view the inside of the eye.

Review the following example. Open the ICD-10-CM codebook and locate the main term "detachment."

EXAMPLE: *A patient is diagnosed with a partial retinal detachment with giant tear of the left eye.*

Alphabetic Index to Diseases:
Detachment → retina → with retinal break → giant → H33.03-

Tabular List:
H33.032 → retinal detachment with giant retinal tear, left eye

Correct code:
H33.032

CODING TIP Many of the diagnosis codes related to conditions/diseases of the eye include laterality in the code. If the laterality is not documented, it is recommended that the provider is queried instead of selecting a unspecified code.

EXAMPLE: *A 68-year-old patient experiences sudden vision loss with the sensation of a veil over his right eye. He is seen by his ophthalmologist the same day. The ophthalmologist examines the patient and diagnoses him with proliferative vitreo-retinopathy with retinal detachment. The patient is scheduled for laser therapy to be performed that afternoon.*

Alphabetic Index:
Detachment → retina → serous → traction → H33.4 -

Tabular List:
H33.4 → Traction detachment of the retina, right eye → H33.41

Correct code:
H33.41

Diabetic Retinopathy

This condition may occur in people with type 1 and type 2 diabetes. This condition is among the leading causes of blindness. Diabetes affects the retina because high blood glucose levels make the walls of small blood vessels thicker but weaker and, therefore, more prone to deformity and leakage.

The types of retinopathy are as follows:

- Background diabetic retinopathy (nonproliferative)

- Proliferative diabetic retinopathy

Nonproliferative diabetic retinopathy is seen in the early stages of the disease. In the nonproliferative stage, microaneurysms form, and small capillaries in the retina break and leak, which is referred to as retinal hemorrhage. The area around each break in the capillaries swells, forming small pouches in which blood

proteins are deposited. Small retinal hemorrhages may distort parts of the field of vision, or, if they are near the macula, they may blur vision. Blind spots are common. As the disease progresses, more vessel leakage occurs. The disease progresses from mild to moderate to severe nonproliferative retinopathy.

This disease becomes proliferative in the advanced stages characterized by new blood vessel formation in the retina due to ischemia from damaged vessels. Nonproliferative retinopathy can lead to total or near-total blindness.

Diabetic macular edema is caused by leakage from the retinal blood vessels, which can cause swelling of the retina. The central portion of the retina swells, which impairs vision. Plaque or exudates may develop in the posterior pole of the retina due to the breakdown of retinal vasculature, which causes loss of vision. Diabetic macular edema is a common complication of diabetic retinopathy and can occur during any stage of the disease.

Proliferative diabetic retinopathy is coded based on whether the diabetes due to an underlying condition (E08.-), is drug or chemical induced (E09.-), Type 1 (E.10-), Type 2 (E11.0-), or other specified diabetes mellitus (E13.-). Review Figure 6.16.

FIGURE 6.16 Excerpt from the Tabular List: *E10.3- Type 1 Diabetes Mellitus with Ophthalmic Complications*

E10	diabetes mellitus
E10.3	Type diabetes mellitus with ophthalmic complications
✓6ᵗʰ E10.35	Type 1 diabetes mellitus with proliferative diabetic retinopathy
E10.351	Type 1 diabetes mellitus with proliferative diabetic retinopathy with macular edema
E10.359	Type 1 diabetes mellitus with proliferative diabetic retinopathy without macular edema

Review the following example:

CODING TIP Don't forget to code in the appropriate category when selecting the appropriate code.

EXAMPLE: *A 67-year-old patient has had type 2 diabetes mellitus for 10 years. She has been on insulin for blood sugar control for the past 3 months. Her blood sugar was doing well on insulin and diet. After visiting her family physician, she is referred to an ophthalmologist with a suspected condition related to the diabetes mellitus. The ophthalmologist examines the patient and determines that she has diabetic retinopathy that is nonproliferative, with macular edema. The condition is moderate. After taking a comprehensive history, the ophthalmologist recommends surgery and the physician schedules surgery for the same day.*

Alphabetic Index:
Diabetes → *Type 2* → *diabetic* → *retinopathy* → *nonproliferative* → *moderate* → *with macular edema* → *E11.331*

Tabular List:
E11.341 → *Type 2 diabetes mellitus with moderate nonproliferative diabetic retinopathy with macular edema*

The documentation indicates the patient is on insulin but is a type 2 patient. In addition to coding for the diabetic retinopathy, an additional code should be selected for the long-term insulin use. There is an instructional note under category E11.- to use and additional code (Z79.4) to report the insulin use.

Tabular List:
Z79.4 Long-term insulin use

Correct code sequencing:
E11.341, Z79.4

GLAUCOMA (H40-H42)

Glaucoma is a disorder in which increasing pressure in the eyeball damages the optic nerve and causes a loss of vision. Usually, glaucoma has no known cause; however, it sometimes runs in families. If the outflow channels are open, the disorder is called open-angle glaucoma. If the iris blocks the channels, the disorder is called closed-angle glaucoma.

In glaucoma, intraocular pressure is measured in the anterior chamber using a procedure called tonometry. Glaucoma produces a loss of peripheral vision or blind spots in the visual field.

In open-angle glaucoma, fluid drains too slowly from the anterior chamber. Pressure gradually rises—almost always in both eyes—causing optic nerve damage and a slow, progressive loss of vision. Vision loss begins at the edges of the visual field and, if not treated, eventually spreads to all parts of the visual field, ultimately causing blindness.

This is the most prevalent form of glaucoma. It is common after age 35 years but occasionally occurs in children. The condition tends to run in families and is most common in people with diabetes or nearsightedness (myopia). Open-angle glaucoma develops more often and may be more severe in blacks than in whites.

Closed-angle glaucoma is caused by the closure of the anterior angle by contact between the iris and the inner surface of the trabecular (supporting or anchoring strand of connecting tissue) meshwork. This condition is characterized in 4 stages or phases:

- Latent angle closure that displays little or no symptoms

- Intermittent angle closure characterized by intermittent, rapidly rising intraocular pressure with throbbing pain in or around the eye

- Acute angle closure, displaying characteristics similar to intermittent angle closure, but as the intraocular pressure continues to increase, the cornea becomes swollen and steamy with excruciating ocular pain. This condition is classified as a medical emergency.

- Chronic angle closure, an irreversible increase of intraocular pressure resulting from progressive damage to the angle structures

Glaucoma appears in category (H40-H42) and is coded to the fourth and fifth characters. Instructional notes should be followed carefully when coding this category. The following are examples:

EXAMPLE: *A 57-year-old patient is diagnosed as having open angle glaucoma due to right eye trauma.*

Alphabetic Index:
Glaucoma → *secondary trauma* → *H40.3-*

Tabular List:
H40.31 → *Glaucoma secondary to eye trauma, right eye*

Correct code:
H40.31

EXAMPLE: *A patient is diagnosed with Lowe's syndrome with glaucoma*

Open the ICD-10-CM codebook to the Alphabetic Index and reference the code in the Tabular list when selecting the correct code.

Alphabetic Index:
Glaucoma → *Lowe's syndrome* → *E72.03 [H42]*

Notice in the alphabetic index that two codes are required; one code for the condition and one code to identify the glaucoma.

Now review Figure 6.17 an excerpt from the Tabular List E72.0-

FIGURE 6.17   Excerpt from the Tabular List: *E72*

E72.0 Disorders of amino-acid transport
E72.00 Disorders of amino-acid transport, unspecified
E72.01 Cystinuria
E72.02 Hartnup's disease
E72.03 Lowe's syndrome
Use an additional code for associated glaucoma (H42)
E72,04 Cystinosis
E72.09 other disorders of amino-acid transport

The first listed or principal diagnosis in this patient encounter is E72.03. The secondary diagnosis is H42.

Review the Tabular List, category H42. Now review Figure 6.18.

FIGURE 6.18   Excerpt from the Tabular List: *H42*

H42 Glaucoma in diseases classified elsewhere
Code first underlying condition such as
amyloidosis (E85. -)
aniridia (Q13.1)
Lowe's syndrome (E72.03)
Reiger's anomaly (Q13.81)
specified metabolic disorder (E70-E90)
EXCLUDES 1 *glaucoma in:*
diabetes mellitus (E08.39, E09.39, E10.39,
E11.39, E13.39)
onchocerciasis (B73.02)
syphilis (A52.71)
tuberculous (A18.59)

Tabular List:
  E72.03 → *Lowe's syndrome*

  H42 → *Glaucoma in diseases classified elsewhere*

Correct code sequencing:
  E72.03, H42

OTHER DISORDERS OF THE EYE AND ADNEXA (H55-H57)

Intraoperative and postprocedural ophthalmologic complications are coded in category H59. Complications of care codes are located within the body system chapters with codes specific to the organ and structures of that body system. The complication codes should be

sequenced first followed by the specific complication of symptom if applicable to the patient's condition.

- H59 Intraoperative and postprocedural complications and disorders of eye and adnexa, not elsewhere classified

Review the following example:

EXAMPLE: *A patient who has cataract surgery on the right eye two days ago was experiencing pain in the right eye. Following a slit lamp examination of the affected eye, the physician discovered lens fragments in the right eye and returned patient to the operating room to remove the fragments.*

Open the ICD-10-CM codebook and locate the correct code.

In addition to the specific complication a secondary diagnosis is needed to identify the ocular pain in ICD-10-CM. The complication is more specific as it identifies which eye is affected.

H59.02	Cataract (lens) fragments in eye following cataract surgery
H59.029	Cataract (lens) fragments in eye following cataract surgery, unspecified eye
H59.021	Cataract (lens) fragments in eye following cataract surgery, right eye
H59.022	Cataract (lens) fragments in eye following cataract surgery, left eye
H59.023	Cataract (lens) fragments in eye following cataract surgery, bilateral
H59.029	Cataract (lens) fragments in eye following cataract surgery, unspecified eye

The correct complication code will identify the affected eye and is coded as H59.111 for the right eye. In addition the ocular pain should be coded as a secondary diagnosis.

Review the category H57.1 for ocular pain.

H57.1	Ocular pain
H57.10	Ocular pain, unspecified eye
H57.11	Ocular pain, right eye
H57.12	Ocular pain, left eye
H57.13	Ocular pain, bilateral
H57.8	Other specified disorders of eye and adnexa

The patient encounter in ICD-10-CM would be coded:

H59.021	Cataract (lens) fragments in eye following cataract surgery, right eye
H59.111	Intraoperative hemorrhage and hematoma of right eye and adnexa
H57.11	Ocular pain, right eye

CHECKPOINT EXERCISE 6-3

Using the ICD-10-CM manual, code the following:

1. _____ Leprosy with infective dermatitis of left eyelid

2. _____ Cataract, senile, bilateral

3. _____ Lattice corneal dystrophy, bilateral

4. _____ Proliferative diabetic retinopathy in a patient with uncontrolled type 1 diabetes

5. _____ Optic neuritis

6. _____ After cataract, right eye

7. _____ Scleritis, left eye

8. _____ Blepharospasm, both eyes

9. _____ Eye strain

10. _____ Glaucoma with bilateral central retinal vein occlusion

11. _____ A 53-year-old hyperopic woman with a family history of angle closure glaucoma was previously noted to have an intra-ocular pressure of 22. She returns for further diagnostic evaluation by gonios-copy. After a comprehensive ophthalmic examination, the physician diagnoses narrow-angle glaucoma of both eyes.

12. _____ A 67-year-old man sees his ophthalmolo-gist with sudden loss of vision (right eye) in an otherwise normal eye. The patient is found to have a subretinal hemorrhage in the posterior pole, obscuring exami-nation of the deeper ocular elements. Intravenous fluorescein angiography cannot demonstrate any abnormalities of the posterior pole. The patient undergoes indocyanine-green video angiography, which detects a treatable subretinal neovascular membrane. The subretinal neovascular membrane is treated with laser photocoagulation.

13. _____ A 60-year-old white man, who is noted to have a pigmented choroidal lesion on the right eye, is referred for evaluation and documentation. The dilated examination shows a 5 × 6-mm pigmented choroidal mass in the right eye that is slightly elevated.

14. _____ A 64-year-old with a recent onset of decreased vision is diagnosed with senile cataracts of both eyes and macular drusen.

15. _____ A 32-year-old with a 12-year history of type 1 diabetes has blurred vision and sudden onset of vitreous floaters in the left eye.

CODING TIP Laterality is important in coding diseases of the eye and adnexa.

Chapter 8, Diseases of the Ear and Mastoid Process (H60-H95)

Chapter 8 in the Tabular List includes the following sections:

- Diseases of external ear (H60-H62)
- Diseases of middle ear and mastoid (H65-H75)
- Diseases of inner ear (H80-H83)
- Other disorders of ear (H90-H94)
- Intraoperative and postprocedural complications and disorders of ear and mastoid process, not elsewhere classified (H95)

The ear is the organ of hearing and balance and con-sists of the outer, middle, and inner ear. The outer ear captures sound waves that are converted into mechani-cal energy by the middle ear. The inner ear converts the mechanical energy into nerve impulses, which then travel to the brain. The inner ear also helps main-tain balance.

DISEASES OF THE EXTERNAL EAR (H60-H62)

Otitis Externa

Otitis externa is an infection of the ear canal. The infection may affect the entire canal, as in general-ized external otitis, or just one small area, as with a boil. Otitis externa is often called swimmers' ear because during the summer season, this condition is most common. Generalized otitis externa can be caused by a variety of bacteria or fungi, and boils are usually caused by bacteria, particularly *Staphylococcus*. In general, otitis externa can also be caused by the following:

- Allergies
- Psoriasis
- Eczema
- Scalp dermatitis
- Injuries in the ear canal while cleaning the ear (cotton swabs are the most likely culprit)
- Water or irritants

Otitis externa is coded as category H60, Diseases of external ear. Codes in this category include:

H60.399   Other infective otitis externa, unspecified ear. Use this code only when a more specific code is not available.

H60.33–   Swimmers' ear (a sudden, severe bacterial infection of the outer ear associated with swimming in fresh water) (sixth character is based on laterality)

H60.2–   Malignant otitis externa (severe infection of the outer ear canal with tissue destruction) (sixth character is based on laterality)

H60.55–   Acute reactive otitis externa (sixth character is based on laterality)

Review the following example:

EXAMPLE: *A patient arrives at her family practitioner's office for a routine visit. The patient's only complaint is slight pain in the left ear. After a detailed examination, the physician documents the diagnosis as an acute onset of otitis externa that is chronic.*

Alphabetic Index:
Otitis → *externa* → *acute* → *(noninfective)* → *H60.50-* → *chronic* → *H60.6-*

In this example, both the acute condition and the chronic condition are reported because there is no combination code to identify the otitis externa, which is both acute and chronic.

Tabular List:
H60.501 → *Unspecified acute noninfective otitis externa, right ear*

H60.62 → *Unspecified chronic otitis externa, left ear*

Correct code sequencing:
H60.501, H60.62

CODING TIP When the diagnostic statement indicates both an acute and chronic condition during the same patient encounter, the acute condition is the first listed diagnosis followed by the chronic condition as the secondary diagnosis.

EXAMPLE: *A patient is treated by his primary care physician for impetigo manifested by otitis externa of the right ear.*

Keep in mind when selecting the code for this encounter that the underlying condition is the impetigo and the manifestation in this example is the otitis externa. The impetigo is sequenced first followed by the otitis externa.

Alphabetic Index:
Impetigo → *external ear* → *L01.00 [H62.40]*

The Alphabetic Index indicates the sequencing of this condition as impetigo as the first listed diagnosis and the otitis externa as the secondary diagnosis reported.

Tabular List:
L01.00 → *Impetigo unspecified*

H62.41 Otitis externa in other diseases classified elsewhere, right ear

Correct code sequencing:
L01.00, H62.41

DISEASES OF THE MIDDLE EAR AND MASTOID (H65-H75)

Diseases in this category include otitis media, mastoiditis, tympanic membrane disorder, and disorders of the middle ear mastoid.

Otitis Media

Middle ear disorders may produce symptoms such as the following:

- Pain
- Fullness or pressure in ear
- Discharge of fluid or pus
- Hearing loss
- Vertigo (whirling sensation)

Symptoms may be caused by infection, injury, or pressure in the middle ear from a blocked eustachian tube. Acute otitis media is a bacterial or viral infection. This disorder can develop in persons of all ages but is most common in young children. Otitis media is coded to H65.- and H66.-. This category should be coded to its highest level of specificity. A fourth or fifth digit is required for correct coding.

Review the following example:

EXAMPLE: *A patient is diagnosed with recurrent bilateral acute secretory otitis media.*

Alphabetic Index:
Otitis → *media†* → *secretory* → *see otitis media, nonsuppurative, acute, serous* → *H65.0-*

Tabular List:
H65.006 → *Acute serous otitis media, recurrent, bilateral*

CODING TIP Documentation must include whether the condition is initial or recurrent and laterality when coding in category H65.0–.

Open the ICD-10-CM codebook and code the following patient encounter using both the Alphabetic Index and the Tabular List.

EXAMPLE: *A patient underwent a revision of the mastoidectomy with apicectomy for cholesteatoma of the left middle ear and mastoid. During the procedure, the patient experienced an intraoperative hemorrhage of the left ear and mastoid process.*

Alphabetic Index:
Cholesteatoma ➝ mastoid ➝ H71.2–

Review the example below (Figure 6.19) from the Tabular List.

FIGURE 6.19   Excerpt from the Tabular List: *H71.2–*

H71.2	Cholesteatoma of mastoid
H71.20	Cholesteatoma of mastoid, unspecified ear
H71.21	Cholesteatoma of mastoid, right ear
H71.22	Cholesteatoma of mastoid, left ear
H71.23	Cholesteatoma of mastoid, bilateral

Tabular List:
H71.22 ➝ Cholesteatoma of mastoid, left ear

You're not finished yet. The complication is also coded. Review the options for coding intraoperative and postprocedural complications of the ear (H95.2) in Figure 6.20.

FIGURE 6.20   Excerpt from Tabular List: *H95.2*

H95.2	**Intraoperative hemorrhage and hematoma of ear and mastoid process complicating a procedure**
	EXCLUDES 1 intraoperative hemorrhage and hematoma of ear and mastoid process due to accidental puncture or laceration during a procedure (H95.3-)
H95.21	Intraoperative hemorrhage and hematoma of the ear and mastoid process complicating a procedure on the ear and mastoid process

The most appropriate complication code in this block is H95.21, Intraoperative hemorrhage and hematoma of the ear and mastoid process complicating a procedure of the ear and mastoid process.

First listed diagnosis:
H71.22 ➝ Cholesteatoma of mastoid, left ear

Secondary diagnosis:
H95.21 ➝ Intraoperative hemorrhage and hematoma of ear and mastoid process complicating ear and mastoid process

Correct code sequencing:
H71.22, H95.21

DISEASES OF THE INNER EAR (H80-H83)

Diseases in this category include Ménière's disease, which is a disorder characterized by the following:

- Hearing loss
- Vertigo
- Nausea
- Vomiting
- Pressure in affected ear
- Tinnitus (eg, noise in the ears, buzzing, ringing)

Hearing can progressively worsen as the disease progresses. Ménière's disease is coded as category H81.–. Codes are available in this category for active, inactive, and unspecified.

Review the following example:

EXAMPLE: *A 30-year-old woman complains of ringing in her ears along with nausea and vomiting. She has experienced these symptoms for 3 months, and they have become continuously worse. Her family physician asks an otologist to evaluate the patient's symptoms. The otologist performs a comprehensive history and examination and determines from a hearing test that the patient has Ménière's disease bilaterally.*

Alphabetic Index:
Ménière's ➝ Ménière's disease, syndrome, or vertigo

Tabular List:
H81.03 ➝ Ménière's disease, bilateral

Correct code:
H81.03

OTHER DISORDER OF EAR (H90-H94)

Hearing Loss

Hearing loss can be caused by a number of factors, including the following:

- Loud noise over a period of time
- Loud music
- Equipment noises
- Chronic ear infections
- Age
- Ear damage

Diagnosis coding of hearing loss is accomplished using category H90.–. Hearing loss can be conductive, that is, due to the sound-conducting structures of the external or middle ear, or sensorineural, a defect in the nerve conduction. Hearing loss should be coded up to the fifth-digit subclassification.

CODING TIP Pay close attention when coding hearing loss. The type of hearing loss is crucial to the subclassification selected.

Review the following example:

EXAMPLE: An established patient who has a history of chronic otitis media is seen for follow-up examination by her ear, nose, and throat physician. The patient complains of hearing loss in the left ear and is having difficulty hearing people. A comprehensive audiogram indicates conductive hearing loss of the middle ear.

"Loss" is the main term, and "hearing" and "conductive" are the subterms.

Alphabetic Index:
Loss → hearing → conductive (air) → H90.1 → left ear H90.12

Tabular List:
H90.12 → Conductive hearing loss, unilateral, left ear with unrestricted hear loss on the contralateral side

Correct code:
H90.12

The following is an additional example:

EXAMPLE: An internist requests that an otologist evaluate his patient's hearing loss. The patient complains of tinnitus from listening to rock music. At the time of the consultation, the otologist removes bilateral cerumen impactions. At the same visit, a comprehensive audiogram is performed, showing bilateral high-frequency sensorineural hearing loss.

Hint: There is more than one diagnosis in this encounter.

First listed diagnosis:
Sensorineural hearing loss bilateral

Alphabetic Index:
Loss → hearing → sensorineural NOS → H90.5

Tabular List:
H90.5 → unspecified sensorineural hearing loss

Secondary diagnosis:
Tinnitus

Alphabetic Index:
Tinnitus → see subcategory H93.–

Tabular List:
H93.13 → Tinnitus, bilateral

CHECKPOINT EXERCISE 6-4

Using the ICD-10-CM codebook, code the following:

1. _____ Ankylosis of malleus bilateral

2. _____ Stenosis of eustachian tube, left ear

3. _____ Adhesive otitis, bilateral

4. _____ Deafness, conductive, mixed

5. _____ Fistula of middle ear

6. _____ Perforation of left eardrum

7. _____ Bilateral atrophic ear with tinnitus

8. _____ Malignant positional vertigo bilaterally

9. _____ Cholesteatoma of both ears

10. _____ Acute tympanitis of right ear

11. _____ A 45-year-old woman with classic Ménière's disease in both ears has disabling episodic vertigo despite appropriate medical treatment. After extensive counseling about treatment options, she undergoes an endolymphatic sac operation. After surgery, she experiences some mild vertigo and fluctuation of hearing, but eventually returns to work.

12. _____ A patient presents with recurring spells of vertigo refractory to medical management.

13. _____ Malignant otitis externa of the right ear

14. _____ Benign paroxysmal positional vertigo

15. _____ Myringitis bullosa hemorrhagica

Tertiary diagnosis:
Cerumen impaction

Alphabetic Index:
Impaction, impacted → cerumen (ear) (external) → H61.2

Tabular List:
H61.23 → Impacted cerumen, bilateral

Correct code sequencing:
H90.5, H93.13, H61.23

Did you get the correct answer? If you did, congratulations! If you missed a diagnosis, go back and reread the scenario, review the Alphabetic Index, and return to the Tabular List.

Test Your Knowledge

Code the following diagnosis coding statements:

1. _____ Ménière's disease (bilateral) in a 29-year-old woman

2. _____ Acute sinusitis due to *Haemophilus influenzae*

3. _____ A 45-year-old woman with schizotypal personality disorder

4. _____ Meningitis with typhoid fever in a 45-year-old man returning from the African jungle

5. _____ A 77-year-old man with Axenfeld's anomaly with glaucoma bilaterally

6. _____ Paralytic blepharoptosis of both eyes

7. _____ Bleeding esophageal varices due to alcoholic cirrhosis of the liver

8. _____ Retained foreign body of the lens in left eye

9. _____ Type 1 diabetes mellitus with polyneuropathy

10. _____ Tobacco use

11. _____ Manic bipolar depressive disorder

12. _____ Panic attack

13. _____ Thrombophlebitis of the iliac vein

14. _____ Chronic alcoholism in remission

15. _____ Psychoneurosis

16. _____ Petit mal epilepsy

17. _____ A 45-year-old man with gastritis and alcohol dependence who continues to drink on a daily basis

18. _____ Werdnig-Hoffmann disease

19. _____ Bell's palsy

20. _____ Absolute glaucoma both eyes

CHAPTER 7

Diseases of the Circulatory and Respiratory Systems (I00-J99)

LEARNING OBJECTIVES

- Understand basic coding guidelines for the circulatory system
- Review guidelines and examples in the respiratory system
- Properly sequence ICD-10-CM codes in the circulatory and respiratory systems
- Assign ICD-10-CM codes to the highest level of specificity
- Successfully complete checkpoint exercises and test your knowledge exercises

Chapter 9 in the Tabular List includes the following sections:

- Acute rheumatic fever (I00-I02)
- Chronic rheumatic heart disease (I05-I09)
- Hypertensive disease (I10-I15)
- Ischemic heart disease (I20-I25)
- Pulmonary heart diseases and diseases of pulmonary circulation (I26-I28)
- Other forms of heart disease (I30-I52)
- Cerebrovascular disease (I60-I69)
- Diseases of the arteries, arterioles, and capillaries (I70-I79)
- Diseases of the veins and lymphatic vessels and lymph nodes, not elsewhere classified (I80-I89)
- Other and unspecified disorders of the circulatory system (I95-I99)

The cardiovascular system is made up of the heart and blood vessels and supplies blood, nutrients, oxygen, hormones, and immunologic substances via a network of arteries originating in the heart and supplying the body's periphery. Included in the circulatory system are:

- Heart
- Arteries
- Veins
- Lymphatics

Following is a review of some of these conditions and the coding issues in this classification.

Acute Rheumatic Fever (I00-I02)

Rheumatic fever (acute rheumatic fever) is sometimes referred as ARF. This condition is an autoimmune disease that occurs after group A (beta hemolytic) streptococcal throat infection. This condition causes inflammatory lesions in connective tissue in the heart, joints, blood vessels, and subcutaneous tissue. Rheumatic fever can affect the heart, joints, skin, and brain. Some of the signs and/or symptoms include:

- Arthritis in joints
- Heart inflammation
- Nodules under the skin
- Skin rash
- Jerky uncontrollable body movements
- Fever
- Joint pain
- EKG changes

Complications of rheumatic fever include atrial fibrillation, carditis, and heart failure. With the availability of antibiotics in the Unites States, rheumatic fever has become easily treatable if the strep infection is caught early. The streptococcus A infection can be diagnosed by a rapid strep test or culture. Rheumatic fever has become less common in the United States. However, in other parts of the world, rheumatic fever is very common.

Rheumatic Heart Disease (I05-I09)

Rheumatic heart disease is the late effect of rheumatic fever. Common symptoms of this disease includes:

- Breathlessness
- Fatigue
- Palpitations
- Chest pain
- Fainting attacks

Rheumatic fever and heart disease affect about 1,800,000 people in the United States.

Open the ICD-10-CM codebook and select the correct code(s) beginning with the Alphabetic Index and referencing the Tabular List.

Review the following example:

> **EXAMPLE:** *A 10-year-old patient visited the emergency room with high fever and sore throat. This has been ongoing for the past two weeks and appears worse now. The physician took a detailed history and performed a comprehensive examination, performing a rapid strep test. The physician diagnoses the patient with rheumatic fever.*

> **Alphabetic Index:**
> *Fever → rheumatic → I00*

> **Tabular List:**
> *I00 → Rheumatic fever without heart involvement*

> **Correct code:**
> *I00*

Hypertensive Disease (I10-I15)

Hypertension (high blood pressure) is probably the most common condition included in this chapter. Abnormally high pressure in the arteries impacts the health of every body system and organ, thus increasing the risk of problems such as stroke, aneurysm, heart failure, heart attack, and kidney and eye damage, to name but a few. To many people, the word *hypertension* suggests excessive tension, nervousness, or stress. In medical terms, however, hypertension refers to a condition of elevated blood pressure regardless of the cause. It has been called "the silent killer" because it usually does not cause symptoms for many years—until a vital organ is damaged.

Blood pressure varies naturally over a person's life. Infants and children normally have much lower blood pressure than adults. Activity also affects blood pressure, which is higher when a person is active and lower when a person is at rest. Blood pressure also varies with the time of day. It is highest in the morning and lowest at night during sleep.

When blood pressure is checked, two values are recorded. The higher one occurs when the heart contracts (systole); the lower occurs when the heart relaxes between beats (diastole). Blood pressure is written as the systolic pressure followed by a slash and the diastolic pressure, for example, 120/80 mm Hg (millimeters of mercury). This reading would be referred to as "one-twenty over eighty."

High blood pressure is defined as a systolic pressure at rest that averages 140 mm Hg or more, a diastolic pressure at rest that averages 90 mm Hg or more, or both. With high blood pressure, usually both the systolic and the diastolic pressures are elevated.

Essential unspecified hypertension is a condition where the systolic pressure is 140 mm Hg or more, but the diastolic pressure is less than 90 mm Hg—that is, the diastolic pressure is in the normal range. Hypertension is increasingly common with advancing age. In almost everyone, blood pressure increases with age, with systolic pressure increasing until at least age 80 and diastolic pressure increasing until age 55 to 60, then leveling off or even falling. Benign hypertension is a condition where mild elevation in arterial blood pressure is found; however, no apparent organic cause is known. Benign hypertension is relatively symptomless. Malignant hypertension is a rare and particularly severe form of high blood pressure that, if left untreated, usually leads to death in 3 to 6 months.

There are two broad categories of hypertension: primary (or essential) and secondary. Despite many years of active research, there is no unifying hypothesis to account for the pathogenesis of primary hypertension. Unlike secondary hypertension, there is no known cause of primary hypertension.

Secondary hypertension has an identifiable cause whereas primary hypertension has no known cause

(ie, it is idiopathic). Patients with secondary hypertension are best treated by controlling or removing the underlying disease or pathology, although they may still require antihypertensive drugs.

There are many known conditions that can cause secondary hypertension. Some causes for secondary hypertension are listed below:

- Renal artery stenosis
- Chronic renal disease
- Primary hyperaldosteronism
- Stress
- Sleep apnea
- Hyper- or hypothyroidism
- Pheochromocytoma
- Preeclampsia
- Aortic coarctation

Before we review the codes for hypertension, let's review the guidelines for coding hypertension as presented in Table 7.1.

In ICD-9-CM, a hypertension table was available in the Alphabetic Index as a reference for hypertension. In ICD-10-CM, there is no hypetension table to reference. All conditions for hypertension including manifestations are listed in the Alphabetic Index under "hypertension."

TABLE 7.1   Official ICD-10-CM Guidelines for Hypertension

Hypertension	Heart conditions classified to I50.– or I51.4-I51.9 are assigned to a code from category I11, Hypertensive heart disease, when a causal relationship is stated (due to hypertension) or implied (hypertensive). Use an additional code from category I50, Heart failure, to identify the type of heart failure in those patients with heart failure.
	The same heart conditions (I50.–, I51.4-I51.9) with hypertension, but without a stated causal relationship, are coded separately. Sequence according to the circumstances of the admission/encounter.
Hypertensive Chronic Kidney Disease	Assign codes from category I12, Hypertensive chronic kidney disease, when both hypertension and a condition classifiable to category N18, Chronic kidney disease (CKD), are present. Unlike hypertension with heart disease, ICD-10-CM presumes a cause-and-effect relationship and classifies chronic kidney disease with hypertension as hypertensive chronic kidney disease.
	The appropriate code from category N18 should be used as a secondary code with a code from category I12 to identify the stage of chronic kidney disease.
	See Section I.C.14, Chronic kidney disease.
	If a patient has hypertensive chronic kidney disease and acute renal failure, an additional code for the acute renal failure is required.

(continued)

TABLE 7.1   *(continued)*

Hypertensive Heart and Chronic Kidney Disease	Assign codes from combination category I13, Hypertensive heart and chronic kidney disease, when both hypertensive kidney disease and hypertensive heart disease are stated in the diagnosis. Assume a relationship between the hypertension and the chronic kidney disease, whether or not the condition is so designated. If heart failure is present, assign an additional code from category I50 to identify the type of heart failure.
	The appropriate code from category N18, Chronic kidney disease, should be used as a secondary code with a code from category I13 to identify the stage of chronic kidney disease.
	See Section I.C.14, Chronic kidney disease.
	The codes in category I13, Hypertensive heart and chronic kidney disease, are combination codes that include hypertension, heart disease, and chronic kidney disease. The "Includes" note at I13 specifies that the conditions included at I11 and I12 are included together in I13. If a patient has hypertension, heart disease, and chronic kidney disease, then a code from I13 should be used, not individual codes for hypertension, heart disease, and chronic kidney disease or codes from I11 or I12.
	For patients with both acute renal failure and chronic kidney disease, an additional code for acute renal failure is required.
Hypertensive Cerebrovascular Disease	For hypertensive cerebrovascular disease, first assign the appropriate code from categories I60-I69, followed by the appropriate hypertension code.
Hypertensive Retinopathy	Subcategory H35.0, Background retinopathy and retinal vascular changes, should be used with code I10, Essential (primary) hypertension, to include the systemic hypertension. The sequencing is based on the reason for the encounter.
Hypertension, Secondary	Secondary hypertension is due to an underlying condition. Two codes are required: one to identify the underlying etiology and one from category I15 to identify the hypertension. Sequencing of codes is determined by the reason for admission/encounter.
Hypertension, Transient	Assign code R03.0, Elevated blood pressure reading without diagnosis of hypertension, unless patient has an established diagnosis of hypertension.
	Assign code O13.–, Gestational [pregnancy-induced] hypertension without significant proteinuria, or O14.–, Pre-eclampsia, for transient hypertension of pregnancy.
Hypertension, Controlled	This diagnostic statement usually refers to an existing state of hypertension under control by therapy. Assign the appropriate code from categories I10-I15, Hypertensive diseases.
Hypertension, Uncontrolled	Uncontrolled hypertension may refer to untreated hypertension or hypertension not responding to current therapeutic regimen. In either case, assign the appropriate code from categories I10-I15, Hypertensive diseases.

Source: ICD-10-CM Official Guidelines for Hypertension

Hypertension can be the cause of various forms of heart and/or vascular disease or it can be related to some heart conditions. Use caution when coding conditions in this category. Always use both the Alphabetic Index and the Tabular List when assigning a code.

As previously indicated, hypertensive disease is located in categories I10-I15. Category I10 to I15 is used only when a diagnosis of hypertension is documented in the medical record. In the Tabular List there are instructional notes to use an additional code to identify the following:

- Exposure to environmental tobacco smoke (Z77.22)
- History of tobacco use (Z87.891)
- Occupational exposure to environmental tobacco smoke (Z57.31)
- Nicotine dependence (F17.–)
- Tobacco use (Z72.0)

Review the following example:

EXAMPLE: A patient visits his internist for his 3-month follow-up visit. He has been treated for essential hypertension for more than 10 years. The patient's current blood pressure is 140/100 mm Hg. A detailed history and examination are performed, and the physician adjusts the patient's medication, reviews previous blood pressure readings, and asks the patient to follow up in one month to see if the blood pressure is under control. The documentation indicates hypertension without good control.

Review what we know about this encounter. We know the patient had been previously diagnosed with hypertension. However, we do not know what type of hypertension the patient is being treated for and we do know that no other conditions are documented that are associated with the hypertension. Proceed as follows:

Alphabetic Index:
Hypertension (essential) → *I10*

Tabular List:
I10 → *Hypertension, Hypertensive*

Correct code:
I10

Now review the category, Hypertensive heart disease. As was mentioned earlier, many conditions are "due to" or a "result of" hypertension. Hypertensive heart disease refers to the secondary effects on the heart when the patient sustains systemic hypertension over a prolonged period. When the diagnostic statement indicates heart condition due to hypertension or hypertensive heart disease, use a code from category I11. When coding in category I11 and heart failure is documented in the medical record, an additional code is required to identify the type of heart failure in category I50.–. As stated in the guidelines, only use a code from category I11 when a causal relationship is stated, for example, "due to hypertension." Remember, if a causal relationship is not stated, the same heart conditions are coded separately and not reported in this category.

Review Figure 7.1.

FIGURE 7.1   Excerpt from the Tabular List: *I11*

✓4th I11   Hypertensive heart disease
[INCLUDES]   any condition in I51.4-I51.9 due to hypertension
    I11.0   Hypertensive heart disease with heart failure
        Hypertensive heart failure
        Use additional code to identify type of heart failure (I50.-)
    I11.9   Hypertensive heart disease without heart failure
        Hypertensive heart disease NOS

Open the ICD-10-CM codebook and select the appropriate code. As always begin with the Alphabetic Index and select the correct code from the Tabular List.

Review the following example:

EXAMPLE: *An established patient arrives for his follow-up appointment with his family physician. The physician performs a detailed history and examination. The patient has a history of hypertensive heart disease and benign hypertension with cardiovascular disease. The diagnosis remains unchanged.*

Alphabetic Index:
Hypertension → *due to* → *heart disease* → *hypertension* → *I11.9*

Tabular List:
I11.9 → *hypertensive heart disease without heart failure*

Correct code:
I11.9

There is no mention of heart failure in the note, and the selection of I11.9 indicates "Without heart failure." Code I11.0 would be selected only if the documentation supports "With heart failure."

Hypertension with Chronic Kidney Disease (I12.–)

The ICD-10-CM guidelines require a code from category I12 if the hypertension is associated with chronic kidney disease (CKD). The guidelines also indicate "if the condition is classifiable to category N18." CKD is classified in category N18. However, if hypertension has a causal relationship to the chronic kidney disease, it is not coded in category N18 but in category I12.

In addition to coding for the hypertension with CKD, the stage of the CKD must be reported as an additional diagnosis from category N18.–.

Open the ICD-10-CM codebook and use both the Alphabetic Index and the Tabular List to code this patient encounter.

EXAMPLE: *A patient is admitted to the hospital with chronic kidney disease in stage 4 due to malignant hypertension.*

Alphabetic Index:
Hypertension → *kidney* → *stage 1 through stage 4 chronic kidney disease* → *I12.9*

Tabular List:
I12.9 → *Hypertensive chronic kidney disease with stage 1 through stage 4 chronic kidney disease, or unspecified chronic kidney disease*

But wait! The instructional note under I12.9 instructs the user to "use additional code to identify stage of chronic kidney disease (N18.1-N18.4, N18.9)."

Turn to category N18.– in the ICD-10-CM codebook and locate the code for CKD.

Now review Figure 7.2.

FIGURE 7.2   Excerpt from the Tabular List: *N18.–*

N18   Chronic Kidney Disease (CKD)
      N18.1   Chronic kidney disease, stage 1
      N18.2   Chronic kidney disease stage 2 (mild)
      N18.3   Chronic kidney disease stage 3 (moderate)
      N18.4   Chronic kidney disease stage 4 (severe)
      N18.6   End stage renal disease
      N18.9   Chronic kidney disease, unspecified

After reviewing Figure 7.2, it is clear that the stage 4 chronic kidney disease is reported with N18.4, which is the secondary diagnosis.

First listed diagnosis:
I12.9 → Hypertensive chronic kidney disease with stage 1 through stage 4 chronic kidney disease, or unspecified chronic kidney disease

Secondary diagnosis:
N18.4 → Chronic kidney disease, stage 4 (severe)

Correct code sequencing:
I12.9, N18.4

Hypertensive Heart and Chronic Kidney Disease (I13.–)

The ICD-10-CM guidelines instruct the user to "assign codes from combination category I13, Hypertensive heart and chronic kidney disease, when both hypertensive kidney disease and hypertensive heart disease are stated in the diagnosis." Also, as with hypertension with CDK, a code from category N18.– should be assigned to identify the CDK. Also with hypertensive heart and CDK, you can assume a causal relationship using the combination code(s) from category I13.–. Don't forget, if heart failure is documented, a code from category I50– must be reported for the failure.

Open the ICD-10-CM codebook and use both the Alphabetic Index and the Tabular List to code this patient encounter.

EXAMPLE: *A patient with hypertensive renal sclerosis was admitted for acute renal failure and treated with dialysis. The patient's blood pressure worsened upon admission, and the physician order an IV hypertensive drug to lower the patient's blood pressure more quickly.*

What do we know about this patient encounter? The patient has hypertensive renal sclerosis. The main term is "sclerosis, renal." However, when referencing the Alphabetic Index, you realize that the instructional note directs the user to "see hypertension cardiorenal." We also know that the patient is in acute renal failure. Now try to locate the correct code.

Alphabetic Index:
Hypertension → cardiorenal → with stage 5 or end stage renal disease I13.11

Tabular List:
I13.11 → Hypertensive heart and chronic kidney disease without heart failure, with stage 5 chronic kidney disease or end stage renal disease

Now you need to locate the correct code for the end stage renal disease in category N18.–.

Tabular List:
N18.6 → End stage renal disease

First listed diagnosis:
I13.11 Hypertensive heart and chronic kidney disease without heart failure, with stage 5 chronic kidney disease or end stage renal disease.

Secondary diagnosis:
N18.6 End stage renal disease

Correct code sequencing:
I13.11, N18.6

EXAMPLE: *A patient is admitted to the hospital with acute diastolic heart failure due to hypertension with renal failure. The patient has end stage renal disease and is currently on dialysis.*

CODING TIP   You may assign an additional code from category I50.– to identify the type of heart failure. More than one code from category I50.– may be assigned if the patient has systolic or diastolic failure and congestive heart failure. Review Figure 7.3.

FIGURE 7.3   Excerpt from the Alphabetic Index: *Congestive Heart Failure*

Failure, heart, congestive (compensated) (decompensated) I50.9
    diastolic (congestive (I50.30)
    acute (congestive) I50.31
    and (on) chronic (congestive) I50.33
    chronic (congestive) I50.32
    and (on) acute (congestive) I50.33
    combined with systolic (congestive) I50.40
    acute (congestive) I50.41
    and (on) chronic (congestive) I50.43
    chronic (congestive) I50.42
    and (on) acute (congestive) I50.43

In the example above, it is stated that the congestive heart failure and kidney disease were due to hypertension. The Official ICD-10-CM Guidelines state that certain heart conditions are assigned to a code from category I13.– when a causal relationship is stated (due to hypertension) or implied (hypertensive). The same heart conditions with hypertension, but without a stated causal relationship, are coded separately. However, hypertension with the existence of kidney disease presumes a causal relationship, so these two conditions are combined into a code from category I13.–. You would also code the acute diastolic heart failure because the ICD-10-CM guidelines indicate under category I13.– to "use an additional code to specify type of heart failure" (I50.– if known).

Alphabetic Index:
Hypertension ➡ cardiorenal ➡ with stage 5 or end stage renal disease ➡ with heart failure ➡ I13.2

Tabular List:
I13.2 ➡ Hypertensive heart and chronic kidney disease with heart failure, with stage 5 chronic kidney disease or end stage renal disease.

Now you need to locate the correct code for the end stage renal disease in category N18.–.

Tabular List:
N18.6 ➡ End stage renal disease

An additional code from category I50.– must be reported for the heart failure as well. We know the patient has acute diastolic heart failure in addition to hypertensive heart and renal disease. Turn to category I50.– in the Tabular List. Review the following:

Tabular List:
I50.31 ➡ Acute diastolic (congestive) heart failure

First listed diagnosis:
I13.11 Hypertensive heart and chronic kidney disease without heart failure, with stage 5 chronic kidney disease or end stage renal disease.

Secondary diagnosis:
N18.6 End stage renal disease

Correct code sequencing:
I13.2, N18.6, I50.31

Category I15 indicates hypertension as secondary. Secondary means the hypertension was caused by another condition; therefore, hypertension is not the primary cause. The Official ICD-10-CM Guidelines state that when hypertension is secondary, two codes are required: one to identify the underlying condition and one from category I15 to identify the hypertension.

Review the following example:

> **EXAMPLE**: A patient is diagnosed with secondary hypertension due to renal occlusion. In this encounter, the renal occlusion is the cause of the hypertension, so the encounter is coded as shown here.

Alphabetic Index:
Occlusion ➡ Renal artery ➡ N28.0

Tabular List:
N28.0 ➡ Renal artery occlusion

We're not finished yet. We must still identify the hypertension as secondary. The renal artery occlusion is causing the hypertension and, if treated, may result in resolving the hypertension. Review the main term "hypertension" in the Alphabetic Index and locate "secondary." You will notice that NEC appears under secondary. Because the encounter did not indicate what type of hypertension, code the encounter as hypertension, unspecified (405.91). Now verify the code in the Tabular List to make sure the appropriate hypertension code has been selected.

Alphabetic Index:
Hypertension ➡ Secondary ➡ renovascular ➡ I15.0

Tabular List:
I15.0 ➡ Renovascular hypertension

First listed diagnosis:
N28.0 Renal artery occlusion

Secondary diagnosis:
I15.0 Secondary renovascular hypertension

Correct code sequencing:
N28.0, I15.0

CODING TIP High blood pressure in the absence of a diagnosis of hypertension should be coded R03.0, Elevated blood pressure reading without diagnosis of hypertension.

CODING TIP Category I50.–, Heart failure, includes associated pulmonary edema. Hypertensive heart disease is classified as I11.–. Hypertensive heart disease and renal failure are classified as I13.–.

Using your ICD-10-CM codebook, code the following:

1. _____ Malignant hypertension due to primary aldosteronism

2. _____ Hypertension, uncontrolled

3. _____ Secondary, benign hypertension due to renal artery occlusion

4. _____ Hypertension due to encepalopathy

5. _____ Chronic arteriosclerotic nephritis

6. _____ Hypertensive heart failure

7. _____ High blood pressure

8. _____ Rheumatic heart failure due to hypertension

9. _____ A patient in her fifth month of pregnancy diagnosed with hypertension with severe edema

10. _____ Pulmonary hypertension

11. _____ Benign hypertension secondary to Cushing's disease

12. _____ Malignant cardiorenal hypertension

13. _____ Malignant hypertension due to a brain tumor

14. _____ Hypertensive cardiomegaly

15. _____ A new patient sees the family physician for a routine checkup. After taking the patient's blood pressure, standing, sitting, and lying down, the readings are 160/100, which indicate hypertension. The documentation in the medical record indicated essential hypertension.

Ischemic Heart Disease (I20-I25)

Ischemic heart disease (IHD), or myocardial ischemia, is a disease characterized by ischemia (reduced blood supply) of the heart muscle, usually due to coronary artery disease (atherosclerosis of the coronary arteries). This category includes myocardial infarction (sometimes referred to as heart attack), angina pectoris, and all other forms (acute and chronic) of ischemic heart disease. Myocardial infarction is a medical emergency

in which the blood supply is restricted or cut off, causing some of the heart's muscle (myocardium) to die from lack of oxygen. Myocardial infarction usually occurs when a blockage in a coronary artery is restricted or cuts off the blood supply to the region of the heart. The heart's ability to keep pumping after a heart attack is related to the extent and location of the damaged tissue (infarction).

Understanding terminology is important when coding in this category.

Following is a review of some common terms:

Angina	Spasmodic, choking, or suffocative pain in the chest due to lack of oxygen in the heart muscles
Coronary occlusion	Complete obstruction of an artery of the heart, usually from progressive atherosclerosis, sometimes complicated by thrombosis
Embolism	Clot that forms in the heart, breaks away, and lodges in the coronary artery
Infarction	An area of coagulation necrosis in tissue due to local ischemia resulting from obstruction of circulation to the area, most commonly by a thrombus or embolus
Ischemia	Deficiency of blood supply usually due to functional constriction or actual obstruction of a blood vessel
Myocardial	Pertaining to the muscular tissue of the heart
NSTEMI	Acronym for nonST segment elevation myocardial infarction, which is a type of heart attack.
STEMI	Acronym for ST segment elevation myocardial infarction, which is a type of heart attack.
Thrombosis	An aggregation of blood factors frequently causing vascular obstruction at the point of its formation

Coding guidelines for ischemic heart disease I21.– include mention of hypertension.

ANGINA (I20)

Under the term "angina" in the Index of Diseases, you will find other noncardiac listings (eg, angina abdominal, angina intestinal, angina tonsil). For the purpose of discussing this category of codes, the term "angina" pertains to chest pain or discomfort occurring when an area of the heart is deprived of oxygen, for example, from coronary artery disease. However, this is not the only cause of angina. Some of the other causes are:

- Abnormalities of the aortic valve
- Aortic valve stenosis
- Hypertrophic subaortic stenosis
- Arterial spasm

The term "angina pectoris" is derived from both Greek (strangling) and Latin (chest) and translates to "a strangling feeling in the chest due to a lack of blood, thus a lack of oxygen supply of the heart muscle, generally due to obstruction or spasm of the heart's blood vessels." Angina pectoris (Prinzmetal angina) may occur when the patient is at rest. This disorder sometimes occurs because of abnormalities of the coronary arteries (aortic stenosis) and valve insufficiencies. The patient usually experiences chest pain. However, other symptoms include chest pressure, heaviness, burning, aching, or a painful feeling that can be felt in the chest, shoulders, arms, throat, neck, jaw, or back.

Some of the most common types of angina include the following:

- *Unstable angina* can be the first sign of a heart attack. The pain occurs while at rest, with more frequent episodes, and it may last longer or occur with minimal or no activity. Typically, medication is the treatment of choice. However, with the unstable nature of this type of angina, it could progress to a myocardial infarction.

- *Stable angina* symptoms present only during exertion or stress and subside with rest.

- *Angina Prinzmetal* occurs when the patient is at rest; it is a variant of angina pectoris. It is often referred to as unstable angina. This condition is associated with ST-segment elevations on an EKG. Symptoms include decreased blood flow to the heart's muscles due to a coronary artery spasm that is close to the blockage. Typically, patients with this type of angina also have coronary artery disease.

Review the following example:

EXAMPLE: *A 62-year-old female patient with a history of angina returns to her family physician for a 6-month follow-up visit. The patient's complete history is reviewed and updated by the nurse. The patient has used tobacco for more than 25 years, but quit smoking 3 years ago. The physician performs a detailed examination and documents anginal syndrome as the diagnosis.*

Alphabetic Index:
Angina (attack) (cardiac) (chest) (heart) (pectoris) (syndrome) (vasomotor) I20.9

Tabular List:
I20.9 ➞ Angina pectoris, unspecified

Because the specific type of angina is not documented, the unspecified code must be assigned. They type of angina that is coded in this category, anginal syndrome, is listed. I20.9 is the correct code to report for the angina. In addition, the patient has a history of tobacco use; it is reported with Z87.891.

Alphabetic Index:
History (personal) ➞ tobacco use ➞ Z87.891

Tabular List:
Z87.891 ➞ Personal history of nicotine dependence

Correct code sequencing:
I20.9, Z87.891

ACUTE MYOCARDIAL INFARCTION

When a person suffers a heart attack, symptoms include shortness of breath, chest discomfort, and crushing chest pain that can spread to the neck or shoulder. A common diagnostic tools is the EKG. If part of the heart muscle is damaged, the EKG will indicate an elevation of the ST segment, or ST elevation. When a heart attack is diagnosed based on the EKG ST elevation, this is referred to as STEMI. Treatment involves giving the patient aspirin and performing a coronary angiogram. This type of patient typically has a blood clot occluding the blood vesel. This clot can be removed and the artery can be widened with a stent.

With NSTEMI, the symptoms are the same for a patient with the ST elevation, but the EKG does not show elevation changes as it does with STEMI. The patient typically has a history of angina, but the EKG may show no abnormality. However, the diagnosis is typically confirmed by blood tests that indicate a rise in cardiac enzymes in the blood. Patient's with this type of heart attack typically are taken to a cath (catheter) lab for an angiography. The patient is likely have a nonocculsive narrowing of a coronary artery.

Acute myocardial infarction (category I21-I22) is site specific:

- Anterior wall (I21.0–)
- Inferior wall (I21.1–)
- Other sites (I21.2–)

Review the official guidelines for reporting a myocardial infarction (heart attack) in Table 7.2.

CODING TIP The guidelines for assigning the correct I22 (subsequent) code are the same as for the initial AMI. The documentation in the patient's chart should indicate what area of the heart muscle is affected.

For categories I21.– to I21.–, a fifth character is required. In addition, the instructional note indicates to use an additional code to identify other circumstances such as tobacco use, dependence, or body mass index (BMI). Review Figure 7.4 for category I21.–.

FIGURE 7.4   Excerpt from the Tabular List: *I21.–*

I21   ST elevation (STEMI) and non-ST elevation (NSTEMI) myocardial infarction
     INCLUDES   cardiac infarction
     coronary (artery) embolism
     coronary (artery) occlusion
     coronary (artery) rupture
     coronary (artery) thrombosis
     infarction of heart, myocardium, or ventricle
     myocardial infarction specified as acute or with a stated
         duration of 4 weeks (28 days) or less from onset
     Use additional code, if applicable, to identify:
       exposure to environmental tobacco smoke (Z77.22)
       history of tobacco use (Z87.891)
       occupational exposure to environmental tobacco
         smoke (Z57.31)
       status postadministration of tPA (rtPA) in a different
         facility within the last 24 hours prior to
         admission to current facility (Z92.82)
       tobacco dependence (F17.-)
       tobacco use (Z72.0)
     Use additional code, if known, to identify:
       body mass index (BMI) (Z68.-)
     EXCLUDES 2   old myocardial infarction (I25.2)
         postmyocardial infarction syndrome
           (I24.1)
         subsequent myocardial infarction
           (I22.-)
I21.0   ST elevation (STEMI) myocardial infarction of
       anterior wall
     I21.01   ST elevation (STEMI) myocardial infarction
         involving left main coronary artery
     I21.02   ST elevation (STEMI) myocardial infarction
         involving left anterior descending coronary
         artery
     I21.09   ST elevation (STEMI) myocardial infarction
         involving other coronary artery of anterior
         wall
         Acute transmural myocardial infarction of
           anterior wall
         Anteroapical transmural (Q wave)
           infarction (acute)
         Anterolateral transmural (Q wave)
           infarction (acute)
         Anteroseptal transmural (Q wave)
           infarction (acute)
         Transmural (Q wave) infarction (acute)
           (of) anterior (wall) NOS

Code the following example:

EXAMPLE: *A 60-year-old patient is admitted to the hospital after suffering from acute pain and collapsing at home. The emergency department physician performs a comprehensive history and examination, obtaining most of the patient's history from the family. This is the first episode of this nature that the patient has experienced. The patient is transferred to the coronary care unit in the hospital. A cardiologist is asked to take over the patient's care. The cardiologist examines the patient in the coronary care unit, reviews the EKG, and determines that the patient has suffered an acute mycardial of the inferolateral transmural Q wave infarction.*

How would you code this encounter? First, let's review what we know about this patient.

- This is the first episode of this nature for the patient.
- The diagnosis is acute myocardial infarction.
- The area affected is the inferior wall.

Based on this information, the following steps should be taken:

Alphabetic Index:
Infarct, infarction (Main term) → *Myocardium, myocardial* → *involving the coronary artery of the inferior wall* → *I21.19*

Tabular List:
I21.19 → *ST elevation (STEMI) myocardial infarction involving other coronary artery of inferior wall*

Correct code:
I21.19

Remember that a fifth character is required to complete the process.

Review the following example, referencing both the Alphabetic Index and the Tabular List, and select the correct code(s).

EXAMPLE: *The patient is seen by the emergency department physician with a prior history of coronary artery disease. The patient presents today stating that his chest pain started yesterday evening and has been somewhat intermittent. The severity of the pain has progressively increased. He describes the pain as a sharp and heavy pain that radiates to his neck and left arm. He ranks the pain a 7 on a scale of 1 to 10. He admits some shortness of breath and diaphoresis. He denies any fever or chills. He states the pain is somewhat worse with walking and seems to be relieved with rest. There is no change in pain with positioning. He states that he took 3 nitroglycerin tablets sublingually over the past hour, which he states has partially relieved his*

TABLE 7.2   ICD-10-CM Official Guidelines for Coding and Reporting Myocardial Infarction

Acute myocardial infarction (AMI) ST elevation myocardial infarction (STEMI) Non-ST elevation myocardial infarction (NSTEMI)	The ICD-10-CM codes for AMI identify the site, such as anterolateral wall or true posterior wall. Subcategories I21.0-I21.2 and code I21.4 are used for STEMI. Code I21.4, Non-ST elevation (NSTEMI) myocardial infarction, is used NSTEMI and nontransmural MIs.
If NSTEMI evolves to STEMI, assign the STEMI code. If STEMI converts to NSTEMI due to thrombolytic therapy, it is still coded as STEMI.	When the patient requires continued care for the myocardial infarction, codes from category I21 may continue to be reported for the duration of 4 weeks (28 days) or less from onset, regardless of the health care setting, including when a patient is transferred from the acute care setting to the post-acute care setting if the patient is still within the 4-week time frame. For encounters after the 4-week time frame and when the patient requires continued care related to the myocardial infarction, the appropriate aftercare code should be assigned, rather than a code from category I21. Otherwise, code I25.2, Old myocardial infarction, may be assigned for old or healed myocardial infarction not requiring further care.
Acute myocardial infarction, unspecified	Code I21.3, ST elevation (STEMI) myocardial infarction of unspecified site, is the default for the unspecified term "acute myocardial infarction." If only STEMI or transmural MI without the site is documented, query the provider as to the site or assign code I21.3.
AMI documented as nontransmural or subendocardial but site provided	If an AMI is documented as nontransmural or subendocardial, but the site is provided, it is still coded as a subendocardial AMI.
Subsequent acute myocardial infarction	A code from category I22, Subsequent ST elevation (STEMI) and nonST elevation (NSTEMI) myocardial infarction, is to be used when a patient who has suffered an AMI has a new AMI within the 4-week time frame of the initial AMI. A code from category I22 must be used in conjunction with a code from category I21. The sequencing of the I22 and I21 codes depends on the circumstances of the encounter. If a patient who is in the hospital due to an AMI has a subsequent AMI while still in the hospital, code I21 would be sequenced first as the reason for admission, with code I22 sequenced as a secondary code. If a patient has a subsequent AMI after discharge for care of an initial AMI, and the reason for admission is the subsequent AMI, the I22 code should be sequenced first followed by the I21. An I21 code must accompany an I22 code to identify the site of the initial AMI and to indicate that the patient is still within the 4-week time frame of healing from the initial AMI.

pain. The patient ranks his present pain a 4 on a scale of 1-10 on the pain scale. The most recent episode of pain has lasted one hour. He had a previous acute MI two weeks ago and was in the critical care unit at this hospital. The emergency department physician references the patient's previous course of hospital treatment including all diagnostic testing and medical treatment, noting that he had suffered an acute MI of the left main coronary wall. The ER physician performs an EKG, and notifies the patient's cardiologist who has come to the ER to see the patient. The cardiologist diagnoses the patient with a subsequent acute MI with a coronary artery embolism of the anterior wall.

Here is what we know about this patient.

- The patient had a previous MI of the left main coronary wall two weeks ago.

- The cardiologist has diagnosed the patient with an acute MI today with a coronary artery embolism of the anterior wall.

Alphabetic Index:
Infarct, Infarction → myocardium, myocardial → ST elevation → anterior wall → I22.0

Tabular List:
I22.0 → Subsequent ST elevation (STEMI) myocardial infarction of anterior wall

But you're not finished yet. The instructional note for the subsequent mycardial infarction category (I22.–) requires a code from category I21.– to identify the previous MI.

First listed diagnosis:
I22.0 Subsequent ST elevation (STEMI) myocardial infarction of anterior wall

Secondary diagnosis:
I21.01 ST Elevation (STEMI) myocardial infaction involving left main coronary artery

Correct code sequencing:
I22.0, I21.01

CORONARY ARTERY DISEASE (I25.–)

Coronary artery disease is a condition in which fatty deposits accumulate in the cells lining the wall of a coronary artery and obstruct blood flow. For the heart to contract and pump normally, the myocardium requires a continuous supply of oxygen-enriched blood from the coronary arteries. When the obstruction of a coronary artery worsens, ischemia to the heart muscle will develop, resulting in heart damage. The major cause of myocardial infarction and angina is coronary artery disease.

Diagnosis codes in this category include:

- Coronary atherosclerosis
- Arterisclerotic heart disease (ASHD)
- Coronary artery stricture
- Aneurysm of the heart and cornary vessels
- Arteriovenous aneurysm
- Chronic coronary insufficiency
- Iatrogenic hypotension

Review the following example:

> ***EXAMPLE:*** *An 84-year-old male discharged home from rehab setting after CVA and benign hypertension with ASHD of the native coronary arteries, requiring warfarin sodium. The hypertension is controlled adequately. Home health agency is providing weekly nursing visit, protime draws, and faxing blood sugar records. Patient is progressing well with PT and OT. Nutrition seems adequate.*

Open the ICD-10-CM codebook and select the appropriate diagnosis code(s).

Alphabetic Index:
Arteriosclerosis, arteriosclerotic ⟶ coronary ⟶ I25.10

Tabular List:
I25.10 ⟶ Ateriosclerosis heart disease of native coronary artery without angina pectoris

But wait! Because hypertension is also a diagnosis identified in the example above, hypertension must be coded as well.

Alphabetic Index:
Hypertension ⟶ Benign ⟶ I10

Tabular List:
Hypertension ⟶ I10

Correct coding sequence:
I25.10, I10

HEART FAILURE (I50)

Heart failure is sometimes referred to as congestive heart failure. This is a serious condition in which the quantity of blood pumped by the heart each minute is not sufficient to meet the body's requirement for oxygen and nutrients. With this condition, the heart's ability to keep up with its workload is diminished. Congestive heart failure is more common in older adults but it can occur in younger people as well.

Other conditions may contribute to heart failure, so use caution when selecting the appropriate diagnosis code. The codes are defined as left and right heart failure and are determined by which ventricle is affected and whether it is diastolic, systolic, and/or a combination of both. Codes for heart failure include associated pulmonary edema.

- Right heart failure
- Left heart failure
- Systolic heart failure
- Diastolic
- Systolic and diastolic

Heart failure unspecified is nonspecific and should only be used when every effort has been exhausted in determining a more definitive diagnosis.

Review the following examples, referencing both the Alphabetic Index and the Tabular List, and select the correct code(s).

> ***EXAMPLE:*** *A patient is diagnosed with congestive heart failure.*

Alphabetic Index:
Failure (Main term) ⟶ Congestive ⟶ I50.9

Tabular List:
I50.9 ⟶ Heart failure, unspecified

Correct code:
I50.9

> ***EXAMPLE:*** *A patient is diagnosed with left heart failure after cardiac surgery.*

Alphabetic Index:
Failure ⟶ Heart ⟶ Following ⟶ Cardiac surgery I97.13–

Tabular List:
I97.130 ⟶ Postprocedural heart failure following cardiac surgery

The note below category I50 indicates to "code first heart failure following surgery (I97.13–)."

Alphabetic Index:
Failure ➞ heart ➞ ventricular ➞ left ➞ I50.1

Tabular List:
I50.1 ➞ Left Ventricular Failure

Correct code sequencing:
I97.130, I50.1

Two codes would be necessary in this example: I97.130 to identify the heart failure following the cardiac surgery and I50.1 for the left ventricular failure.

A subclassification is used to identify whether the heart failure is diastolic, systolic, or a combination. Review these subcategories in Figure 7.5.

FIGURE 7.5   Excerpt from the Tabular List: I50.–

I50.2   Systolic (congestive) heart failure
EXCLUDES 1   Combined systolic (congestive) and diastolic (congestive heart failure (I50.4-)
    I50.20   Unspecified systolic (congestive) heart failure
    I50.21   Acute systolic (congestive) heart failure
    I50.22   Chronic systolic (congestive) heart failure
    I50.23   Acute on chronic systolic (congestive) heart failure
I50.3   Diastolic (congestive) heart failure
EXCLUDES 1   Combined systolic (congestive) and diastolic (congestive) heart failure (I50.4-)
    I50.30   Unspecified diastolic (congestive) heart failure
    I50.31   Acute diastolic (congestive) heart failure
    I50.32   Chronic diastolic (congestive) heart failure
    I50.33   Acute on chronic diastolic (congestive) heart failure
I50.4   Combined systolic and diastolic heart failure
    I50.40   Unspecified combined systolic (congestive) and diastolic (congestive) heart failure
    I50.41   Acute combined systolic (congestive) and diastolic (congestive) heart failure
    I50.42   Chronic combined systolic (congestive) and diastolic (congestive) heart failure
    I50.43   Acute on chronic combined systolic (congestive) and diastolic (congestive) heart failure

---

Review the following example, referencing both the Alphabetic Index and the Tabular List, and select the correct code(s).

EXAMPLE: A patient was admitted to the hospital with chest pain. After the physician examined the patient and performed an EKG, the physician confirmed the patient's diagnosis as acute combined systolic and diastolic heart failure.

Alphabetic Index:
Failure (heart) congestive ➞ diastolic (congestive)
Combined with systolic (I50.4–)

The next step is to review the Tabular List for the fifth-digit subclassification, which identifies the condition. Review the following:

Tabular List:
I50.41 Acute combined systolic (congestive) and diastolic (congestive) heart failure

Correct code:
I50.41 Acute systolic and diastolic heart failure

Cerebrovascular Disease (I60-I69)

The word *cerebrovascular* is made up of two parts "cerebro," which refers to the large part of the brain, and "vascular," which means arteries and veins. Together, cerebrovascular refers to blood flow in your brain. The term "cerebrovascular disease" covers acute stroke and other diseases that may lead to stroke, such as carotid stenosis and aneurysms.

More than 700,000 Americans suffer a major cerebrovascular event, usually a stroke, each year. Stroke is the third leading cause of death in the United States and the number one cause of disability, with more than 3,000,000 people currently living with permanent brain damage caused by such an event. On average, someone in the United States suffers a stroke every 53 seconds, and every 3.3 minutes someone dies of a stroke.

Stroke occurs when the blood flow to the brain is somehow disrupted and brain cells lose their supply of nutrients. This happens when the brain receives too little, or too much, blood. If this problem is not fixed within a short time, usually hours, brain cells die and the individual will be left with permanent brain damage. Once brain cells die, they cannot be regrown or revitalized. There are two types of stroke: ischemic and hemorrhagic. Ischemic stroke is more common and occurs when blood flow to the brain is blocked. Hemorrhagic stroke is less common, but more deadly, and occurs when there is bleeding into or around the brain itself. Hemorrhagic stroke includes both intracerebral hemorrhage and subarachnoid hemorrhage.

The heart pumps blood up to the brain through two sets of arteries: the carotid arteries and the vertebral arteries. The carotid arteries can be found in the front of the neck and are what is felt when a pulse is taken just under your jaw. The carotid artery splits into the external and internal arteries near the top the neck, with the external carotid artery supplying blood to the face and the internal carotid artery going into the skull. Once in the skull, the internal carotid artery branches to form two large arteries, the anterior cerebral and middle cerebral arteries, and several smaller arteries, the ophthalmic, posterior communicating, and anterior choroidal arteries. These arteries supply blood to the front two-thirds of the brain.

The vertebral arteries come up along side the spinal column and cannot be felt from the outside. The vertebral arteries join to form a single basilar artery near the brain stem, which is located near the base of the skull. The vertebrobasilar system sends many small branches into the brain stem and branches off to form the posterior cerebellar and posterior meningeal arteries, which supply the back third of the brain. The jugular and other veins bring blood out of the brain.

Because the brain relies on only two sets of major arteries for its blood supply, it is very important that these arteries remain healthy. Often, when an ischemic stroke occurs, the carotid or vertebral artery system is blocked with a fatty buildup called plaque, allowing little or no blood to flow to the brain. During a hemorrhagic stroke, an artery in or on the surface of the brain has ruptured or is leaking, causing bleeding and damage in or around the brain.

SIGNS AND SYMPTOMS OF STROKE

There are warning signs of an impending stroke; a stroke often does not strike unannounced.

- Prior stroke. Stroke can strike a person twice. Suffering one stroke, regardless of its severity, increases your chances of suffering a second stroke.

- Transient ischemic attack (TIA). A TIA is a temporary cerebrovascular disruption that leaves no permanent damage. These are recognizable events and can be a predictor of a future, more devastating stroke.

- Headache. A severe, sudden, unusual headache can be a sign of a hemorrhagic stroke and requires immediate medical attention.

Symptoms of TIA include:

- Visual disturbances, including blocked or loss of vision in one eye, blurry vision, or "graying"

- Weakness, numbness, or clumsiness in one arm or hand

- Language problems, including slurred speech or speaking jibberish

- Facial droop/weakness

- Unusual dizziness, vertigo, and overall numbness may also indicate a vertebrobasiliar TIA

CODING ISSUES

Diagnosis codes in this category include:

- Subdural hemorrhage

- Thrombosis of the arteries

- Transient cerebral ischemia

- Hypertensive encephalopathy

- Stroke/CVA

- Cerebral aneurysm

- Speech and language deficits that include:
  - Aphasia impairment or inability to communicate by speaking, writing, or signing
  - Dysphasia-impaired speech, marked by inability to sequence language

- Hemiplegia

- Monoplegia

- Other effects of cerebrovasuclar disease including:
  - Facial weakness
  - Vertigo
  - Late effects

Review the Table 7.3 for coding cerebrovascular conditions.

Review the following example, referencing both the Alphabetic Index and the Tabular List, and select the correct code(s).

EXAMPLE: A 72-year-old woman suffered an acute right CVA resulting in a left spastic hemiplegia, which is her dominant side. She has been hospitalized the past 3 days for the CVA. Although she can move her left arm, she has no functional use of it because her increased muscle tone results in a flexion synergy in which she adducts her shoulder, flexes her elbow, and pulls her hand into a tight fist. In order to diminish the spasticity during her daily activities, the provider applies deep pressure to the patient's biceps. The provider then internally rotates the patient's upper arm, extends the elbows, pronates the forearm, and extends the patient's fingers and thumb. This combination of movements releases the spasm, and with manual guidance from the provider, the patient is able to practice grasping, holding, and releasing large objects.

Notice that in this example, the patient has a right CVA and a left spastic hemiplegia (paralysis of the left side of the body).

Alphabetic Index:
Disease ➡ cerebrovascular ➡ acute ➡ I67.8

Tabular List:
I67.8 ➡ Other specified cerebrovascular diseases

Hemiplegia is mentioned. Do you code it? Open the ICD-10-CM codebook to the Alphabetic Index under Hemiplegia and find out.

Alphabetic Index:
Hemiplegia ➡ following ➡ cerebral infarction I69.35–

Because the hemiplegia is a sequelae to the CVA, you would report an additional code with a sixth character in this classification (I69.35–).

Tabular List:
I69.352 ➡ Hemiplegia and hemiparesis following cerebral infarction affecting left dominant side

Correct code sequencing:
I67.8, I69.352

TABLE 7.3   Official Guidelines for Coding and Reporting Cerebrovascular Accident

Atherosclerotic Coronary Artery Disease and Angina	ICD-10-CM has combination codes for atherosclerotic heart disease with angina pectoris. The subcategories for these codes are I25.11, Atherosclerotic heart disease of native coronary artery with angina pectoris, and I25.7, Atherosclerosis of coronary artery bypass graft(s) and coronary artery of transplanted heart with angina pectoris.
	When using one of these combination codes, it is not necessary to use an additional code for angina pectoris. A causal relationship can be assumed in a patient with both atherosclerosis and angina pectoris, unless the documentation indicates the angina is due to something other than the atherosclerosis.
	If a patient with coronary artery disease is admitted due to an acute myocardial infarction (AMI), the AMI should be sequenced before the coronary artery disease.
	See Section I.C.9, Acute myocardial infarction (AMI).
Intraoperative and Postprocedural Cerebrovascular Accident	Medical record documentation should clearly specify the cause-and-effect relationship between the medical intervention and the cerebrovascular accident in order to assign a code for intraoperative or postprocedural cerebrovascular accident.
	Proper code assignment depends on whether it was an infarction or hemorrhage and whether it occurred intraoperatively or postoperatively. If it was a cerebral hemorrhage, code assignment depends on the type of procedure performed.
Sequelae of Cerebrovascular Disease Category I69, Sequelae of Cerebrovascular Disease	Category I69 is used to indicate conditions classifiable to categories I60-I67 as the causes of "late effects" (neurologic deficits), themselves classified elsewhere. These late effects include neurologic deficits that persist after initial onset of conditions classifiable to categories I60-I67.
	The neurologic deficits caused by cerebrovascular disease may be present from the onset or may arise at any time after the onset of the condition classifiable to categories I60-I67.
Codes from Category I69 with Codes from I60-I67	Codes from category I69 may be assigned on a health care record with codes from I60-I67, if the patient has a current cerebrovascular disease and deficits from an old cerebrovascular disease.
Code Z86.73	Assign code Z86.73, Personal history of transient ischemic attack (TIA), and cerebral infarction without residual deficits (and not a code from category I69) as an additional code for history of cerebrovascular disease when no neurologic deficits are present.

CHECKPOINT EXERCISE 7-2

Using your ICD-10-CM codebook, code the following:

1. _____ Myoendocarditis

2. _____ An 80-year-old female with new onset atrial fibrillation has a two-hour history of excruciating abdominal pain. Emergent angiography reveals an embolus occluding her superior mesenteric artery.

3. _____ Cardiomyopathy with myotonia atrophica

4. _____ Nocturnal angina

5. _____ Ventricular aneurysm

6. _____ Posterobasal infarction

7. _____ Hypotension

8. _____ Acute myocardial infarction, 68-year-old female patient 4 weeks ago; readmitted to the hospital because of hypertension

9. _____ Cerebrovascular accident

10. _____ Initial episode of acute myocardial infarction of the atrium in a 70-year-old man

11. _____ A 56-year-old woman hospitalized with acute inferior myocardial infarction with a history of smoking suddenly develops severe congestive heart failure on day 3 after infarction. The patient has not smoked for 6 years.

12. _____ Angina pectoris

13. _____ Congestive heart failure

14. _____ A 70-year-old male complains of a swollen left lower extremity. Noninvasive studies rule out DVT in the left leg, but Doppler signals suggest a more central obstruction to venous return. An abdominal and pelvic CT scan reveals a 5-cm isolated common iliac artery aneurysm compressing the iliac vein.

15. _____ A 70-year-old female arrives in the ED with a severely painful arm and numbness of her hand. Symptom onset was sudden and occurred 3 hours prior to arrival. Exam reveals a cold and pulseless limb. Cardiac rhythm is irregular, and ECG confirms atrial fibrillation not present on a study performed one month earlier. An emergent embolectomy is performed.

Diseases of the Respiratory System (J00-J99)

Chapter 8 in the Tabular List includes the following sections:

- Acute upper respiratory infections (J00-J06)
- Influenza and pneumonia (J09-J18)
- Other acute lower respiratory infections (J20-J22)
- Other diseases of the upper respiratory tract (J30-J39)
- Chronic lower respiratory diseases (J40-J47)
- Lung diseases due to external agents (J60-J70)
- Suppurative and necrotic conditions of the lower respiratory tract (J85-J86)
- Other diseases of the pleura (J90-J94)
- Intraoperative and postprocedural complications and disorders of the respiratory system, not elsewhere classified (J95)
- Other diseases of the respiratory system (J96-J99)

Diseases of the respiratory system are located in Chapter 8 of the Tabular List. If an infectious organism or agent is the cause of the disease, there will be an instructional note to "use additional code to identify the infectious agent." Most of these infectious organisms can be found in Chapter 1 of ICD-10-CM, Infectious and Parasitic Diseases.

The respiratory system begins with the nose and mouth and continues through airways to the lungs, where oxygen from the atmosphere is exchanged for carbon dioxide from the body's tissues. The lungs, the largest part of the respiratory system, look like large pink sponges that almost fill the chest. The left lung is a little smaller than the right lung because it shares space with the heart in the left side of the chest. Each lung is divided into lobes (sections). There are three in the right lung and two in the left.

Among the most common symptoms of respiratory disorders are:

- Cough
- Shortness of breath
- Chest pain
- Wheezing
- Stridor (a crowing sound when breathing)
- Hemoptysis (coughing up blood)

- Cyanosis (bluish discoloration)

- Finger clubbing

- Respiratory failure

Following is a review of the most common conditions and diseases in this chapter.

ACUTE UPPER RESPIRATORY INFECTIONS (J00-J06)

Conditions in this classification include:

- Acute rhinitis

- Acute nasopharyngitis (common cold)

- Acute sinusitis

- Acute pharyngitis

- Acute tonsillitis

- Acute laryngitis

- Acute upper respiratory infection

- Acute bronchitis

Review Figure 7.6, which is an excerpt from the Alphabetic Index for the main term.

FIGURE 7.6   Excerpt from the Alphabetic Index: *Sinusitis*

Sinusitis (accessory) (chronic) (hyperplastic) (nonpurulent)
            (purulent) (nasal) J32.9
    acute J01.90
    ethmoidal J01.20
        recurrent J01.21
    frontal J01.10
        recurrent J01.11
    involving more than one sinus, other than pansinusitis J01.80
        recurrent J01.81
    maxillary J01.00
        recurrent J01.01
    pansinusitis J01.40
        recurrent J01.41
        recurrent J01.91
    specified NEC J01.80
        recurrent J01.81
    sphenoidal J01.30

Open the ICD-10-CM codebook and select the correct code(s), referencing first the Alphabetic Index and the Tabular List.

Review the following example:

EXAMPLE: This patient was referred for evaluation and treatment of chronic sinusitis. This is a 55-year-old female who states she started having severe sinusitis about two to three months ago with facial discomfort, nasal

congestion, eye pain, and postnasal drip symptoms. She states she really has sinus problems, but this infection has been rather severe and she notes she has not had much improvement with antibiotics. She currently is not taking any medication for her sinuses. She also has noted that she is having some problems with ear popping and fullness. She tried Allegra without much improvement, and she believes the Allegra may have caused problems with balance to worsen. She believes she has some degree of allergy symptoms. The physician diagnosed the patient with acute and chronic sinusitis. She was placed on Veramyst nasal spray, two sprays each nostril daily and even twice daily if symptoms are worsening. A Medrol Dosepak was prescribed as directed. The patient was given instruction on use of nasal saline irrigation to be used twice daily and Clarinex 5 mg daily was recommended.

Alphabetic Index:
    Sinusitis ➞ acute ➞ J01.90

Tabular List:
    J01.90 ➞ Acute sinusitis, unspecified

Notice in the instructional note under J01 that there is an Excludes 2 note indicating that if chronic sinusitis is documented it can also be reported in category J32.0-J32.8.

Tabular List:
    J32.9 ➞ Chronic sinusitis, unspecified

Because the type of sinusitis is not specified, an unspecified code(s) is used.

Correct code sequencing:
    J01.90, J32.9

CODING TIP Remember, if the patient has an acute condition that is also chronic, the acute condition is reported as the first listed diagnosis.

The common cold is listed under "cold" in the Alphabetic Index (J00), whereas nasopharyngitis (acute) is listed as nasopharyngitis.

Open the ICD-10-CM codebook and select the correct code(s), referencing first the Alphabetic Index and the Tabular List.

Review the following example:

EXAMPLE: A 16-year-old girl visits her family physician with complaints of sore throat, chronic cough, sneezing, and pain in ears and nose. After an expanded problem-focused history and examination, her family physician diagnoses the condition as acute rhinitis and prescribes over-the-counter medication for relief.

Alphabetic Index:
 Rhinitis ➞ with ➞ sore throat ➞ nasopharyngitis
 ➞ J00

Tabular List:
 J00 ➞ acute nasopharyngitis (common cold)

Correct code:
 J00

CODING TIP Do not forget to code the infectious organism (agent) when coding diseases of the respiratory system.

INFLUENZA AND PNEUMONIA (J09-J18)

Codes for pneumonia and influenza can be found in two chapters: Chapter 9 and in Chapter 1 in the ICD-10-CM Tabular List, Certain Infectious and Parasitic Diseases. Pneumonia is an infection of the lungs that involves the small air sacs (alveoli) and the tissues around them.

Pneumonia is a group of illnesses, each caused by a different microscopic organism. Usually pneumonia starts after organisms are inhaled into the lungs, but sometimes the infection is carried to the lungs in the bloodstream or it migrates to the lungs directly from a nearby infection.

The most common causes are bacteria and viruses. Some bacterial causes include:

- *Streptococcus pneumoniae*

- *Staphylococcus aureus*

- Legionnella

- *Haemophilus influenzae*

- Fungi

- *Mycoplasma pneumoniae* (common in older children and younger adults)

Viruses include:

- Influenza (flu)

- Chickenpox

Common symptoms of pneumonia are:

- Cough, producing sputum

- Chest pain

- Chills

- Fever

- Shortness of breath

CODING TIP Pneumonia is coded in both Chapters 1 and 9 in the ICD-10-CM Tabular List.

- Chapter 1: Certain Infectious and Parasitic Diseases

- Chapter 9: Diseases of the Respiratory System

Review laboratory reports and x-rays to determine underlying infection and manifestation.

Pneumonia can normally be diagnosed and confirmed with a chest x-ray, which helps to determine the organism causing the disease. Sputum collection and blood specimens are also good diagnostic tools for the physician to use to identify the organism causing the pneumonia.

Pneumonia can be complicated to code. Make sure to determine the cause of the pneumonia before attempting to select the appropriate code. The Tabular List will be helpful in directing you to the underlying condition.

Review Table 7.4 for coding influenza.

TABLE 7.4	Official Guidelines for Coding and Reporting Influenza
Influenza due to certain identified viruses	Code only confirmed cases of avian influenza (code J09.0–, Influenza due to identified avian influenza virus) or novel H1N1 or swine flu, code J09.1–. This is an exception to the hospital inpatient guideline Section II, H (Uncertain Diagnosis).
	In this context, "confirmation" does not require documentation of positive laboratory testing specific for avian or novel H1N1 (or swine flu) influenza. However, coding should be based on the provider's diagnostic statement that the patient has avian influenza.
	If the provider records "suspected or possible or probable avian influenza," the appropriate influenza code from category J10, Influenza due to unspecified influenza virus, should be assigned. A code from category J09, Influenza due to certain identified influenza viruses, should not be assigned.

Source: Official ICD-10-CM Guidelines for Influenza

Open the ICD-10-CM codebook and select the correct code(s), referencing first the Alphabetic Index and the Tabular List, for the following examples.

EXAMPLE: *A 30-year-old established patient visits her family physician with complaints of fever, chills, and sore throat. The physician performs an expanded problem-focused history and examination and suspects pneumonia. To confirm the diagnosis, the physician orders posteroanterior and lateral chest x-rays, collects sputum, and orders a complete blood cell count. The tests ordered come back positive for pneumonia caused by Staphylococcus aureus.*

Alphabetic Index:
Pneumonia ➡ *Due to (in) Staphylococcus* ➡ *aureus* ➡ *J15.21*

Tabular List:
J15.21 ➡ *Pneumonia due to Staphylococcus aureus*

Correct code:
J15.21 Pneumonia due to Staphylococcus aureus

EXAMPLE: *A patient is diagnosed with pneumonia in whooping cough.*

In this example, the first listed diagnosis is whooping cough and the secondary diagnosis is pneumonia.

Alphabetic Index:
Pneumonia ➡ *In* ➡ *Whooping cough A37.91*

Tabular List:
A37.91 ➡ *Whooping cough, unspecified species with pneumonia*

Correct code:
A37.91

In the example above, the patient encounter is not coded in the respiratory system (Chapter 9) in ICD-10-CM. Intead, it is coded using a combination code in Chapter 1, which includes both pneumonia and whooping cough.

EXAMPLE: *A 35-year-old patient visits his physician with complaints of sore throat, runny nose, coughing, congestion, and overall aching. He can only talk in a whisper, which has been ongoing for 5 days. During the examination, the patient mentions he forgot to get his flu shot this year. After an expanded problem-focused history and examination, the physician diagnoses influenza with laryngitis.*

Alphabetic Index:
Influenza, influenza ➡ *with laryngitis* ➡ *J11.1*

Tabular List:
J11.1 ➡ *Influenza due to unidentified influenza virus with other respiratory manifestations* ➡ *influenzal laryngitis NOS*

Correct code:
J11.1

PNEUMONIA DUE TO SARS-ASSOCIATED CORONAVIRUS

Severe acute respiratory syndrome (SARS) is a recognized febrile severe lower respiratory illness that is caused by infection with a novel coronavirus, SARS-associated coronavirus (SARS-CoV). During the winter of 2002 through the spring of 2003, the World Health Organization received reports of more than 8000 SARS cases and nearly 800 deaths worldwide. According to the Centers for Disease Control and Prevention, since 2004 there were only a few cases in the United state and there appears to be no further spread of the disease currently. However, the United States is vulnerable to more widespread, disruptive outbreaks in other countries and people who travel to other countries should be aware of this syndrome.

Many studies have been undertaken to evaluate whether there are specific laboratory and/or clinical parameters that can distinguish SARS-CoV disease from other febrile respiratory illnesses. Researchers are also working on the development of laboratory tests to improve diagnostic capabilities for SARS-CoV and other respiratory pathogens. To date, however, no specific clinical or laboratory findings can distinguish with certainty SARS-CoV disease from other respiratory illnesses rapidly enough to inform management decisions that must be made soon after the patient presents to the health care system.

The vast majority of patients with SARS-CoV disease:

- Have a clear history of exposure either to a SARS patient(s) or to a setting in which SARS-CoV transmission is occurring

- Develop pneumonia

Laboratory tests are helpful but do not reliably detect infection early in the illness.

Common symptoms of SARS-CoV include flu-like symptoms, fever, chills, cough, headache, and myalgia. The symptoms may range from mild to more severe forms of respiratory illness. The diagnosis of SARS-CoV is based on 3 elements:

- Clinical presentation

- Laboratory test results

- Epidemiological exposure

Open the ICD-10-CM codebook and select the correct code(s), referencing first the Alphabetic Index and the Tabular List.

Review the following examples:

> **EXAMPLE:** *This 35-year-old patient fell ill two days after returning from a trip to the Far East. She visit her family physician with cough, headache, and severe shortness of breath. A chest x-ray was ordered, which confirmed the presence of infiltrates indicative of pneumonia. After a comprehensive history and examination the physician diagnosed the patient with pneumonia due to SARS.*
>
> **Alphabetic Index:**
> Pneumonia ➝ due to SARS-associated coronavirus ➝ J12.81
>
> **Tabular List:**
> J12.81 ➝ Pneumonia due to SARS-associated coronavirus
>
> **Correct code:**
> J12.81

Review the following example:

> **EXAMPLE:** *A passenger arriving in Chicago on a plane from Ontario was diagnosed with SARS. All 159 passengers on board were taken to the hospital emergency department and admitted for laboratory testing and observation. No evidence of SARS was found in any of the other passengers on board the flight.*
>
> **Alphabetic Index:**
> Exposure ➝ to ➝ communicable diseases, NEC ➝ Z20.89
>
> **Tabular List:**
> Z20.89 ➝ Contact with and (suspected) exposure to other communicable diseases
>
> **Correct code:**
> Z20.89

Because there is not a classification specifically for SARS, you would report the exposure as a "not elsewhere classified" disease.

Because laboratory evidence did not confirm SARS in the remaining passengers, a Z code is used to identify the exposure to the disease.

CODING TIP When a patient has been exposed to SARS, but nothing in the laboratory findings indicates the disease is present, use Z20.89-Exposure to SARS-associated coronavirus.

OTHER DISEASES OF THE UPPER RESPIRATORY TRACT (J30-J39)

Other diseases of the upper respiratory tract include:

- Nasal polyps
- Chronic sinusitis
- Chronic diseases of the tonsils and adenoids
- Chronic laryngitis
- Allergic rhinitis

Combination coding is common with diseases of the respiratory system. Open the ICD-10-CM codebook and select the correct code(s), referencing first the Alphabetic Index and the Tabular List.

Review the following example:

> **EXAMPLE:** *A 7-year-old patient visits his family physician. His mother says that her son is complaining of a sore throat and ear pain and has been running a temperature of 100°F for more than 3 days. He has had previous episodes of tonsillitis and adenoiditis. After a detailed history and examination, the physician diagnoses a recurrence of tonsillitis and adenoiditis, which has become chronic. The physician prescribes an oral antibiotic for the patient and discusses removal of the tonsils and adenoids when the infection has subsided. The patient is to return to the office in one week for a recheck.*

Open the ICD-10-CM codebook and look for the correct code(s). The Tabular List provides one code for chronic tonsillitis and adenoiditis. It would be incorrect to use both 474.00 and 474.01 when a combination code is available.

> **Alphabetic Index:**
> Tonsillits ➝ with ➝ adenoiditis ➝ J35.03
>
> **Tabular List:**
> J35.03 ➝ Chronic tonsillitis and adenoiditis
>
> **Correct code:**
> J35.03

Open the ICD-10-CM codebook and select the correct code(s), referencing first the Alphabetic Index and the Tabular List.

Review the following example:

> **EXAMPLE:** *This patient is a 67-year-old female with a history of left true vocal cord nodule with hoarseness and history of occasional tobacco use. The patient underwent a suspension microdirect laryngoscopy, with a left true vocal cord stripping of nodule.*

For this example, you will need 3 codes for the patient encounter.

Alphabetic Index:
Nodule → vocal cord → J38.2

History (personal) tobacco use → Z87.891

Hoarseness → R49.0

First listed diagnosis:
J38.2 → Nodules of vocal cords

Secondary diagnosis:
R49.0 → dysphonia → hoarseness

Tertiary diagnosis:
Z87.891 → Personal history of tobacco use

Correct code sequencing:
J38.2, R49.0, Z87.891

CHRONIC OBSTRUCTIVE PULMONARY DISEASE (J44.–)

Chronic obstructive pulmonary disease (COPD) refers to two closely related respiratory disorders that gradually take a person's breath away: chronic bronchitis and/or emphysema associated with airflow obstruction. A person with COPD sometimes has both chronic bronchitis and emphysema or may just have one of these diseases. The explanations in the following paragraphs may help you understand chronic bronchitis and emphysema.

Chronic bronchitis is a long-standing inflammation of the airways that produces a lot of mucus, causing wheezing and infections. It's considered chronic if someone has coughing and mucus on a regular basis for at least 3 months a year and for two years in a row.

Emphysema is a disease that destroys the air sacs and/or the smallest breathing tubes in the lungs. Simply put, the lungs lose elasticity, similar to an overused rubber band. This causes the air sacs to become enlarged, thus making breathing difficult.

Nothing can reverse the lung damage that occurs with COPD. In the beginning stages of COPD, a person may have only a mild shortness of breath and occasional coughing spells. Many people don't know they have COPD at first. Initial symptoms can include a general feeling of illness, increasing shortness of breath, coughing, and wheezing. But as the disease progresses, symptoms become increasingly more severe.

The overwhelming cause of COPD is smoking. In fact, approximately 90% of COPD patients have a history of smoking.

CHECKPOINT EXERCISE 7-3

Using the ICD-10-CM codebook, code the following:

1. _____ Nasal polyp

2. _____ Chronic ethmoidal sinusitis

3. _____ Laryngoplegia

4. _____ Chronic laryngitis with laryngotracheitis

5. _____ Pneumonia in anthrax

6. _____ Retropharyngeal abscess

7. _____ Pneumonia

8. _____ Tonsillar tag

9. _____ Acute pulmonary edema due to an unknown chemical

10. _____ Pneumonia due to coccidioidomycosis

11. _____ A 50-year-old male undergoes an epiglottic flap for glottic stenosis after a vertical hemilaryngectomy.

12. _____ A 72-year-old man undergoes a diagnostic fiberoptic bronchoscopy for evaluation of hemoptysis.

13. _____ A patient presents with symptoms of high fever, gastrointestinal pain, headache, myalgia, and dry cough. The physician diagnoses the patient with Legionnaires' disease

14. _____ Chronic nasopharyngitis

15. _____ Allergic rhinitis due to cat dander

Other risk factors include:

- Heredity

- Second-hand smoke

- Exposure to air pollution at work and in the environment

- A history of childhood respiratory infections

The primary symptom of COPD is shortness of breath accompanied by a cough or wheezing. Because COPD is often a combination of emphysema and chronic bronchitis associated with airflow obstruction, it's important to understand the symptoms of each of these conditions. Symptoms of emphysema include cough, shortness of breath, and a limited exercise tolerance. Symptoms of chronic bronchitis associated with airflow obstruction include chronic cough, increased mucus, frequent clearing of the throat, and shortness of breath. Keep in mind, not all types of chronic bronchitis are associated with COPD.

In the later stages of the disease, someone with COPD could suffer from severe shortness of breath, coughing, excessive amounts of sputum (mucus), wheezing, recurrent infections, swollen ankles, and a bluish skin tint. At advanced stages, people with COPD may need constant care and supplemental oxygen in order to breathe.

Conditions in this classification include:

- Bronchitis
- Emphysema
- Asthma
- Bronchiectasis
- Extrinsic allergic alveolitis
- Chronic airway obstruction, not elsewhere classified

Coding Issues

When coding COPD, accurate identification of the specific condition attributed to the airway obstruction along with any associated acute conditions such as acute bronchiectasis is necessary. When the diagnosis in the medical record states "COPD" without associated conditions, it is coded as J44.9, Chronic airway obstruction, unspecified. Use this code only when a more specific diagnosis code cannot be assigned. Accurate coding of COPD and related conditions is critical.

If an acute lower respiratory infection is present (J44.0), an additional code should be used to identify the infection, if known. The code set also states that asthma should be coded in addition to these codes, if applicable. Other codes that may be reported are:

- History of tobacco use (Z87.891)
- Exposure to environmental tobacco smoke (Z77.22)
- Tobacco use (Z72.0)

Review the ICD-10-CM guidelines for reporting COPD and asthma in Table 7.5.

TABLE 7.5 Official Guidelines for Coding and Reporting Chronic Obstructive Pulmonary Disease [COPD] and Asthma

Acute exacerbation of chronic obstructive bronchitis and asthma	The codes in categories J44 and J45 distinguish between uncomplicated cases and those in acute exacerbation. An acute exacerbation is a worsening or a decompensation of a chronic condition.
	An acute exacerbation is not equivalent to an infection superimposed on a chronic condition, though an exacerbation may be triggered by an infection.
Acute respiratory failure, acute respiratory failure as principal diagnosis	A code from subcategory J96.0, Acute respiratory failure, or subcategory J96.2, Acute and chronic respiratory failure, may be assigned as a principal diagnosis when it is the condition established after study to be chiefly responsible for occasioning the admission to the hospital and the selection is supported by the Alphabetic Index and the Tabular List. However, chapter-specific coding guidelines (such as obstetrics, poisoning, HIV, newborn) that provide sequencing direction take precedence.
Acute respiratory failure as secondary diagnosis	Respiratory failure may be listed as a secondary diagnosis if it occurs after admission or if it is present on admission but does not meet the definition of principal diagnosis.
Sequencing of acute respiratory failure and another acute condition	When a patient is admitted with respiratory failure and another acute condition (eg myocardial infarction, cerebrovascular accident, aspiration pneumonia), the principal diagnosis will not be the same in every situation. This applies whether the other acute condition is a respiratory or nonrespiratory condition. Selection of the principal diagnosis will be dependent on the circumstances of admission. If both the respiratory failure and the other acute condition are equally responsible for occasioning the admission to the hospital, and there are no chapter-specific sequencing rules, the guideline regarding two or more diagnoses that equally meet the definition for principal diagnosis (see Section II, C) may be applied in these situations.
	If the documentation is not clear as to whether acute respiratory failure and another condition are equally responsible for occasioning the admission, query the provider for clarification.

Source: Official ICD-10-CM Guidelines for Hypertension

Open the ICD-10-CM codebook and select the correct code(s), referencing first the Alphabetic Index and the Tabular List.

Review the following example:

> **EXAMPLE:** *A 66-year-old male with **decompensated COPD**, hypertension, and a history of smoking 40 packs of cigarettes per year has a 3-cm peripheral nodule in the right upper lobe. He is scheduled for a diagnostic thoracoscopy and biopsy using a left lateral position. Anesthesia with an inhalational agent and muscle relaxant, double-lumen endotracheal tube, and arterial blood pressure monitoring is planned.*

> **Alphabetic Index:**
> *Pulmonary* ➞ *see condition* ➞ *disease* ➞ *pulmonary* ➞ *obstructive (difuse)* ➞ *with* ➞ *bronchitis (chronic)* ➞ *acute exacerbation J44.1*

> **Tabular List:**
> *J44.1* ➞ *Chronic obstructive pulmonary disease with (acute) exacerbation*

> **Correct code:**
> *J44.1*

What is the rationale for selecting J44.1? When reviewing the Tabular List under J44.–, the guidance under the subclassification lists the following conditions:

- Asthma with chronic obstructive pulmonary disease

- Chronic asthmatic (obstructive) bronchitis

- Chronic bronchitis with airway obstruction

- Chronic bronchitis with emphysema

- Chronic emphysematous bronchitis

- Chronic obstructive asthma

- Chronic obstructive bronchitis

- Chronic obstructive tracheobronchitis

Because the condition mentioned in the example above indicates decompensated COPD, J44.1 would be the appropriate diagnosis code.

Open the ICD-10-CM codebook and select the correct code(s), referencing first the Alphabetic Index and the Tabular List.

Review the following example:

> **EXAMPLE:** *A 45-year-old patient is diagnosed with emphysema with chronic obstructive bronchitis and is admitted to the hospital. After a detailed history with a detailed examination, the physician determines the patient's condition has not currently exacerbated.*

> **Alphabetic Index:**
> *Disease* ➞ *bronchitis* ➞ *with* ➞ *emphysematous (obstructive)* ➞ *J44.9*

> **Tabular List:**
> *J44.9* ➞ *Chronic obstructive pulmonary disease, unspecified*

> **Correct code:**
> *J44.9*

ASTHMA (J45.–)

Asthma (J45.–) is a condition in which the airways are narrowed because hyperreactivity to certain stimuli produces inflammation; the airway narrowing is reversible. Asthma attacks vary in frequency and severity. Some people with asthma are symptom-free most of the time, with an occasional, brief, mild episode of shortness of breath. Others cough and wheeze most of the time and have severe attacks after viral infections, exercise, or exposure to allergens or irritants. Crying or hearty laughing may also bring on symptoms.

An asthma attack may begin suddenly with:

- Wheezing

- Coughing

- Shortness of breath

People with asthma usually first notice shortness of breath, coughing, or chest tightness. The attack may be over in minutes or it may last for hours or days. Itching on the chest or neck may be an early symptom, especially in children. A dry cough at night or while exercising may be the only symptom. During an asthma attack, shortness of breath may become severe, creating a feeling of anxiety.

Coding Issues

Diagnosis codes are selected with the use of category J45–. Documentation for asthma includes:

- Severity of disease (mild intermittent, moderate, persistent, etc.)

- If an exacerbation is documented

- If status asthmaticus is documented

When reviewing the Tabular List, note that a fifth-character subclassification is required to code to the highest level of specificity (see Figure 7.7).

FIGURE 7.7   Excerpt from the Tabular List: *J45 Asthma*

J45   **Asthma**
[INCLUDES]   **Allergic (predominantly) asthma**
       Allergic bronchitis NOS
       Allergic rhinitis with asthma
       Atopic asthma
       Extrinsic allergic asthma
       Hay fever with asthma
       Idiosyncratic asthma
       Intrinsic nonallergic asthma
       Nonallergic asthma
Use additional code to identify:
       exposure to environmental tobacco smoke (Z77.22)
       exposure to tobacco smoke in the perinatal period
          (P96.81)
       history of tobacco use (Z87.891)
       occupational exposure to environmental tobacco smoke
          (Z57.31)
       tobacco dependence (F17.-)
       tobacco use (Z72.0)
[EXCLUDES 1]   detergent asthma (J69.8)
       eosinophilic asthma (J82)
       lung diseases due to external agents (J60-J70)
       miner's asthma (J60)
       wheezing NOS (R06.2)
       wood asthma (J67.8)
[EXCLUDES 2]   asthma with chronic obstructive pulmonary
       disease
          chronic asthmatic (obstructive) bronchitis
             chronic obstructive asthma

✓5th J45.2 Mild intermittent asthma
       J45.20   Mild intermittent asthma,
                uncomplicated
                Mild intermittent asthma NOS
       J45.21   Mild intermittent asthma with
                (acute) exacerbation
       J45.22   Mild intermittent asthma with
                status asthmaticus

✓5th J45.3 Mild persistent asthma
       J45.30   Mild persistent asthma,
                uncomplicated
                Mild persistent asthma NOS
       J45.31   Mild persistent asthma with (acute)
                exacerbation
       J45.32   Mild persistent asthma with status
                asthmaticus

✓5th J45.4 Moderate persistent
       J45.40   Moderate persistent, uncomplicated
                Moderate persistent asthma NOS
       J45.41   Moderate persistent with (acute)
                exacerbation
       J45.42   Moderate persistent with status
                asthmaticus

✓5th J45.5 Severe persistent
       J45.50   Severe persistent, uncomplicated
                Severe persistent asthma NOS
       J45.51   Severe persistent with (acute)
                exacerbation
       J45.52   Severe persistent with status
                asthmaticus
       J45.9   Other and unspecified asthma

Open the ICD-10-CM codebook and select the correct code(s), referencing first the Alphabetic Index and the Tabular List.

Review the following examples:

EXAMPLE: A 12-year-old female patient visits a pulmonologist because she has experienced 3 asthma attacks during a one-week period. Neither her oral medication nor her inhaler seem to help much. The physician performs an expanded problem-focused history and examination, reviews the previous patient notes, and decides to increase the dosage of her oral medication and change the inhaler dosage. The physician instructs the patient's mother on signs and symptoms and asks that the patient return in two weeks to monitor her progress. The patient's mother is also asked to call the office if another episode occurs. The physician diagnoses the patient with mild intermittent asthma with acute exacerbation.

Alphabetic Index:
Asthma, asthmatic (bronchial) (catarrh) (spasmodic) → mild intermittent → with → exacerbation (acute) → J45.21

Tabular List:
J45.21 Mild intermittent asthma with (acute) exacerbation

Correct code:
J45.21

EXAMPLE: A patient is diagnosed with asthma with an acute exacerbation of the chronic obstructive pulmonary disease.

Alphabetic Index:
Asthma, asthmatic (bronchial) (catarrh) (spasmodic) J45.909 → with chronic obstructive pulmonary disease (COPD) → with exacerbation → J44.1

Tabular List:
J44.1 → Chronic obstructive pulmonary disease with (acute) exacerbation

Correct code:
J44.1

CODING TIP Make sure the documentation in the medical record supports the code selection. If the diagnosis is not specific enough to code, clarify the diagnosis with the physician.

ACUTE RESPIRATORY DISTRESS SYNDROME (J80)

This is a type of lung failure resulting from many different disorders that cause fluid accumulation in the lungs (pulmonary edema). This syndrome is a medical emergency that can occur in people who previously had normal lungs. Despite the fact that it is sometimes called adult respiratory distress syndrome, this condition can occur in children. Acute respiratory distress syndrome is coded to classification J80, and there is only one code in the subclassification.

Open the ICD-10-CM codebook and select the correct code(s), referencing first the Alphabetic Index and the Tabular List.

Review the following example:

CODING TIP A 47-year-old female was hospitalized for shortness of breath and chest pain. After a full battery of diagnostic tests, the physician diagnoses the patient with acute respiratory distress syndrome.

> **Alphabetic Index:**
>   *Syndrome* → *Respiratory distress* → *Acute* → *J80*
>
> **Tabular List:**
>   *J80* → *Acute respiratory disress syndrome*
>
> **Correct code:**
>   *J80*

ACUTE RESPIRATORY FAILURE (J96.–)

Respiratory failure is a condition that affects breathing function or the lungs themselves and can result in failure of the lungs to function properly. The main tasks of the lungs and chest are to get oxygen from the air that is inhaled into the bloodstream and, at the same to time, to eliminate carbon dioxide (CO_2) from the blood through air that is breathed out. In respiratory failure, the level of oxygen in the blood becomes dangerously low and/or the level of CO_2 becomes dangerously high. There are two ways in which this can happen. Either the process by which oxygen and CO_2 are exchanged between the blood and the air spaces of the lungs (a process called "gas exchange") breaks down or the movement of air in and out of the lungs (ventilation) does not take place properly.

Several different abnormalities of breathing function can cause respiratory failure. The major categories, with specific examples of each, are:

▪ *Obstruction of the airways.* Examples are chronic bronchitis with heavy secretions, emphysema, cystic fibrosis, or asthma (a condition in which it is very hard to get air in and out through narrowed breathing tubes).

▪ *Weak breathing.* This can be caused by drugs or alcohol, which depress the respiratory center; extreme obesity; or sleep apnea, where patients stop breathing for long periods while sleeping.

▪ *Muscle weakness.* This can be caused by a muscle disease called myasthenia, muscular dystrophy, polio, a stroke that paralyzes the respiratory muscles, injury of the spinal cord, or Lou Gehrig's disease.

▪ *Lung diseases, including severe pneumonia.* Pulmonary edema, or fluid in the lungs, can be the source of respiratory failure. Also, it can often be a result of heart disease, respiratory distress syndrome, pulmonary fibrosis and other scarring diseases of the lung, radiation exposure, burn injury when smoke is inhaled, or widespread lung cancer.

▪ *An abnormal chest wall.* This is a condition that can be caused by scoliosis or severe injury of the chest wall.

A majority of patients with respiratory failure suffer from shortness of breath. The patient may become confused and disoriented and find it impossible to carry out their normal activities or do their work. Marked CO_2 excess can cause headaches and, in time, a semiconscious state or even coma. Low blood oxygen causes the skin to take on a bluish tinge. It also can cause an abnormal heart rhythm (arrhythmia). Physical examination may show a patient who is breathing rapidly, is restless, and has a rapid pulse. Lung disease may cause abnormal sounds heard when listening to the chest with a stethoscope: wheezing in asthma, "crackles" in obstructive lung disease. A patient with ventilatory failure is prone to gasp for breath and may use the neck muscles to help expand the chest.

Diagnosis

If a patient is treated for acute respiratory failure, a code from J96.0– is reported as the first listed diagnosis. If the reason for the encounter chiefly to be responsible for treatment is the primary reason for care, a code from J96.0- may be listed as the first listed or principal diagnosis. Respiratory failure may be listed secondary if it is present on admission and not the first listed/principal diagnosis. Review the guidelines for coding respiratory failure in Table 7.6.

CODING TIP Based on the ICD-10-CM Guidelines, if the documentation is not clear as to whether acute respiratory failure and another condition are equally responsible for occasioning the admission, query the provider for clarification.

TABLE 7.6   Official ICD-10-CM Guidelines for Coding and Reporting Respiratory Failure

Acute respiratory failure as principal diagnosis	A code from subcategory J96.0, Acute respiratory failure, or subcategory J96.2, Acute and chronic respiratory failure, may be assigned as a principal diagnosis when it is the condition established after study to be chiefly responsible for occasioning the admission to the hospital and the selection is supported by the Alphabetic Index and the Tabular List.
	However, chapter-specific coding guidelines (such as obstetrics, poisoning, HIV, newborn) that provide sequencing direction take precedence.
Acute respiratory failure as secondary diagnosis	Respiratory failure may be listed as a secondary diagnosis if it occurs after admission or if it is present on admission but does not meet the definition of principal diagnosis.
Sequencing of acute respiratory failure and another acute condition	When a patient is admitted with respiratory failure and another acute condition, (eg myocardial infarction, cerebrovascular accident, aspiration pneumonia), the principal diagnosis will not be the same in every situation. This applies whether the other acute condition is a respiratory or nonrespiratory condition.
	Selection of the principal diagnosis will be dependent on the circumstances of admission.
	If both the respiratory failure and the other acute condition are equally responsible for occasioning the admission to the hospital, and there are no chapter-specific sequencing rules, the guideline regarding two or more diagnoses that equally meet the definition for principal diagnosis *(Section II, C.)* may be applied in these situations.

Source: Official ICD-10-CM Guidelines for Influenza

CHECKPOINT EXERCISE 7-4

Using the ICD-10-CM codebook, code the following:

1. _____ Recurrent bronchiectasis

2. _____ Acute chemical bronchitis

3. _____ Pleurisy

4. _____ Millar's asthma

5. _____ Pyocele turbinate sinusitis

6. _____ Silicotic fibrosis of lung

7. _____ Mediastinal emphysema

8. _____ Bronchiolitis due to respiratory syncytial virus (RSV)

9. _____ Patient with acute bronchitis and cystic fibrosis

10. _____ Acute nontransmural infarction

11. _____ Influenza with acute bronchitis

12. _____ Emphysema with acute bronchitis with exacerbation

13. _____ Chronic ethmoidal sinusitis

14. _____ Upper respiratory infection

15. _____ A 66-year-old male has unexplained dyspnea that interferes with his ability to work and exercise. A complex pulmonary stress test is ordered after other studies fail to identify the cause of dyspnea.

EXAMPLE: *A 74-year-old male was admitted to the emergency department with symptoms of shortness of breath and disorientation. The ER physician examined the patient and called a pulmonologist in for a consult. The pulmonologist admitted the patient to perform further testing. The patient also indicated he was experiencing headache and confusion over the past few days. After examination and review of diagnostic tests ordered, the pulmonologist diagnosed the patient with acute respiratory failure with acute hypoxia. The patient was transferred to the critical unit and put on a ventilator.*

Open your ICD-10-CM codebook and code this patient encounter.

Alphabetic Index:
Failure → respiration, respiratory → acute → with → hypoxia → J96.01

Tabular List:
J96.01 → Acute respiratory failure with hypoxia

Correct code:
J96.01

Test Your Knowledge

1. _____   Bilateral carotid occlusion

2. _____   COPD with asthma in a 65-year-old male cigarette smoker

3. _____   A 67-year-old woman with acute pericarditis

4. _____   An 85-year-old man with COPD, emphysema, and benign hypertension

5. _____   A patient diagnosed with acute unstable angina with a personal history of myocardial infarction

6. _____   Acute lobar pneumonia

7. _____   Aortic stenosis

8. _____   Acute subendocardial infarction, initial episode

9. _____   Congestive heart failure

10. _____   Mitral valve insufficiency

11. _____   Angina pectoris

12. _____   Respiratory failure due to congestive heart failure

13. _____   Chronic pulmonary edema

14. _____   A 67-year-old female with atrial fibrillation fails an attempt at trans-thoracic cardioversion to return sinus rhythm. She then undergoes transvenous intracardiac cardioversion.

15. _____   A 55-year-old male is hospitalized for unstable angina pectoris. Coronary angiography reveals two severe discrete stenoses in the proximal segments of the right and left anterior descending coronary arteries.

16. _____   Acute laryngitis

17. _____   A 62-year-old man with recurrent ventricular tachycardia has undergone a comprehensive electrophysiologic study and is found to have inducible ventricular tachycardia.

18. _____   Bill, a 67-year-old male with coronary artery disease status post-myocardial infarction and chronic obstructive pulmonary disease, was found to have a 5.8-cm diameter abdominal aortic aneurysm.

19. _____   A patient admitted to critical care with severe chest pain and shortness of breath was diagnosed as having acute subendocardial infarction that was complicated by respiratory failure.

20. _____   Sarah, a 42-year-old established patient, was diagnosed by her family physician with Pleurobronchopneumonia. The physician sent the patient to the hospital for admission.

Diseases of the Digestive, Musculoskeletal, and Genitourinary Systems and Skin and Subcutaneous Tissues (K00-N99)

LEARNING OBJECTIVES

- Understand coding guidelines for the Musculoskeletal and Genitoruinary systems

- Understand coding guidelines for skin and subcutaneous tissue

- Properly sequence ICD-10-CM codes in the digestive, musculoskeletal, and genitourinary systems and skin and subcutaneous tissue

- Assign ICD-10-CM codes to the highest level of specificity

- Successfully complete checkpoint exercises and "Test Your Knowledge" exercises

Diseases of the Digestive System (K00-K94)

Chapter 11 in the Tabular List includes the following sections:

- Diseases of Oral Cavity and Salivary Glands (K00-L14)

- Diseases of Esophagus, Stomach, and Duodenum (K20-K31)

- Diseases of the Appendix (K35-K38)

- Hernia (K40-K46)

- Noninfectious Enteritis and Colitis (K50-K52)

- Other Diseases of Intestines (K55-K63)

- Diseases of the Peritoneum and Retroperitoneum (K65-K68)

- Disease of Liver (K70-K77)

- Disorders of Gallbladder, Biliary Tract, and Pancreas (K80-K87)

- Other Diseases of the Digestive System (K90-K94)

Diseases of the digestive system are located in Chapter 11 of the Tabular List. The digestive system is responsible for receiving food, breaking it down into nutrients (a process called digestion), absorbing the nutrients into the bloodstream, and eliminating the indigestible parts of food from the body. The digestive tract consists of the:

- Mouth
- Throat
- Esophagus
- Stomach
- Small intestine
- Large intestine
- Rectum
- Anus

The digestive system also includes organs that lie outside the digestive tract:

- Pancreas
- Liver
- Gallbladder

Codes are categorized in a manner that follows the same path as the digestive system, starting with disorders of the teeth. Pay special attention when coding in this chapter. As with previous chapters, a fifth-digit assignment is necessary with many of the codes. Make sure to read all "includes" and "excludes" notes in this chapter. Following is a review of the most common diagnoses.

DISEASES OF THE ORAL CAVITY AND SALIVARY GLANDS (K00-K14)

The oral cavity is formed by an array of tissues that function in or are associated with the processes that are performed with what we typically refer to as our mouth. The organs found within the oral cavity, are the tongue, and the glands which empty their secretory products into the oral cavity (salivary glands). The oral cavity is lined by a stratified squamous epithelium. The epithelial lining is divided into two broad types:

- Masticatory epithelium covers the surfaces involved in the processing of food (tongue, gingivae, and hard palate). The epithelium is keratinized to different degrees depending on the extent of physical forces exerted on it.

- Lining epithelium, that is, nonkeratinized stratified squamous epithelium, covers the remaining surfaces of the oral cavity.

Salivary Gland Disorders

Salivary glands are found in and around the mouth and throat. The major salivary glands are the parotid, submandibular, and sublingual glands. These glands secrete saliva into the mouth; the parotid through tubes that drain saliva, called salivary ducts, near the upper teeth; the submandibular under the tongue; and the sublingual through many ducts in the floor of the mouth.

In addition to these glands, there are many tiny glands called minor salivary glands located in the lips, inner cheek area (buccal mucosa), and extensively in other linings of the mouth and throat. Salivary glands produce the saliva used to moisten the mouth, initiate digestion, and help as a protection from tooth decay.

Category K11.– includes diseases of the salivary glands. Some of the conditions in this classification include:

- Atrophy: wasting away or necrosis of salivary gland tissue

- Hypertrophy: overgrown or overdeveloped salivary gland tissue

- Retention cyst of the salivary gland; dilated salivary gland cavity filled with mucous

- Stenosis

- Obstruction: Obstruction of the flow of saliva most commonly occurs in the parotid and submandibular glands, usually because stones have formed. Symptoms typically occur when eating. Saliva starts to flow but cannot exit the ductal system, leading to swelling of the involved gland and significant pain, sometimes with infection. Unless stones totally obstruct saliva flow, the major glands will swell during eating and then gradually subside after eating, only to enlarge again at the next meal. Infection can develop in the pool of blocked saliva, leading to more severe pain and swelling in the glands. If untreated for a long time, the glands may become abscessed.

It is possible for the duct system of the major salivary glands that connects the glands to the mouth to be abnormal. These ducts can develop small constrictions, which decrease salivary flow, leading to infection and obstructive symptoms.

Salivary gland enlargement can occur in autoimmune diseases such as human immunodeficiency virus (HIV) and Sjögren's syndrome where the body's immune system attacks the salivary glands, causing significant inflammation. Dry mouth or dry eyes are common. This may occur with other systemic diseases such as rheumatoid arthritis. Diabetes may cause enlargement of the salivary glands, especially the parotid glands. Alcoholics may have salivary gland swelling, usually on both sides.

Review the following example. Open up the ICD-10-CM codebook, referencing both the Alphabetic Index and the Tabular List to locate the correct code.

> **EXAMPLE:** *A patient presented with severe pain in the mouth. After the physician examined the patient and x-rays were taken, the patient was diagnosed with sialolithiasis (calculus of the salivary gland).*
>
> **Alphabetic Index:**
> Calculus ➞ salivary (duct) (gland) ➞ K11.5
>
> **Tabular List:**
> K11.5 ➞ Sialolithiasis ➞ Calculus of salivary gland or duct
>
> **Correct code:**
> K11.5

Diseases of the oral soft tissues, excluding lesions specific for gingivae and tongue, are classified in K12.– (stomatitis and related lesions). These conditions include:

- Stomatitis
- Canker sores
- Cellulitis of the floor of the mouth
- Cysts
- Diseases of the lips
- Hyperplasia of oral mucosa

Stomatitis, or viral stomatitis, is a common infection in children between ages one and two years. The child will typically run a fever and drool and will be very uncomfortable. Sores on the tongue or around the mouth are common.

The herpes labialis virus (cold sores) typically produces sores near the front of the mouth, lips, and tongue. Another herpes-related virus that tends to affect the rear of the mouth around the tonsils, referred to as herpangina, is not caused by the herpes virus but by a related herpes-type bug called coxsackie virus.

Canker sores, aphthous stomatitis, or aphthous ulcers are not thought of as being associated with fever. They simply appear. Herpetic stomatitis is a contagious viral illness caused by herpes virus hominis (also herpes simplex virus, HSV) that is diagnosed mainly in children. This condition probably represents their first exposure to herpes virus and can result in a systemic illness characterized by high fever (often as high as

104°F), blisters, ulcers in the mouth, and inflammation of the gums. The inside of the cheeks and tongue frequently develop ulcers 1 to 5 mm in diameter with a grayish-white base and a reddish perimeter.

These ulcers are very painful and cause drooling, difficulty swallowing, and decrease in food intake even though the patient may be hungry.

Symptoms of stomatitis include:

- Fever; may precede appearance of blisters and ulcers by one or two days
- Irritability
- Blisters in the mouth, often on the tongue or cheeks
- Ulcers in the mouth, often on the tongue or cheeks; these form after the blister pops
- Swollen gums
- Pain inside the mouth
- Drooling
- Difficulty swallowing (dysphagia)

Review the following example:

> **EXAMPLE:** *A worried mother brought her two-year-old daughter to the family physician. The mother stated the child was drooling and had been running a slight fever; the mother noticed sores in the child's mouth. After a detailed history and examination, the physician diagnosed the patient with ulcerative stomatitis, prescribed antiviral medication, and asked the mother to bring the child back for a follow-up visit in two weeks or to call if the symptoms were not relieved.*

Open the ICD-10-CM codebook and select the appropriate diagnosis code, referencing both the Alphabetic Index and the Tabular List. The main term in this example is "ulcer."

> **Alphabetic Index:**
> Ulcer ➞ stomatitis ➞ K12.1
>
> **Tabular List:**
> K12.1 ➞ Other forms of stomatitis ➞ ulcerative stomatitis
>
> **Correct code:**
> K12.1 Ulcerative stomatitis

DISEASES OF THE ESOPHAGUS, STOMACH, AND DUODENUM (K20-K31)

The esophagus is the channel that leads from the throat (pharynx) to the stomach. The walls of the esophagus propel food to the stomach with waves of muscular contractions called peristalsis. There is a band of muscle called the upper esophageal sphincter near the junction of the throat and the esophagus. Slightly above the junction of the esophagus and the stomach, there is another band of muscle called the lower esophageal sphincter. During swallowing, the sphincters relax so that food can pass to the stomach. The most common symptoms of esophageal disorders are dysphagia, chest pain, and back pain.

Categories K20-K22 encompass the diseases of the esophagus. Some of the common conditions in this category include:

- Ulcers
- Inflammation
- Reflux
- Rupture
- Perforation
- Spasms

Gastroesophageal reflux disease (GERD) refers to the backward flow of acid from the stomach up into the esophagus. People experience heartburn, also known as acid indigestion, when excessive amounts of stomach acid flow back into the esophagus. GERD is caused by incomplete closure of the sphincter. The squamous epithelial lining of the esophagus becomes irritated and inflamed. In some patients, the lining may become ulcerated and scarred.

Open the ICD-10-CM codebook and select the appropriate diagnosis code, referencing both the Alphabetic Index and the Tabular List for the following examples.

> **EXAMPLE:** *A patient with a history of gastrointestinal acid reflux disease returns to his gastroenterologist for a follow-up examination. The patient has been taking Prilosec for 6 months, with little relief. The patient missed the previous appointment 3 months ago. After a detailed history and examination, the physician schedules the patient for a diagnostic endoscopy to be performed the same day. After the procedure, the physician determines that the patient's condition has now worsened and diagnoses reflux esophagitis.*

Alphabetic Index:
   Esophagitis ➡ *Reflux K21.0*

Tabular List:
   K21.0 ➡ *Gastro-esophageal reflux disease with esophagitis*

Correct code:
   K21.0

> **EXAMPLE:** *A 48-year-old female patient with a history of esophageal reflux returns to her internist for follow-up. The patient states that she is feeling much better now that the physician has prescribed Zantac for the reflux. She has had no further problems with chronic heartburn and is doing well. The physician advises her to continue on the medication and to follow up in 3 months or to call if the medication fails to provide relief.*

Alphabetic Index:
   Reflux (Main term) ➡ *Gastro-esophageal* ➡ *K21.9*

Tabular List:
   K21.9 ➡ *Gastro-esophageal reflux disease without esophagitis* ➡ *esophageal reflux NOS*

Correct code:
   K21.9

Esophagitis is a common medical condition usually caused by gastroesophageal reflux. Less frequent causes include infectious esophagitis (in patients who are immunocompromised), radiation esophagitis, and esophagitis from direct erosive effects of ingested medication or corrosive agents.

Reflux esophagitis develops when gastric contents are passively regurgitated into the esophagus. Gastric acid, pepsin, and bile irritate the squamous epithelium, leading to erosion and ulceration of the esophageal mucosa. Eventually, a columnar epithelial lining may develop. This lining is a premalignant condition termed Barrett esophagus.

Esophageal reflux symptoms occur monthly in 33 to 44% of the general population; 7 to 10% have daily symptoms. Moderate to severe symptoms of this condition produce morbidity secondary to pain and anxiety.

Serious complications include esophageal strictures, Barrett esophagus, and adenocarcinoma. Aspiration of gastric contents occurs more often in children and may be associated with bronchospasm, pneumonitis, and apnea. The most common complaint is heartburn (dyspepsia), a burning sensation in the mid chest caused by contact of stomach acid with inflamed esophageal mucosa. Symptoms often are maximal while supine, when bending over, when wearing tight clothing, or after large meals.

Other common symptoms include upper abdominal discomfort, nausea, bloating, and fullness. Less common symptoms include dysphagia, odynophagia, cough, hoarseness, wheezing, and hematemesis.

The patient may experience chest pain indistinguishable from that of coronary artery disease. Pain often is midsternal, with radiation to the neck or arm, and may be associated with shortness of breath and diaphoresis. Chest pain may be relieved with nitrates if esophageal spasm is involved, further confounding diagnostic evaluation.

Infants with reflux are at greater risk of aspiration. Symptoms include weight loss, regurgitation, excessive crying, back arching, respiratory distress, and apnea.

Common factors that increase the risk of reflux esophagitis include:

- Pregnancy

- Obesity

- Scleroderma

- Smoking

- Ingestion of alcohol, coffee, chocolate, and fatty or spicy foods

- Certain medications (eg, beta-blockers, nonsteroidal anti-inflammatory drugs [NSAIDs], theophylline, nitrates, alendronate, calcium channel blockers)

- Mental retardation requiring institutionalization

- Spinal cord injury

- Being immunocompromised

- Radiation therapy for chest tumors

Pill esophagitis is thought to be secondary to chemical irritation of the esophageal mucosa from certain medications (eg, iron, potassium, quinidine, aspirin, steroids, tetracyclines, NSAIDs), especially when swallowed with too little fluid.

Review the following example:

EXAMPLE: A 45-year-old male patient with esophageal reflux was admitted from the emergency room to the hospital with dysphagia, wheezing, and hematemesis. A gastroenterologist was contacted to see the patient. The physician was unable to establish a diagnosis based on the examination of the patient and performed a diagnostic endoscopy. The endoscopy revealed that the patient had acute esophagitis. In addition to the acute esophagitis, the physician diagnosed the patient with an esophageal ulcer that was due to constant ingestion of aspirin.

Open the ICD-10-CM codebook and code this patient encounter.

Alphabetic Index:
　　Esophagitis ➝ *K20.9*

Tabular List:
　　K20.9 ➝ *acute* ➝ *Esophagitis, NOS*

Because there is not a more specific code in ICD-10-CM to report the acute esophagitis, the Alphabetic Index instructions are followed.

But wait! The physician also diagnosed the patient with an esophageal ulcer. Code K20.9 does not describe this condition, so an additional diagnosis code is needed.

Alphabetic Index:
　　Main term ➝ *ulcer* ➝ *esophagus (peptic)* ➝ *due to ingestion* ➝ *aspirin* ➝ *K22.10*

Tabular List:
　　K22.10 ➝ *Ulcer of esophagus without bleeding*

First listed diagnosis:
　　K20.9 Esophagitis (acute), NOS

Secondary diagnosis:
　　K22.10 Ulcer of esophagus without bleeding

Correct code sequencing:
　　K20.9, K22.10

Note: Because there is not a code to identify the esophagitis as acute in ICD-10-CM, the only option is K20.9, which is unspecified.

Barrett's Syndrome

Barrett's syndrome, or Barrett's esophagus, is a disorder secondary to chronic gastroesophageal reflux damage to the mucosa. Barrett's esophagus, which has been associated with GERD, has a tendency to progress to adenocarcinoma. Obesity and GERD appear to be the most significant risk factors for developing Barrett's esophagus. This disorder is classified in Other Specified Disorders of the Esophagus as K22.–. Some conditions or diseases can be referenced in the Alphabetic Index by their name. In this instance, the main term in the Alphabetic Index is "Barrett's."

Open the ICD-10-CM codebook and select the appropriate diagnosis code, referencing both the Alphabetic Index and the Tabular List for the following example.

EXAMPLE: A 50-year-old woman with chronic dysphagia and recurrent GERD undergoes endoscopic evaluation. The scope is advanced from the esophagus into the stomach and duodenum to complete the evaluation, with particular attention to the gastroesophageal junction. The physician diagnoses the patient with Barrett's esophagus with low-grade dysplasia.

Alphabetic Index:
Main term: Barrett's syndrome ➔ see Barrett's esophagus ➔ with low-grade dysplasia ➔ K22.710

Tabular List:
K22.710 ➔ Barrett's esophagus with low grade dysplasia

Correct code:
K22.710

Ulcers (K25-K28)

Ulcers are a common disorder treated by many practitioners. An ulcer is a focal area of the stomach or duodenum that has been destroyed by digestive juices and stomach acid. Most ulcers are very small, but they can cause tremendous discomfort and pain. Ulcers in the stomach are called gastric ulcers, and ulcers in the duodenum are called duodenal ulcers. In general, ulcers in the stomach and duodenum are referred to as peptic ulcers, or PUD. Although people often attribute ulcers to stress, there are actually two major causes of ulcers:

- *Helicobacter pylori* (*H pylori*)
- Regular use of NSAIDs

Complications of this disease include:

- Hemorrhage (bleeding ulcer)
- Anemia
- Fatigue
- Bloody or black stools
- Nausea (with bleeding ulcers)
- Perforation (a hole in the wall of the stomach or duodenum)
- Chronic inflammation and swelling of gastric and duodenal tissues
- Vomiting and weight loss

Ulcers are coded using the following categories:

- K25 Gastric ulcer
- K26 Duodenal ulcer
- K27 Peptic ulcer
- K28 Gastrojejunal ulcer

These codes are combination codes that identify complications of ulcers (bleeding and perforation).

A secondary code is not required unless the patient has multiple complications. Information required in documentation includes:

- Acute or chronic
- Hemorrhage
- Perforation
- Hemorrhage with perforation
- Without hemorrhage or perforation

Review Figure 8.1, which is an illustration of "gastric ulcer" in the Tabular List.

FIGURE 8.1   Excerpt from the ICD-10-CM Tabular List: *K25*

K25 Gastric ulcer
[INCLUDES] erosion (acute) of stomach
pylorus ulcer (peptic)
stomach ulcer (peptic)
Use additional code to identify:
alcohol abuse and dependence (F10.-)
[EXCLUDES 1] acute gastritis (K29.0-)
peptic ulcer NOS (K27.-)

K25.0 Acute gastric ulcer with hemorrhage
K25.1 Acute gastric ulcer with perforation
K25.2 Acute gastric ulcer with both hemorrhage and perforation
K25.3 Acute gastric ulcer without hemorrhage or perforation
K25.4 Chronic or unspecified gastric ulcer with hemorrhage
K25.5 Chronic or unspecified gastric ulcer with perforation
K25.6 Chronic or unspecified gastric ulcer with both hemorrhage and perforation
K25.7 Chronic gastric ulcer without hemorrhage or perforation
K25.9 Gastric ulcer, unspecified as acute or chronic, without hemorrhage or perforation

Open the ICD-10-CM codebook and select the appropriate diagnosis code, referencing both the Alphabetic Index and the Tabular List for the following example.

EXAMPLE: *A patient was admitted by his family physician with an acute gastric ulcer that had perforated.*

Alphabetic Index:
Ulcer gastric ➡ see ulcer stomach ➡ stomach ➡ acute with perforation ➡ K25.1

Tabular List:
K25.1 Acute gastric ulcer with perforation

Correct code:
K25.1

Open the ICD-10-CM codebook and select the appropriate diagnosis code, referencing both the Alphabetic Index and the Tabular List for the following two examples.

EXAMPLE: A 42-year-old patient with a history of gastric ulcers arrives at the emergency department with complaints of nausea, vomiting, and rectal bleeding. The emergency department physician contacts the general surgeon on call, who diagnoses the patient with acute gastric ulcer perforation with bleeding. The patient is taken to surgery for repair of the perforated ulcer.

We must first determine the diagnosis. According to the medical record documentation, the patient has a history of gastric ulcers. But the condition has now deteriorated. The final diagnosis is the definitive diagnosis or the reason for the visit to the emergency department, which is acute gastric perforated ulcer with bleeding.

Alphabetic Index:
Ulcer (Main term) ➡ Gastric—see Ulcer, stomach ➡ Ulcer, stomach (eroded) (peptic) (round) ➡ Acute ➡ with hemorrhage and perforation K25.2

Tabular List:
K25.2 Acute gastric ulcer with both hemorrhage and perforation

Correct code:
K25.2

EXAMPLE: A 58-year-old patient was diagnosed with a duodenal ulcer 3 years ago. He has been visiting his physician for the past 3 months complaining of nausea, vomiting, weight loss, inability to digest food, and overall feeling of fatigue. The patient states that the Prilosec he is taking for his condition makes little difference. The physician schedules the patient for a diagnostic endoscopy the same week. The diagnostic endoscopy shows pyloric ulcer, acute, with hemorrhage.

Alphabetic Index:
Ulcer (Main term) ➡ duodenum ➡ acute ➡ with ➡ hemorrhage ➡ K26.0

Tabular List:
K26.0 ➡ Acute duodenal ulcer with hemorrhage

If you selected K26.0 as the diagnosis, congratulations! If you were unsuccessful, go back and reread the documentation and try again.

Gastritis (K29.–)

Gastritis is inflammation of the stomach lining in which the lining resists irritation and can usually withstand very strong acid.

There are several types of gastritis:

- Acute stress gastritis is caused by a sudden severe illness or injury. The injury may not even be to the stomach.

- Chronic erosive gastritis can result from irritants such as drugs, especially aspirin and other NSAIDs, Crohn's disease; and bacterial and viral infections.

- Viral or fungal gastritis may develop in people with a prolonged illness or an impaired immune system.

- Eosinophilic gastritis may result from an allergic reaction to roundworm infestation.

- Atrophic gastritis results when antibodies attack the stomach lining, causing it to become very thin and lose many or all of the cells that produce acid and enzymes.

- Menetrier's disease is a form of gastritis whose cause is not known.

- Plasma cell gastritis is another form of gastritis with an unknown cause.

Symptoms vary, depending on the type of gastritis; however, a person with gastritis has indigestion and discomfort in the upper abdomen. Gastritis and duodenitis are classified as K29.– and require a fifth character when codes are assigned in this category to identify "with or without bleeding."

Use caution when making a selection. Open the ICD-10-CM codebook and locate the following diagnosis code using both the Alphabetic Index and the Tabular List.

EXAMPLE: A gastroenterolgist performed an endoscopy on a 47-year-old alcoholic patient in remission. The patient was experiencing bloating, stomach pains, and nausea. Based on the endoscopy performed, the phsycian diagnosed the patient with alcoholic gastritis with hemorrhage.

Alphabetic Index:
Gastritis ➡ alcoholic ➡ with bleeding ➡ K29.21

Tabular List:
K29.21 ➡ Alcoholic gastritis with bleeding

However, you're not finished yet. Review the instructional notes under category K29.2, which indicate that an additional code is required to identify the alcohol abuse or dependence with category F10.–.

Turn to category F10 and reference the code choices. A patient who is an alcoholic is considered alcohol dependent. We know that this patient is in remission. Category F10.2 is used to report an alcohol-dependent individual. Review Figure 8.2.

FIGURE 8.2   Excerpt from the Tabular List: *F10.2–*

F10.2 **Alcohol dependence**
   EXCLUDES 1   alcohol abuse (F10.1-)
      alcohol use, unspecified (F10.9-)
   EXCLUDES 2   toxic effect of alcohol (T51.0-)
      F10.20   Alcohol dependence, uncomplicated
      F10.21   Alcohol dependence, in remission
      F10.22   Alcohol dependence with intoxication
   Acute drunkenness (in alcoholism)
   EXCLUDES 1   alcohol dependence with withdrawal
      (F10.23-)

The following fifth-character subclassification in F10.2 identifies whether the patient has an uncomplicated condition related to the alcohol dependence, is in remission, or is intoxicated.

The correct code selection for the example above is F10.21.

First listed diagnosis:
   K29.21 Alcoholic gastritis with bleeding

Secondary diagnosis:
   F10.21 Alcohol dependence, in remission

Correct code sequencing:
   K29.21, F10.21

Other Diseases of Stomach and Duodenum (K31.–)

Surgical gastrostomy is a method of direct enteral feeding access. Surgical gastrostomy or jejunostomy is frequently performed when patients are undergoing laparotomy for related or unrelated abdominal problems. Complication of gastrostomy is coded in subclassification Z43.1. Codes in this category include closure of artificial openings, passage of sounds or bougies through artificial openings, cleansing the artificial opening, and removal of catheter from the artifical opening. Gastrostomy status is reported with code Z93.1. If the patient has an infection, this is reported with code K94.22 (gastrostomy infection). When coding K94.22, pay attention to the instructional notes

that direct the coder to use an additional code to specify the type of infection and the organism, which includes cellulitis of the abdominal wall (L03.311) or sepsis (A40-A41).

Open the ICD-10-CM codebook and locate the following diagnosis code, using both the Alphabetic Index and the Tabular List for this example.

   EXAMPLE: *A 65-year-old male presents with the inability to eat orally. Attempts to relieve the obstruction by flexible endoscopy, dilatation, and laser therapy are unsuccessful. The patient is malnourished and needs enteral nutritional support. The decision is made to perform a laparoscopic feeding gastrostomy on 2/16/xx. He is discharged two days postoperatively with instructions for wound care and gastrostomy feeding techniques. Three days later on 2/22/xx the patient is back in the hospital with symptoms of a sudden onsent of a spiking fever and chills. The patient is transferred to the critical care unit and IV fluids are given to fight the septicemia due to a staph infection.*

Alphabetic Index:
   Infection ➝ *gastrostomy* ➝ *K94.22*

Tabular List:
   K94.22 ➝ *gastrostomy infection*

But wait! The septicemia and staph infection must also be coded. The instructional notes in the tabular list indicate that an additional code is required to specify the type of infection and its organism.

Alphabetic Index:
   Main term ➝ *Septecemia* ➝ *see sepsis* ➝ *sepsis* ➝ *staphylococcal* ➝ *A41.2*

Tabular List:
   A41.2 ➝ *Sepsis due to unspecified staphyococcus*

Correct code(s):
   First listed diagnosis, K94.22 Infection of gastrostomy Secondary diagnosis, A41.2 Staphylococcal septicemia unspecified

DISEASE OF APPENDIX (K35-K38)

The appendix is a 3½-inch-long tube of tissue that extends from the large intestine. It contains lymphoid tissue and may produce antibodies. It is interesting to note that no one is absolutely certain of its function. People live without an appendix, with no apparent consequences.

The most common disease in this classification is appendicitis, which is an inflammation of the appendix. It is a medical emergency that requires prompt surgery to remove the appendix. Left untreated, an inflamed appendix will eventually burst, or perforate, causing infection into the abdominal cavity. This can lead to peritonitis, a serious infection of the abdominal cavity's lining (the peritoneum) that can be fatal unless it is treated quickly with strong antibiotics.

Sometimes a pus-filled abscess forms outside of the appendix. Fibrous scar tissue then "walls off" the appendix from the rest of the abdomen, preventing the spread of infection. An abscessed appendix is a less urgent situation; unfortunately, it cannot be identified without surgery. For this reason, all cases of appendicitis are treated as emergencies.

In the United States, 1 in 15 people develop appendicitis. Although it can strike at any age, appendicitis is rare in individuals under age 2 and most common in those who are between the ages 10 and 30.

The symptoms of appendicitis include:

- Dull pain near the navel or the upper abdomen that becomes sharp as it moves to the lower right abdomen

- Loss of appetite

- Nausea and/or vomiting soon after abdominal pain begins

- Temperature of 99 to 102°F

- Constipation or diarrhea

- Gas

Other symptoms that could appear are:

- Dull or sharp pain anywhere in the upper or lower abdomen, back, or rectum

- Painful urination

- Vomiting that precedes the abdominal pain

CODING TIP K37 is a generalized code and it is not to be used in an acute care setting.

Review the following example:

> ***EXAMPLE:*** *A 50-year-old patient visits his family physician complaining of nausea and abdominal pain that is sometimes dull but sometimes sharp. The physician performs a detailed history and examination. The physician refers the patient to a general surgeon for consultation. After examining the patient, the general surgeon immediately sends him to the hospital and performs an appendectomy the same day. The patient is released the following day. The diagnosis documented on the operative report indicates acute appendicitis with peritonitis.*

> ***Alphabetic Index:***
> *Appendicitis (Main term)* → *Acute* → *With* → *peritonitis* → *with perforation or rupture* → *K35.2*

> ***Tabular List:***
> *K35.2* → *Acute appendicitis with generalized peritonitis*

> ***Correct code:***
> *K35.2*

HERNIA (K40-K46)

There are various types of hernias. *Inguinal hernias* make up approximately 75% of abdominal wall hernias. With an inguinal hernia, a loop of intestine pushes through an opening in the abdominal wall into the inguinal canal, the passageway through which the testes descend into the scrotum. Inguinal hernias are very common and occur in males. There are two different types of inguinal hernias, direct and indirect. Both occur in the groin area and are similar in appearance, as a bulge in the inguinal area. An indirect hernia descends from the abdomen into the scrotum; this type of hernia can occur at any age. A direct inguinal hernia, which occurs inside of the site of the indirect hernia where the abdominal wall is thinner, will protrude into the scrotum. A direct hernia tends to occur in the middle aged or elderly person because the abdominal wall weakens with age.

An *incisional hernia* is caused by a flaw in the abdominal wall and creates an area of weakness in which the hernia may develop. An incisional hernia can return even when repaired.

A *femoral hernia* is the path through which the femoral artery, vein, and nerve leave the abdominal cavity to enter the thigh. A femoral hernia causes a bulge to develop below the inguinal crease in the mid-thigh area. This type of hernia typically occurs in women and carries the risk of becoming reducible and strangulated. In this context, "reducible" means pushed back in place and "strangulated" means having the blood supply cut off.

An *umbilical hernia,* which typically occurs at birth, is a protrusion of the umbilicus ("bellybutton"). This type of hernia occurs when the abdominal wall does not close completely at birth. This type of hernia is less than half an inch across and often closes on its own. If the hernia is larger and does not close, a repair may be necessary, usually when the child is between 2 and 4 years of age. Umbilical hernias can occur in older children and adults because the abdominal wall may be weak for some time.

Epigastric hernias occur between the naval and lower part of the rib cage, at the midline of the abdomen.

This type of hernias is composed of fatty tissue and rarely contains intestine. Epigastric hernias are typically painless; however, it may not be possible to push this type of hernia back into the abdomen.

A *spigelian hernia* occurs along the edge of the rectus abdominus muscle through the spigelian fascia, which is located on one side of the middle abdomen. This type of hernia is rare.

A *diaphragmatic hernia* is a birth defect. It occurs when there is an abnormal opening in the diaphragm and is caused by improper joining of structure during fetal development. The abdominal organs, which include the stomach, spleen, part of the liver, kidney, and small intestine, appear in the chest cavity, preventing the lung tissue on the affected side from fully developing.

Following is a review of some of the codes in category K40-K46. Note that a fifth character is required for most codes in these subclassifications, which include inguinal hernias, femoral hernias, and ventral hernias. Review Figure 8.3.

FIGURE 8.3   Fifth-Digit Classification for Bilateral Inguinal Hernias

K40.0 Bilateral inguinal hernia, with obstruction, without
          gangrene
       Inguinal hernia (bilateral) causing obstruction without gangrene
       Incarcerated inguinal hernia (bilateral) without gangrene
       Irreducible inguinal hernia (bilateral) without gangrene
       Strangulated inguinal hernia (bilateral) without gangrene
  K40.00 Bilateral inguinal hernia, with obstruction,
            without gangrene, not specified as recurrent
            Bilateral inguinal hernia, with obstruction,
            without gangrene NOS
  K40.01 Bilateral inguinal hernia, with obstruction,
            without gangrene, recurrent
K40.1 Bilateral inguinal hernia, with gangrene
  K40.10 Bilateral inguinal hernia, with gangrene, not
            specified as recurrent
            Bilateral inguinal hernia, with gangrene NOS
  K40.11 Bilateral inguinal hernia, with gangrene,
            recurrent
K40.2 Bilateral inguinal hernia, without obstruction or
          gangrene
  K40.20 Bilateral inguinal hernia, without obstruction or
            gangrene, not specified as recurrent
            Bilateral inguinal hernia NOS
  K40.21 Bilateral inguinal hernia, without obstruction or
            gangrene, recurrent

The fifth-character subclassification is based on whether the hernia is unilateral or bilateral and whether it is recurrent or not specified as recurrent. Make sure the documentation is specific. If unclear, ask the physician for clarification. K40.0 Example of Bilateral Inguinal Hernia Coding.

Diagnosis codes range from K40.0- to K46.9. Documentation required includes:

- Site of hernia
- Laterality when appropriate
- If gangrene or obstruction is present
- If condition is recurrent

Hernias are categorized by type of hernia, as follows:

- Inguinal (K40.0–)
- Femoral (K41.0–)
- Umbilical (K42.0–)
- Ventral (K43.0–)
- Diaphragmatic (K 44.0–)
- Other abdominal hernia (K45.0–)
- Unspecified abdominal hernia (K46.0–)

Combination coding is used to identify gangrene or obstruction. Documentation indicating that the hernia is "strangulated" and/or "incarcerated" is classified as an obstruction. Incisional ventral hernia is classified as recurrent.

CODING TIP An incisional ventral hernia is always classified as recurrent.

Open the ICD-10-CM codebook using both the Alphabetic Index and the Tabular List to select the correct code(s) in the next two examples. Keep in mind that when reporting a hernia diagnosis, the main term in the Alphabetic Index is "hernia" then type of hernia.

> ***EXAMPLE:*** *The patient, a 63-year-old male, presented to the general surgeon with complaints of a bulge in the left groin. The patient stated that he noticed this bulge and had pain for approximately two weeks prior to the appointment. Upon examination in the office, the patient was found to have a left inguinal hernia consistent with tear, and was scheduled for surgery the following day.*
>
> ***Alphabetic Index:***
>   *Hernia → inguinal → unilateral → no specified as recurrent → K40.90*
>
> ***Tabular List:***
>   *K40.90 → Unilateral inguinal hernia, without obstruction or gangrene, not specified as recurrent → Inguinal hernia NOS → Unilateral inguinal hernia NOS*
>
> ***Correct code:***
>   *K40.90*

EXAMPLE: A 3-year-old patient was diagnosed with a strangulated umbilical hernia with obstruction. The patient was taken to the operating room for the hernia repair. A standard curvilinear umbilical incision was made, and dissection was carried down to the hernia sac using a combination of Metzenbaum scissors and Bovie electrocautery. The sac was cleared of overlying adherent tissue, and the fascial defect was delineated. The fascia was cleared of any adherent tissue for a distance of 1.5 cm from the defect. The sac was then placed into the abdominal cavity, and the defect was closed primarily using simple interrupted 0 Vicryl sutures. The umbilicus was then reformed using 4-0 Vicryl to tack the umbilical skin to the fascia. The wound was then irrigated using sterile saline, and hemostasis was obtained using Bovie electrocautery. The skin was approximated with 4-0 Vicryl in a subcuticular fashion. The skin was prepped with benzoin, and Steri-Strips were applied. A dressing was then applied.

Alphabetic Index:
 Hernia ➞ strangulated ➞ see also hernia by site, with obstruction ➞ umbilical ➞ with obstruction ➞ K42.0

Tabular List:
 K42.0 Umbilical hernia with obstruction, without gangrene ➞ Strangulated umbilical hernia, without gangrene

Correct code:
 K42.0

Hiatal hernia is found in category K44.–. Following are descriptions of general types of hiatal hernias.

A *hiatal hernia* is an abnormal bulging of a portion of the stomach through the diaphragm; it is coded as K44.9, Diaphragmatic hernia. A hiatal hernia with obstruction is coded as K44.0, and a hiatal hernia with gangrene is coded as K44.1.

A *sliding hiatal hernia* exists when the junction between the esophagus and the stomach (which is normally below the diaphragm) protrudes above the diaphragm.

A *paraesophageal hiatal hernia* exists when the junction between the esophagus and stomach is in the normal place below the diaphragm, but a portion of the stomach is pushed above the diaphragm and lies beside the esophagus. This type of hernia generally produces no symptoms. However, the hernia may be trapped or pinched by the diaphragm, which results in a loss of blood supply. Trapping is serious and painful. The condition is called strangulation and requires immediate surgery.

The cause of hiatal hernia is usually unknown; it may be a birth defect or the result of an injury. People who have a sliding hiatal hernia usually have either no symptoms or minor ones.

Review the following example and see Figure 8.4.

FIGURE 8.4   Excerpt from the Alphabetic Index: *Hernia, Hiatal*

> Hernia, hernial (acquired) (recurrent) K46.9
> hiatal (esophageal) (sliding) K44.9
>   with
>   gangrene (and obstruction) K44.1
>   obstruction K44.0

EXAMPLE: A 46-year-old patient is diagnosed with a para-esophageal hiatal hernia with obstruction.

Alphabetic Index:
 Hernia (Main term) ➞ Hiatal (esophageal) (sliding) ➞ with ➞ Obstruction K44.0

Tabular List:
 K44.0 ➞ Diaphragmatic hernia with obstruction, without gangrene

Correct code:
 K44.0

NONINFECTIOUS ENTERITIS AND COLITIS (K50-K52)

The major stage of digestion occurs in the small intestine. Predigested material supplied by the stomach (chyme) is further subjected to the action of 3 powerful digestive fluids within the small intestine. These digestive fluids are:

- Pancreatic fluid

- Intestinal enzymes

- Bile

These fluids neutralize gastric acid, ending the gastric phase of digestion. The small intestine is anchored to the spinal column by a vascular membrane called the mesentery. The ileocecal sphincter is a circular muscle at the junction of the small and large intestines. When the sphincter relaxes, the contents of the ileum pass successively through portions of the large intestine.

Some common conditions under this classification include inflammatory bowel disease and irritable bowel syndrome.

INFLAMMATORY BOWEL DISEASE

Inflammatory bowel disease is the general name for several distinct diseases that cause intestinal inflammation.

Two of the most common inflammatory bowel diseases are:

- Ulcerative colitis
- Crohn's disease

Ulcerative colitis causes inflammation and ulcers in the top layers of the large intestinal lining. The inflammation usually occurs in the rectum and lower part of the colon but it may affect the entire colon. Ulcerative colitis usually presents as a pit-like abscess.

Crohn's disease is an inflammatory condition that causes inflammation in the small intestine but it can affect any segment of the gastrointestinal tract. This condition most commonly involves the terminal ileum and colon. It can cause pain and diarrhea. Crohn's disease is different from ulcerative colitis because it causes inflammation deep within the intestines (intestinal wall). Crohn's disease is commonly referred to as enteritis.

Symptoms of Crohn's disease include:

- Abdominal pain
- Diarrhea
- Weight loss
- Rectal bleeding
- Anemia in some patients
- Intestinal blockage

Open the ICD-10-CM codebook, using both the Alphabetic Index and the Tabular List, select the correct code(s).

> **EXAMPLE:** *A 23-year-old has a history of 20-pound weight loss and abdominal pain with recurrent rectal bleeding. A CT scan shows a thickened terminal ileum, which is suggestive of Crohn's disease. An endoscopy is performed to evaluate for Crohn's disease. A normal esophagus and duodenum are visualized. There are multiple superficial erosions or aphthous ulcers in the stomach, along with a few scattered aphthous ulcers in the large intestine, large ulcers, and a very irregular ileocecal valve. The physician documents a diagnosis consistent with Crohn's disease of the large intestine with abscess.*

> **Alphabetic Index:**
> *Disease → Crohn's → see Enteritis, regional → enteritis, regional → large intestine → abscess → K50.114*

> **Tabular List:**
> *K50.114 → Crohn's disease of large intestine with abscess*

> **Correct code:**
> *K50.114*

OTHER DISEASES OF INTESTINES (K55-K63)

Irritable Bowel Syndrome

Irritable bowel syndrome is a common disorder. Symptoms of this disorder include:

- Cramping
- Constipation
- Diarrhea
- Lower abdominal pain
- Gas
- Bloating
- Change in bowel habits

Open the ICD-10-CM codebook, using both the Alphabetic Index and the Tabular List, select the correct code(s) for the next two examples.

> **EXAMPLE:** *A 41-year-old established patient visits his family physician with complaints of diarrhea, gas, cramping, and bloating. The patient has a history of irritable bowel syndrome and diverticulitis. A problem-focused history and examination are performed, and the physician's documentation indicates the diagnosis is spastic colon with acute diverticulitis.*

> **Alphabetic Index:**
> *Spastic, see also spasm → spasm, spastic, spasticity → Colon → with diarrhea → K58.*

> **Tabular List:**
> *K58.0 → Irritable bowel syndrome with diarrhea*

> **Correct code:**
> *K58.0*

However, we're not finished. Review the encounter. There are two diagnoses: irritable bowel syndrome and diverticulitis. The diverticulitis should now be coded.

Alphabetic Index:
Diverticulitis (acute) ➜ K57.92

Tabular List:
K57.92 ➜ Diverticulitis of intestine, part unspecified, without perforation or abscess without bleeding

Correct code:
K57.92

Note: Because there is no indication that hemorrhage or bleeding is present, K57.92 will be the appropriate code.

Correct code sequencing:
K58.0 Irritable bowel syndrome with diarrhea (first listed diagnosis)

K57.92 Diverticulitis of intestine, part unspecified, without perforation or abscess without bleeding (secondary diagnosis)

EXAMPLE: The patient is a 46-year-old female who presents to the emergency department with an approximate one-week history of abdominal pain that has been persistent. She has had no nausea and vomiting. She noticed some bright red blood in her rectum that has been ongoing for the past 3 days. She has had no fevers or chills and no history of jaundice. The patient denies any significant recent weight loss. The physician orders labs and a CT scan. The physician diagnoses the patient with sigmoid diverticulitis, orders medication for the patient, and refers the patient to a gastroenterologist for further care.

Alphabetic Index:
Diverticulitis (Main term) ➜ large intestine ➜ bleeding K57.33

Tabular List:
K57.33 Diverticulitis of large intestine without perforation or abscess with bleeding

Correct code:
K57.33

The most common syndrome in this category is rectal polyps, which is found under "other disorders of the intestine" (K62.0-K62.1). Colorectal cancer is the second most common cancer and the third leading cause of cancer death among American men and women. These cancers arise in the colon. Tumors may also arise in the lining of the very last part of the colon, the rectum. If detected early, colon cancer is treatable.

Cancer of the colon and rectum usually begins as a polyp. Polyps are benign growths in the lining of the large intestine. Although most polyps never become cancerous, virtually all colon and rectal cancers start from these benign growths.

Polyps and cancer develop when there are mutations or errors in the genetic code that controls the growth and repair of the cells lining the colon. In addition, people may inherit genetic diseases in which the risk of colon polyps and cancer is very high.

Two common types of polyps are found in the large intestine:

- *Hyperplastic polyps*: small, completely benign polyps that do not carry a risk of developing into cancer

- *Adenomas*: benign polyps that are considered precursors (the first stage) of colon cancer

Although anyone can get colorectal cancer, it is most common among people over the age of 50. Women have a higher risk of colon cancer, while men are more likely to develop rectal cancer.

Risk factors for colorectal cancer include:

- Polyps

- Diet high in fat and low in fiber

- Family history of polyps or colorectal cancer

- Family history of familial polyposis, a disease in which hundreds of polyps cover the colon

- Inflammatory bowel disease (Crohn's disease or ulcerative colitis)

Symptoms of colorectal cancer include the following:

- A change in bowel habits (constipation or diarrhea)

- Blood on or in the stool that is either bright or dark

- Unusual abdominal or gas pains

- Very narrow stool

- A feeling that the bowel has not emptied completely after passing stool

- Unexplained weight loss

- Fatigue

There are 3 types of screening methods for colorectal cancer:

- *Sigmoidoscopy*: A thin, lighted tube called an endoscope is inserted into the rectum and the lower half of the colon. The inside lining of the colon is viewed through the endoscope.

- *Colonoscopy*: This is the same test as a sigmoidoscopy except that the endoscope is passed through the entire colon.

- *Barium enema*: A chalky white substance (barium) is given as an enema before an x-ray of the colon is taken. The barium highlights the colon and rectum.

Open the ICD-10-CM codebook, using both the Alphabetic Index and the Tabular List, select the correct code(s).

> **EXAMPLE:** *A 58-year-old patient is experiencing severe diarrhea with negative stool culture. Her physician recommends a colonoscopy. With the patient under intravenous sedation, the colonoscope is inserted into the rectum and advanced to the colon and beyond the splenic flexure, maneuvered through the hepatic flexure, and moved down the ascending colon to the cecum. The appendiceal orifice is visualized. The ileocecal valve is entered, and approximately 10 cm of terminal ileum is visualized and photographed; it is within normal limits. The scope is withdrawn from the right colon and pulled back to the transverse, descending sigmoid and rectum; all are adequately visualized, and there is no active colitis. Two rectal polyps are excised by snare technique and sent to pathology. Postoperative diagnosis is benign rectal polyps with no active colitis.*

In order to correctly code this procedure, read the entire procedure description. Do not rely on the postoperative diagnosis to code the encounter. The pathology report should be reviewed before determining the final diagnosis. We know that rectal polyps were removed, sent to pathology, and diagnosed benign. The final diagnosis is rectal polyps.

Alphabetic Index:
Polyp, polypus (Main term) → Rectum → (nonadenomatous) → K62.1

Tabular List:
K62.1 → rectal polyp

Correct code:
K62.1

CODING TIP If the documentation indicates the patient has an adenomatous polyp, it is coded as a neoplasm with D12.8.

OTHER DISEASES OF THE DIGESTIVE SYSTEM

The biliary system includes the organs and duct system that create, transport, store, and release bile into the duodenum (the first part of the small intestine) for digestion. In order to code for the biliary system, a good understanding of the common diseases is important. The biliary system includes the liver, gallbladder, and bile ducts (named the cystic, hepatic, common hepatic,

common bile, and pancreatic). There are many disorders of the biliary system that require clinical care by a physician. These conditions include:

- Gallstones
- Cholangitis
- Cholecystitis
- Biliary cirrhosis/bile duct cancer

Gallstones form when bile stored in the gallbladder hardens into stone-like material. Too much cholesterol, bile salts, or bilirubin (bile pigment) can cause gallstones. Slow emptying of the gallbladder can also contribute to the formation of gallstones.

When gallstones (calculus) are present in the gallbladder itself, it is called *cholelithiasis*. When gallstones are present in the bile ducts, it is called *choledocholithiasis*. Gallstones that obstruct bile ducts can lead to severe or life-threatening infection of the bile ducts, pancreas, or liver. Bile ducts can also be obstructed by cancer or trauma. Cholelithiasis is coded to K80.–. A fifth-character subclassification is required when coding these conditions. The fourth-digit subclassification indicates the type of cholelithiasis, and the fifth digit indicates where obstruction is present. Review Figure 8.5.

FIGURE 8.5   Fifth-Digit Subclassification for Category K80.0–

K80.1	Calculus of gallbladder with other cholecystitis
K80.10	Calculus of gallbladder with chronic cholecystitis without obstruction Cholelithiasis with cholecystitis NOS
K80.11	Calculus of gallbladder with chronic cholecystitis with obstruction
K80.12	Calculus of gallbladder with acute and chronic cholecystitis without obstruction
K80.13	Calculus of gallbladder with acute and chronic cholecystitis with obstruction
K80.18	Calculus of gallbladder with other cholecystitis without obstruction
K80.19	Calculus of gallbladder with other cholecystitis with obstruction

Several conditions may trigger an infection in the bile duct system. The primary cause of cholangitis is an obstruction or blockage somewhere in the bile duct system. Blockage may be from:

- Stones
- Tumor
- Blood clots

- A narrowing that may occur after surgery

- Swelling of the pancreas

- Parasite invasion

Other causes of cholangitis include a backflow of bacteria from the small intestine, bacteremia, or complications following a diagnostic endoscopy. Infection causes pressure to build up in the bile duct.

Symptoms may range from moderate to severe and may include:

- Pain in the right, upper quadrant of the abdomen

- Fever and chills

- Jaundice (yellowing of the skin and eyes)

- Low blood pressure

- Lethargy

- A decreased level of alertness

Open the ICD-10-CM codebook, using both the Alphabetic Index and the Tabular List, select the correct code(s).

> **EXAMPLE:** *A 28-year-old male presents with a history of an intermittent fever, jaundice, and vague upper, right quadrant fullness. CT scan of the abdomen reveals a cystic lesion near the mid portion of the common bile duct and no evidence of metastatic disease. Preoperative ERCP confirms a small calculus of the cystic duct. At laparotomy, the calculus is excised, and frozen section reveals no adenocarcinoma. A primary extrahepatic common duct repair is performed over a T-tube.*

> **Alphabetic Index:**
> *Calculus → cystic duct → see calculus, gallbladder → calculus → gallbladder → K80.20*

> **Tabular List:**
> *K80.20 → Calculus of gallbladder without cholecystitis without obstruction*

Note: Because the goal is to code to the highest level of specificity, a fifth character is required. Because the physician's documentation did not indicate cholecystitis, the code selection K80.20 is most appropriate without mention of obstruction.

> **Correct code:**
> *K80.20 Calculus of gallbladder without cholecystitis without obstruction*

Cholecystitis is an inflammation of the gallbladder wall and nearby abdominal lining. Cholecystitis is usually caused by a gallstone in the cystic duct, the duct that connects the gallbladder to the hepatic duct. Other causes of cholecystitis may include the following:

- Bacterial infection in the bile duct system (The bile duct system is the drainage system that carries bile from the liver and gallbladder into the area of the small intestine called the duodenum.)

- Tumor of the pancreas or liver

- Decreased blood supply to the gallbladder (this sometimes occurs in persons with diabetes)

- Gallbladder "sludge"

Gallbladder sludge is a thick material that cannot be absorbed by bile in the gallbladder and most commonly occurs in pregnant women or individuals who have experienced a rapid weight loss. Cholecystitis may occur quite suddenly or gradually over many years. A typical cholecystitis attack normally lasts two to three days. Some of the symptoms include:

- Intense and sudden pain in the upper quadrant of the abdomen

- Painful recurring attacks for several hours after meals

- Vomiting

- Rigid abdominal muscles on the right side

- Nausea

- Fever and chills

- Jaundice

- Itching (rare)

- Abdominal bloating

- Loose, light-colored bowel movements

Open the ICD-10-CM codebook, using both the Alphabetic Index and the Tabular List, select the correct code(s).

> **EXAMPLE:** *A 50-year-old female presents with a history of nausea, fever, chills, and abdominal bloating over the past month. After a comprehensive history and examination, the physician decides to perform an ERCP, which reveals an obstruction of the bile duct with cholecystitis and acute cholangitis. A resection and primary anastomosis are performed. At operation, the distal bile duct is obliterated with marked fibrosis to the level of the bifurcation of the right and left hepatic ducts, and the right and left hepatic ducts are anastomosed Roux-en-Y to the jejunum. The patient goes to ICU for 48 hours postoperatively, has a subsequent uneventful recovery, and is discharged on the 12th postoperative day.*

Alphabetic Index:

Cholecystitis ➡ *with calculus, stones in bile duct (common) (hepatic) –see calculus, bile duct* ➡ *calculus* ➡ *bile duct* ➡ *with* ➡ *cholecystitis (with cholangitis)* ➡ *with obstruction* ➡ *K80.41*

Tabular List:

K80.41 ➡ *Calculus of bile duct with cholecystitis, unspecified, with obstruction*

Correct code:

K80.41

Another condition that is found in this subclassification is biliary cirrhosis, which is a rare form of liver cirrhosis caused by diseases or defects of the bile ducts. A common symptom is cholestasis, which is an accumulation of bile in the liver. There are two types of biliary cirrhosis:

- Primary biliary cirrhosis: inflammation and destruction of bile ducts in the liver

- Secondary biliary cirrhosis: results from prolonged bile duct obstruction or narrowing or closure of the bile duct

Open the ICD-10-CM codebook, using both the Alphabetic Index and the Tabular List, select the correct code(s).

EXAMPLE: A 47-year-old male with a history of previous chronic alcohol abuse. Two years ago, he completed an alcoholic rehabilitation program and has not had an alcoholic drink since that time and is in remission. He is an attorney and practicing at the present time. His major complaint is constant mid epigastric pain and weight loss over the past 6 months. At operation, there is evidence of cirrhosis of the liver due to the many years of alcohol abuse.

Alphabetic Index:

Main term ➡ *cirrhosis* ➡ *liver* ➡ *alcoholic* ➡ *K70.30*

Tabular List:

K70.3 ➡ *Alcoholic cirrhosis of liver without ascites*

Because the physician's documentation indicates the patient has abused alcohol in the past, the alcohol abuse should be coded as a secondary diagnosis.

Alphabetic Index:

Main term ➡ *alcohol, alcoholic* ➡ *addiction* ➡ *with remission* ➡ *F10.21*

Tabular List:

F10.21 ➡ *Alcohol dependence in remission*

Note that the patient is in remission. Because this example indicates the patient has undergone a treatment program and is in remission, F10.21 is selected.

Correct code sequencing:

K70.3 Alcoholic cirrhosis of liver without ascites (first-listed diagnosis)

F10.21 Alcohol dependence in remission (secondary)

CHECKPOINT EXERCISE 8-1

Using your ICD-10-CM codebook, code the following:

1. _____ Cholecystitis with cholelithiasis

2. _____ Spastic colon

3. _____ Necrosis of intestine

4. _____ Cholecystitis

5. _____ Rectal pain

6. _____ Perirectal cellulitis

7. _____ Recurrent appendicitis

8. _____ Peptic ulcer due to overuse of asprin

9. _____ GERD

10. _____ Diverticulitis of colon with associated hemorrhage

11. _____ A two-year-old male presents with an incarcerated right inguinal hernia.

12. _____ A 65-year-old woman had low anterior resection of a rectal cancer 2 years ago. Multiple diminutive polyps were found in the right colon. These were removed by hot biopsy forceps technique.

13. _____ A 21-year-old female presents in the emergency department with findings consistent with appendicitis. Once a decision to operate has been made, the surgeon stabilizes and prepares the patient for emergency surgery. At operation, an inflamed (nonperforated) appendix is resected.

14. _____ A 23-year-old female with Crohn's disease has two areas of ileal disease. Failing medical treatment, the operation includes laparoscopic assessment of the intestinal tract for active Crohn's disease.

15. _____ A 19-month-old child has an umbilical hernia with incarcerated small bowel and small bowel obstruction.

Diseases of the Skin and Subcutaneous Tissue (L00-L99)

Chapter 12 in the Tabular List includes the following sections:

- Infections of Skin and Subcutaneous Tissue (L00-L08)

- Bullous Disorders (L10-L14)

- Dermatitis and Eczema (L20-L30)

- Papulosquamous Disorders (L40-L45)

- Urticaria and Erythema (L49-L54)

- Radiation-related Disorders of the Skin and Subcutaneous Tissue (L55-L59)

- Disorders of Skin Appenages (L60-L75)

- Intraoperative and Postprocedural Complications of Skin and Subcutaneous Tissue (L76)

- Other Disorders of the Skin and Subcutaneous Tissue (L80-L99)

This category includes some of the following conditions:

- Impetigo

- Furnicles

- Carbuncles or abscesses

- Cellulitis and lymphangitis

A furuncle, or boil, is a skin abscess that is small and solitary, usually caused by a staphylococcal infection of the follicular or sebaceous glands. A carbuncle is a group of confluent furuncles (boils) with associated connecting sinus tracts and multiple openings in the skin. This lesion usually occurs on the back of the neck. Diabetics are especially prone to developing carbuncles because of their reduced resistance to infection.

Cellulitis refers to a spreading acute inflammatory process. This type of inflammation is commonly seen with staphylococcal bacterial infections and is due to the body's inability to confine the organism. Cellulitis is seen in the skin and subcutaneous tissue and is characterized by nonlocalized edema and redness.

CODING ISSUES

Many codes in this category are identified by type of condition and anatomic location on the body. In addition, if an infectious agent is present, the coder is instructed to use an additional code from categories B95-B97 to identify the infectious agent. Pay careful attention to the excludes1 and Excludes 2 notes in these categories.

Open the ICD-10-CM codebook, using both the Alphabetic Index and the Tabular List, select the correct code(s) for the following two examples.

> *EXAMPLE: A 22-year-old male presents to the dermatologist's office with what appears to be a boil. After an expanded problem-focused examination, the physician determines the boil on the patient's neck is a carbuncle and performs an incision and drainage (I&D) in the office.*
>
> ***Alphabetic Index:***
> *Carbuncle → Neck → L02.13*
>
> ***Tabular List:***
> *L02.13 → Carbuncle of neck*
>
> ***Correct code:***
> *L02.13*
>
> *EXAMPLE: A 60-year-old patient is diagnosed with cellulitis of the left great toe due to a staphylococcal infection.*
>
> ***Alphabetic Index:***
> *Cellulitis → Toe → L03.03–*

Notice in this example that laterality is important in selection of the code.

> ***Tabular List:***
> *L03.3– → Cellulitis of toe → left toe → L03.032*

The category note instructs you to use an additional code to identify the organism (B95.8, Staphylococcus, unspecified).

> ***Correct codes:***
> *L03.032, B95.8*

This section excludes certain infections of the skin classified under "Infectious and Parasitic Diseases," such as herpes simplex and herpes zoster, molluscum contagiosum, and viral warts.

DERMATITIS AND ECZEMA (L20-L30)

This section includes codes relating to dermatitis, which is a generic, clinical term used to describe a wide variety of skin conditions, all characterized by inflammation of the skin (commonly called eczema). Dermatitis accounts for about one third of patients who consult a dermatologist. Symptoms include itchy skin that can redden with acute attacks that range from blisters or crusty scales. Types of dermatitis include:

- Contact dermatitis

- Eczema

- Seborrheic dermatitis

- Nummular dermatitis

Contact dermatitis occurs as a delayed hypersensitivity reaction to chemical allergens such as clothing, cosmetics, jewelry, and various metals. Contact dermatitis requires an externally applied inciting agent; dermatitis caused by substances taken internally is classified separately (category 693, Dermatitis due to substances taken internally).

Atopic dermatitis, or eczema, is dermatitis of unknown etiology marked by itching and scratching in an individual with inherently irritable skin. There may be allergic, hereditary, or psychological components. The disease rarely occurs before two months of age and may occur initially quite late in life. In about 70% of all cases there is a family history of the disease.

Seborrheic dermatitis is a common form of dermatitis that occurs at sites of greatest concentration of sebaceous glands: scalp, face, ears, neck, axillae, breasts, umbilicus, and anogenital regions.

Nummular dermatitis occurs more commonly in men than women and typically occurs in patients over age 55. It can be caused by taking hot showers or living in a dry climate.

Open the ICD-10-CM codebook, using both the Alphabetic Index and the Tabular List, select the correct code(s) for the following two examples.

> **EXAMPLE:** *A woman presents to her physician with complaints of an extremely itchy and erythematous rash that appeared on her uncovered arms and legs after she pulled weeds out of her flower garden. The patient had the plants sprayed with an insecticide; after working in the garden, she developed the itchy rash. The physician diagnoses contact dermatitis due to poison ivy and treats the patient appropriately.*

> **Alphabetic Index:**
> Dermatitis ➡ Due to ➡ insecticide ➡ L24.5

> **Tabular List:**
> L24.5 ➡ Irritant contact dermatitis due to other chemical products ➡ irritant contact due to insecticide

> **Correct code:**
> L24.5

> **EXAMPLE:** *A 32-year-old female patient bought some new eye makeup. After using it for the first time, the patient developed a rash and was itching. The itching continued after she removed the makeup. The next morning her rash was worse and her eyelids were red*

and sore. She went to her physician the same morning and was diagnosed with dermatities due to the makeup, was given a topical ointment, and told to discountinue using the product.

> **Alphabetic Index:**
> Dermatitis ➡ irritant ➡ due to ➡ cosmetics L24.3

> **Tabular List:**
> L24.3 ➡ Irritant contact dermatitis due to cosmetics

> **Correct code:**
> L24.3

PAPULOSQUAMOUS DISORDERS (L40-L45)

Two of the most common disorders in this category are psoriasis and urticaria. Psoriasis is a chronic inflammatory disease of the skin of unknown cause that varies greatly in severity and is characterized by thickened areas of skin with silver-colored scales. This condition is not contagious and commonly affects the skin, scalp, elbows, and knees. This condition is considered chronic, and patients have periods of improvement that can be followed by a flare-up.

Urticaria (hives) is an acute patchy eruption of elevated wheals or skin redness with severe itching or stinging. Urticaria can be allergic, idiopathic, thermal, dermatographic (due to applied pressure or friction), vibratory, or cholinergic.

Open the ICD-10-CM codebook, using both the Alphabetic Index and the Tabular List, select the correct code(s).

> **EXAMPLE:** *A 55-year-old female patient seeks help from a dermatologist her family physician referred her to. After taking a comprehensive history and performing a detailed examination, the physician determines the patient has psoriasis vulgaris.*

> **Alphabetic Index:**
> Psoriasis ➡ vulgaris ➡ L40.0

> **Tabular List:**
> L40.0 ➡ psoriasis vulgaris

> **Correct code:**
> L40.0

> **EXAMPLE:** *A 55-year-old patient was experiencing severe itching on the neck and chest, which were sometimes painful. She had been taking a new medication for her blood pressure, and a few days later the patient developed these symptoms. The patient went to a dermatologist to find out why she was itching and her skin was blotchy. The physician diagnosed the patient with hives, changed her blood pressure medication, and gave her a prescription to alleviate her symptoms.*

Alphabetic Index:
    Urticaria ➞ due to ➞ drugs ➞ L50.0

Tabular List:
    L50.0 ➞ Allergic Urticaria

Correct code:
    L50.0

RADIATION-RELATED DISORDERS OF THE SKIN AND SUBCUTANEOUS TISSUE (L55-L59)

Sunburns are classified in category L55 and are coded based on first, second, or third-degree sunburn. A sunburn results from too much sun exposure. Another source of sunburn is related to improper tanning bed usage. Injury can occur within 30 minutes of exposure. Some people burn differently than others depending on the type of skin. A mild case of sunburn results in minor skin redness or irritation. More severe cases, referred to as sun poisoning, may result in burning, blistering, dehydration, and electrolyte imbalance. Common symptoms of sunburn are:

- Fever
- Chills
- Blistering
- Nausea
- Vomiting
- Skin loss or peeling

Actinic keratoses is a condition resulting in a crusty or scaly bump on the skin's surface. They are sometimes referred to as "sun spots, age spots, or solar keratoses." Typically referred to as AKs, these are considered precancerous and are the first step to the development of cancer. Treatment includes cryosurgery, which is freezing the area with liquid nitrogen to eradicate the AK. Curettage is another method where the lesion is scraped and may be submitted to pathology for analysis. Chemical peels are sometimes helpful in removing an AK as is shave excision.

Open the ICD-10-CM codebook, using both the Alphabetic Index and the Tabular List, select the correct code(s).

> *EXAMPLE: A patient with a history of AKs from years of using a tanning bed was taken into the outpatient operating room for an excisional biopsy of two actinic keratoses. A 2-cm AK was excised from the left abdomen and a 1-cm medial actinic keratoses was removed from the arm. After the AKs were removed from both areas, they were closed with a one-layer plastic closure. The patient tolerated the procedure well and was released in good condition.*

Alphabetic Index:
    Actinic keratosis ➞ L57.0

Tabular List:
    L57.0 ➞ Actinic keratoses

Review the instructional notes under category L57. The instructional notes state, "use additional code to identify the source of the ultraviolet radiation." The documentation indicates that the AKs were caused by overuse of a tanning bed. Review W89 and X32 in the Tabular List and determine which is the most appropriate secondary diagnosis.

Tabular List:
    W89 ➞ Exposure to tanning bed ➞ Exposure to man-made visible and ultraviolet light ➞ W89.1 Tanning Bed

There are instructions in this category that a seventh character is required to report:

A   Initial

D   Subsequent

S   Sequela

In this instance, it appears that this is the first encounter for this patient, so the seventh character is "A." However, W89.1 is only 4 characters and 7 are necessary. We will use dummy placeholders in order to code to the seventh character. The code is reported as W89.1xxA.

Correct code sequencing:
    L57.0, W89.1xxA

OTHER DISORDERS OF SKIN AND SUBCUTANEOUS TISSUE (L80-L99)

Chronic ulcers of the skin are long-standing, slow-to-heal ulcers accompanied by sloughing of inflamed necrotic tissue. Codes for decubitus ulcers are classified in L89 and nondecubitus ulcers in L97, both are coded with a sixth character. The fifth character identifies the site of the ulcer, and the sixth character is used for reporting the depth of the ulcer. If gangrene is present, it is reported first as I96. Decubitus ulcers in this category include:

- Bed sores
- Plaster ulcer
- Pressure ulcers
- Pressure sore

Nondecubitus ulcers include:
- Chronic ulcer of the skin
- Nonhealing ulcer of the skin

- Noninfected sinus of the skin

- Trophic ulcer NOS

- Tropical ulcer NOS

- Ulcer of the skin NOS

In order to code decubitus and nondecubitus ulcers, the site and depth must be documented in the medical record. When multiple ulcers are documented in the medical record, only the most severe ulcer of the same site is coded.

Decubitus ulcers may occur at multiple sites. A decubitus ulcer that has become serious and does not respond to treatment may support medical necessity for hospital admission. If the reason for admission is the decubitus ulcer, it should be reported as the principal or first listed diagnosis. Secondary codes for other problems or problems associated with the decubitus ulcer should be reported also.

If the patient has an underlying condition such as diabetes mellitus or atherosclerosis of the lower extremities, it should be coded as the first listed diagnosis followed by the code for the nondecubitus ulcer. The codes for diabetes mellitus and atherosclerosis include extremity ulcers, but L97– will identify the site and depth of the ulcer and should also be reported.

It is common for patients with these conditions to develop these types of ulcers. If there is no underlying cause or condition, the nondecubitus ulcer is listed first. There is an instructional note for both of these categories to code first gangrene if present. Gangrene is necrosis of the tissue.

Specific guidelines exist in ICD-10-CM for coding and reporting pressure ulcers. Review Table 8.1.

Open the ICD-10-CM codebook, using both the Alphabetic Index and the Tabular List, select the correct code(s).

TABLE 8.1   Official Guidelines for Coding and Reporting Pressure Ulcers

Pressure ulcer stage codes Pressure ulcer stages	Codes from category L89, Pressure ulcer, are combination codes that identify the site of the pressure ulcer as well as the stage of the ulcer.
	ICD-10-CM classifies pressure ulcer stages based on severity, which is designated by stages 1 through 4, unspecified stage, and unstageable.
	Assign as many codes from category L89 as needed to identify all the pressure ulcers the patient has, if applicable.
Unstageable pressure ulcers	Assignment of the code for unstageable pressure ulcer (L89.–0) should be based on the clinical documentation. These codes are used for pressure ulcers whose stage cannot be clinically determined (eg, the ulcer is covered by eschar or has been treated with a skin or muscle graft) and pressure ulcers that are documented as deep tissue injury but not documented as due to trauma. This code should not be confused with the codes for unspecified stage (L89.–9). When there is no documentation regarding the stage of the pressure ulcer, assign the appropriate code for unspecified stage (L89.–9).
Documented pressure ulcer stage	Assignment of the pressure ulcer stage code should be guided by clinical documentation of the stage or documentation of the terms found in the Alphabetic Index.
	For clinical terms describing the stages that are not found in the Alphabetic Index and if there is no documentation of the stage, the provider should be queried.
Patients admitted with pressure ulcers documented as healed	No code is assigned if the documentation states that the pressure ulcer is completely healed.
Patients admitted with pressure ulcers documented as healing	Pressure ulcers described as healing should be assigned the appropriate pressure ulcer stage code based on the documentation in the medical record. If the documentation does not provide information about the stage of the healing pressure ulcer, assign the appropriate code for unspecified stage.
	If the documentation is unclear as to whether the patient has a current (new) pressure ulcer or if the patient is being treated for a healing pressure ulcer, query the provider.
Patient admitted with pressure ulcer evolving into another stage during the admission	If a patient is admitted with a pressure ulcer at one stage and it progresses to a higher stage, assign the code for the highest stage reported for that site.

EXAMPLE: *A patient who has been bedridden for several months has developed a bedsore on the left buttock. The physician examines the patient and determines it is a stage 2 pressure ulcer and treats her decubitus ulcer (bedsore) appropriately.*

Alphabetic Index:
Ulcer ➞ *Decubitus* ➞ *see ulcer, pressure by site* ➞ *pressure* ➞ *stage 2* ➞ *buttock* ➞ *L89.3-*

Tabular List:
L89.3– ➞ *pressure ulcer of buttocks* ➞ *L89.32* ➞ *pressure ulcer of left buttock* ➞ *L89.322* ➞ *pressure ulcer of left buttock, stage 3*

Correct code:
L89.322

Review this example. Open the ICD-10-CM codebook and, referencing both the Alphabetic Index and the Tabular List, locate the correct diagnosis code(s),

EXAMPLE: *A 60-year-old patient with type 1 diabetes has a chronic ulcer of the left thigh with muscle necrosis due to the diabetes.*

Alphabetic Index:
Ulcer ➞ *thigh* ➞ *see ulcer lower limb* ➞ *lower limb, thigh* ➞ *with muscle necrosis* ➞ *left* ➞ *L97.123*

Tabular List:
L97.123 non-pressure chronic ulcer of left thigh with necrosis of muscle

You're not finished yet. This patient is a type 1 diabetic patient, and the ulcer is due to the diabetes, that is, it is a manifestation of the diabetes. Reference the instructional note at the beginning of this classification and locate the correct diabetes code and correct sequencing.

Alphabetic Index:
Diabetes, diabetic ➞ *type 1* ➞ *with* ➞ *skin ulcer* ➞ *E10.622*

Tabular List:
E10.622 Type 1 diabetes mellitus with other skin ulcer

A note underneath the diabetes code instructs the coder to "use additional code to identify site of ulcer."

First listed diagnosis:
E10.622 Type 1 diabetes mellitus with other skin ulcer

Secondary diagnosis:
L97.123 Non-pressure chronic ulcer of left thigh with necrosis of muscle

Correct code sequencing:
E10.622, L97.123

CHECKPOINT EXERCISE 8-2

Using your ICD-10-CM codebook, code the following:

1. _____ Cellulitis of left leg and foot due to Staphylococcus

2. _____ Scleroderma systemic

3. _____ Pilonidal cyst

4. _____ Dermatitis due to unspecified substance taken internally

5. _____ Actinic keratosis

6. _____ Urticaria due to cold and heat

7. _____ A patient was diagnosed with Addison's keloid.

8. _____ A patient was experiencing inflammation in the mouth and on the face. The physician determined the patient was suffering from septic granuloma.

9. _____ A one-month-old female patient was diagnosed with cradle cap.

10. _____ A chronic skin condition usually of the face characterized by persistent erythema, engorgement papules, is called rhinophyma.

11. _____ Decubitis ulcer of the ankle

12. _____ Focal hyperhidrosis

13. _____ A 30-year-old male with vitiligo, hands and face, requires extensive tattooing.

14. _____ A 71-year-old non-insulin–dependent, diabetic female presents with chronic, recurring multiple hyperkeratotic lesions on both feet. The lesions are located on the dorsum of the second, third, and fifth toes of both feet and on the plantar aspect of both feet. The patient has tried cutting the lesions with a straight razor and has used over-the-counter acid preparations. The lesions on both feet are pared, and 1/8-inch felt aperture pads are cut and applied to each toe; and 1/4-inch felt pads are cut and applied to the plantar aspect of both feet.

15. _____ A 65-year-old female undergoes the debridement of infected skin from the fourth digital interspace right foot, in office.

Diseases of the Musculoskeletal System and Connective Tissue (M00-M99)

Chapter 13 of the Tabular List includes the following sections:

- Infectious Arthropathies (M00-M02)

- Inflammatory Polyarthropathies (M05-M14)

- Osteoarthritis (M15-M19)

- Other Joint Disorders (M20-M25)

- Dentofacial Anomallies (including malocclusion) and Other Disorders of Jaw (M26-M27)

- Systemic Connective Tissue Disorders (M30-M36)

- Deforming Dorsopathies (M40-M43)

- Spondylopathies (M45-M49)

- Other Dorsopathies (M50-M54)

- Disorders of Muscles (M60-M63)

- Disorders of Synovium and Tendon (M65-M67)

- Other Soft Tissue Disorders (M70-M79)

- Disorders of Bone Density and Structure (M80-M85)

- Other Osteopathies (M86-M90)

- Chrondropathies (M91-M94)

- Other Disorders of the Musculoskeletal System and Connective Tissue (M95)

- Intraoperative and Postprocedural Complications and Disorders of Musculoskeletal System, Not Elsewhere Classified (M96)

- Biomechanical Lesions, Not Elsewhere Classified (M99)

Many conditions in Chapter 13 of ICD-10-CM are results of trauma or previous injury to a site or are recurrent conditions. A current acute injury is reported with an injury code. Also included in this chapter are recurrent bone, joint, and muscle conditions. Most codes in Chapter 13 have site and laterality designations. The site designations for the limbs are:

- Upper arm

- Lower arm

- Upper and lower leg

  - Humerus

  - Ulna

- Femur

- Tibia

- Fibula

When a condition is described stating "arm" or "leg" without further elaboration as to whether the site is upper or lower, the code for the upper arm or lower leg should be used. When the condition is identified by stating more than one bone, joint, or muscle, a code for multiple sites is selected. If a multiple site code is not available and multiple sites are involved, each site is coded separately.

ARTHROPATHIES AND RELATED DISORDERS (M00-M25)

This section includes some of the conditions described in the following paragraphs.

Systemic lupus erythematosus is a chronic autoimmune inflammatory disease involving multiple organ systems and marked by periods of exacerbation and remission. Its name is derived from the characteristic butterfly rash over the nose and cheeks that resembles a wolf's face. The disease is most prevalent in nonwhite women of childbearing age. Patients present with a wide diversity of clinical signs, but polyarthralgia, polyarthritis, glomerulonephritis, fever, malaise, normocytic anemia, and vasculitis of small vessels of the hands and feet causing peripheral neuropathy are the most common.

Arthropathy (any disease of a joint) associated with infections includes arthritis, arthropathy, polyarthritis, and polyarthropathy. The codes under this category require that you code first for the underlying disease.

Rheumatoid arthritis and other inflammatory polyarthropathies include juvenile chronic polyarthritis. Rheumatoid arthritis is a chronic systemic disease marked by inflammatory changes in the joints and related structures that result in crippling deformities. The pathologic changes in the joints are generally thought to be caused by an autoimmune disease.

Osteoarthrosis and allied disorders include degenerative and hypertrophic arthritis or polyarthritis, degenerative joint disease, and osteoarthritis. Osteoarthritis is a type of arthritis marked by progressive cartilage deterioration in synovial joints and vertebrae. Risk factors include aging, obesity, overuse or abuse of joints as in sports or strenuous occupations, and trauma.

Review the following examples. Open the ICD-10-CM codebook, referencing both the Alphabetic Index and the Tabular List, select the correct code(s).

> **EXAMPLE:** *A 53-year-old patient presents with severe pain and swelling of the knee joints. He is diagnosed with localized osteoarthritis of both knees.*
>
> **Alphabetic Index:**
> *Osteoarthritis* ➡ *knees* ➡ *bilateral* ➡ *M17.0*
>
> **Tabular List:**
> *M17.0* ➡ *Bilateral primary osteoarthritis of knee*
>
> **Correct code:**
> *M17.0*

Note: Codes in this category identify laterality.

> **EXAMPLE:** *A 70-year-old patient is diagnosed with rheumatoid myopathy with rheumatoid arthritis of the right and left hip.*

In ICD-10-CM, a combination code or code for multiple sites does not exist, so both codes are reported for the right and left hip.

> **Alphabetic Index:**
> *Myopathy* ➡ *rheumatoid* ➡ *with arthritis* ➡ *M05.45–*
>
> **Tabular List:**
> *M05.451* ➡ *Rheumatoid myopathy with rheumatoid arthritis of right hip*
>
> *M05.452* ➡ *Rheumatoid myopathy with rheumatoid arthritis of left hip*
>
> **Correct code(s):**
> *M05.451, M05.452*

DORSOPATHIES (M40-M54)

Dorsopathy is any disease of the back (dorso-, word root means "back"). This section of codes includes codes for spondylosis (any degenerative condition of the spine), intervertebral disk disorders, lumbago (low back pain), and sciatica (severe pain in the leg along the course of the sciatic nerve felt at the back of the thigh and running down the inside of the leg).

Review these examples. Open the ICD-10-CM codebook and, referencing both the Alphabetic Index and the Tabular List, locate the correct diagnosis code(s).

> **EXAMPLE:** *A woman was diagnosed with cervical spondylosis with spondylogenic compression of the cervical spinal cord (myelopathy).*

> **Alphabetic Index:**
> *Spondylosis* ➡ *Cervical, cervicodorsal, cervicothoracic* ➡ *S13.4*
>
> **Tabular List:**
> *S13.4* ➡ *sprain of ligaments of cervical spine*
>
> *A seventh character is required for this classification*
>
> **Correct code:**
> *S13.4xxA*

Note: This patient encounter is not coded in the Musculoskeletal System section of ICD-10-CM but in the Injuries and Poisonings section.

> **EXAMPLE:** *A patient was experiencing chronic and constant back pain and visited a spine surgeon at the suggestion of her family physician. The surgeon examined the patient and ordered a CT scan followed by an MRI. Based on the test results, the surgeon diagnosed the patient with spondylolydis of the lumbosacral region.*

> **Alphabetic Index:**
> *Spondylolysis (acquired)* ➡ *lumbosacral region* ➡ *M43.07*
>
> **Tabular List:**
> *M43.07* ➡ *Spondylolysis lumbosacral region*
>
> **Correct code:**
> *M43.07*

OTHER SOFT TISSUE DISORDERS (M70-M79)

Rheumatism is a general term for acute and chronic conditions characterized by inflammation, muscle soreness and stiffness, and pain in joints and associated structures. It includes arthritis due to rheumatic fever or trauma, degenerative joint disease, neurogenic arthropathy, hydroarthrosis, myositis, bursitis, fibromyositis, and many other conditions. The term "enthesopathy" appears under category M76 and represents disorders of peripheral ligamentous or muscular attachments.

Review the following examples. Open the ICD-10-CM codebook and, referencing both the Alphabetic Index and the Tabular List, locate the correct diagnosis code(s).

> **EXAMPLE:** *A patient presents with complaints of generalized muscle pain and stiffness in both shoulders. The physician determines that the patient is suffering from myositis due to poor posture.*

> **Alphabetic Index:**
> *Myositis* ➡ *Due to posture* ➡ *see myocitis specified type NEC* ➡ *M60.80–*

In this example, because both shoulders are affected, two codes will be required. In this code subclassification, there is not one code to report the laterality as bilateral.

Tabular List:
   M60.80 ➡ *other myositis* ➡ *M60.811* ➡ *right shoulder*

   M60.812 ➡ *other myositis* ➡ *left shoulder*

Correct code(s):
   M60.811 (right shoulder), M60.812 (left shoulder)

EXAMPLE: *A patient who is experiencing acute pain in the right leg sought treatment from an orthopedic surgeon who diagnosed the patient with Achilles tendinitis of the right leg.*

Alphabetic Index:
   Tendonitis ➡ Achilles ➡ M76.6–

Tabular List:
   M76.6- ➡ *Achilles tendonitis* ➡ *right leg* ➡ *M76.61*

Correct code:
   M76.61

MUSCLE WEAKNESS (M62.81)

Weakness may be subjective (the person feels weak but has no measurable loss of strength) or objective (measurable loss of strength as noted in a physical exam). Weakness may be generalized (total body weakness) or localized to a specific area, side of the body, limb, or muscle.

Common Causes of Muscle Weakness

Measurable weakness may result from a variety of conditions including metabolic, neurologic, and primary muscular diseases and toxic disorders. Causes of muscle weakness include:

- Metabolic
  - Addison's disease
  - Thyrotoxicosis
- Neurologic
  - Stroke (often localized or focal weakness)
  - Bell's palsy (weakness of one side of the face)
  - A nerve impingement syndrome such as a slipped disk in the spine
  - Multiple sclerosis
  - Amyotrophic lateral sclerosis (ALS or Lou Gehrig's disease; focal developing to generalized)
  - Cerebral palsey (focal weakness associated with spasticity)
  - Guillain-Barre syndrome

- Primary Muscular Diseases
  - Muscular dystrophy (Duchenne)
  - Becker muscular dystrophy
  - Myotonic dystrophy
  - Dermatomyositis
- Toxic
  - Organophosphate poisoning (insecticides, nerve gas)
  - Paralytic shellfish poisoning
  - Botulism
- Other
  - Myasthenia gravis (an autoimmune disorder that interferes with the transmission of nerve impulses to muscle)
  - Poliomyelitis (an infectious disease that damages motor neurons)
  - Dermatomyositis/polymyositis (autoimmune diseases leading to proximal muscle weakness, muscle pain, and sometimes skin rashes)

Review the following example. Open the ICD-10-CM codebook and, referencing both the Alphabetic Index and the Tabular List, locate the correct diagnosis code(s).

EXAMPLE: *A 45-year-old female visits her family physician complaining of muscle weakness in both knees. She indicates she does not know the source. The patient has no other symptoms. After a comprehensive history and physical examination are performed, the physician diagnoses the patient with muscle weakness and schedules additional testing.*

Alphabetic Index:
   Weakness ➡ muscle ➡ M62.81

Tabular List:
   M62.8 ➡ *specified disorders of muscle* ➡ *M62.81 generalized muscle weakness*

Correct code:
   M62.81

OSTEOPATHIES AND CHONDROPATHIES (M80-M94)

This section of codes includes some of the following conditions:

- Osteoporosis
- Osteomalacia
- Stress fractures
- Pathological fractures

- Dysplasia

- Osteitis

- Disorder of bone density and structure

Osteoporosis

There are two categories of codes in ICD-10-CM. They are:

- M80 Osteoporosis with current pathologic fracture

- M81 Osteoporosis without current pathologic fracture

Osteoporosis is a systemic condition where all bones of the musculoskeletal system are affected. Category M81 is reported for patients who do not currently have a pathologic fracture due to the osteoporosis but may have had a pathologic fracture in the past. For patients with a history of fractures as a result of osteoporosis, the status code Z87.310 is reported. Category M80 is reported for a patient who has a current pathologic fracture. A traumatic fracture care code is not reported for a patient with known osteoporosis who suffers a fracture, even if the patient has a minor fall or trauma, if that fall would not usually break a normal healthy bone.

Review Figure 8.6, which is an excerpt from ICD-10-CM for osteoporosis without pathological fracture.

FIGURE 8.6   Excerpt from the ICD-10-CM Tabular List: *M81*

M81 Osteoporosis without current pathological fracture
    Use additional code to identify:
    major osseous defect, if applicable (M89.7-)
    personal history of osteoporosis fracture (Z87.310)
    EXCLUDES 1   osteoporosis with current pathological fracture
            (M80.-)
    Sudeck's atrophy (M89.0)
    M81.0 Age-related osteoporosis without current
            pathological fracture
    Involutional osteoporosis without current pathological
            fracture
    Osteoporosis NOS
    Postmenopausal osteoporosis without current pathological
            fracture
    Senile osteoporosis without current pathological fracture
    M81.6 Localized osteoporosis [Lequesne]
    EXCLUDES 1   Sudeck's atrophy (M89.0)
    M81.8 Other osteoporosis without current pathological
            fracture
                Drug-induced osteoporosis without current
                        pathological fracture
                Idiopathic osteoporosis without current
                        pathological fracture
                Osteoporosis of disuse without current
                        pathological fracture
                Postoopherectomy osteoporosis without
                        current pathological fracture
                Postsurgical malabsorption osteoporosis
                        without current pathological fracture
                Post-traumatic osteoporosis without current
                        pathological fracture

Osteomyelitis is an inflammation of the bone, especially the marrow, caused by a pathogenic organism. Symptoms include pain in the affected part, fever, sweats, leukocytosis, rigid overlying muscles, inflamed skin, and pain on pressure over the affected part. This code provides instructions to use a fifth digit to identify the causative organism, such as Staphylococcus.

Osteochondropathies are diseases of the bone and cartilage. Osteochrondrosis is a disease that causes degenerative changes in the ossification centers of the epiphyses of bones, particularly during periods of rapid growth in children. The process continues to the stage of avascular and aseptic necrosis, and there is slow healing and repair.

Review Table 8.2.

Curvatures of the spine include kyphosis (also known as "hunchback"), which is an abnormal increase in the outward curvature of the thoracic spine; lordosis (also known as "swayback"), which is an abnormal increase in the forward curvature of the lower or lumbar spine; and scoliosis, which is an abnormal lateral or sideways curvature of the spine.

Review the following examples. Open the ICD-10-CM codebook and, referencing both the Alphabetic Index and the Tabular List, locate the correct diagnosis code(s).

> *EXAMPLE: A patient is treated with medication for post-menopausal osteoporosis. The patient had a pathologic fracture one year ago, and the physician is following her condition every 3 months.*
>
> **Alphabetic Index:**
>   *Osteoporosis → age related → M81.0*
>
> **Tabular List:**
>   *M81.0 → Age-related osteoporosis without current pathological fracture*

You also need to report the personal history of the healed osteoporosis fracture. There is an instructional note indicating that the history should be coded.

> **Secondary diagnosis:**
>   *Z87.310 Personal history of (healed) osteoporosis fracture*
>
> **Correct code sequencing:**
>   *M81.0, Z87.310*

CODING TIP Code the personal history of a healed osteoporosis fracture, when the condition exists, using Z98.310.

TABLE 8.2 Official Guidelines for Coding and Reporting Fractures in ICD-10-CM

Site and laterality	Most of the codes within Chapter 13 have site and laterality designations. The site represents the bone, joint, or the muscle involved. For some conditions where more than one bone, joint, or muscle is usually involved, such as osteoarthritis, there is a "multiple sites" code available. For categories where no multiple site code is provided and more than one bone, joint, or muscle is involved, multiple codes should be used to indicate the different sites involved.
Bone versus joint	For certain conditions, the bone may be affected at the upper or lower end (eg, avascular necrosis of bone, M87, Osteoporosis, M80, M81). Though the portion of the bone affected may be at the joint, the site designation will be the bone, not the joint.
Acute traumatic versus chronic or recurrent musculoskeletal conditions	Many musculoskeletal conditions are a result of previous injury or trauma to a site or are recurrent conditions. Bone, joint, or muscle conditions that are the result of a healed injury are usually found in Chapter 13. Recurrent bone, joint, or muscle conditions are also usually found in Chapter 13. Any current, acute injury should be coded to the appropriate injury code from Chapter 19. Chronic or recurrent conditions should generally be coded with a code from Chapter 13. If it is difficult to determine from the documentation in the record which code is best to describe a condition, query the provider.
Coding of pathologic fractures	Seventh character A is for use as long as the patient is receiving active treatment for the fracture. Examples of active treatment are: surgical treatment, emergency department encounter, evaluation and treatment by a new physician. Seventh character D is to be used for encounters after the patient has completed active treatment. The other seventh characters, listed under each subcategory in the Tabular List, are to be used for subsequent encounters for treatment of problems associated with the healing, such as malunions, nonunions, and sequelae.
	Care for complications of surgical treatment for fracture repairs during the healing or recovery phase should be coded with the appropriate complication codes.
	See Section I.C.19, Coding of traumatic fractures.
Osteoporosis	Osteoporosis is a systemic condition, meaning that all bones of the musculoskeletal system are affected. Therefore, site is not a component of the codes under category M81, Osteoporosis without current pathological fracture.
	The site codes under category M80, Osteoporosis with current pathological fracture, identify the site of the fracture, not the osteoporosis.
Osteoporosis without pathological fracture	Category M81, Osteoporosis without current pathological fracture, is used for patients with osteoporosis who do not currently have a pathologic fracture due to the osteoporosis, even if they have had a fracture in the past. For patients with a history of osteoporosis fractures, status code Z87.310, Personal history of (healed) osteoporosis fracture, should follow the code from M81.
Osteoporosis with current pathological fracture	Category M80, Osteoporosis with current pathological fracture, is for patients who have a current pathologic fracture at the time of an encounter. The codes under M80 identify the site of the fracture. A code from category M80, not a traumatic fracture code, should be used for any patient with known osteoporosis who suffers a fracture, even if the patient had a minor fall or trauma, if that fall or trauma would not normally break a normal healthy bone.

Source: ICD-10-CM Official Guidelines for Chapter 13, Diseases of the Musculoskeletal System and Connective Tissue

EXAMPLE: *A patient is diagnosed with chronic inflammation (osteomyelitis) of the right shoulder due to recurrent staphylococcal infections of the bone.*

Alphabetic Index:
Osteomyelitis ➞ acute ➞ scapula ➞ M86.01–

Tabular List:
M86.011 ➞ *Acute hematogenous osteomyelitis right shoulder*

A note at the beginning of this category indicates that an additional code is needed to identify the infectious agent, Staphylococcus in B95-B97.

Tabular List:
B95.8 ➞ *Unspecified staphylococcus as the cause of the disease classified elsewhere*

Correct codes:
M86.011, B95.8

Nontraumatic Compartment Syndrome

Nontraumatic compartment syndrome is coded in category M79.–. Compartment syndromes are classified either as traumatic or nontraumatic and may be acute or chronic. Compartment syndromes due to trauma are not coded in this category. Compartment syndromes, whether they are traumatic or nontraumatic, involve compression of the nerves and blood vessels within an enclosed space. This leads to impaired blood flow and damage to muscles and nerves.

Pathological Fractures

A traumatic fracture is a break in normal, healthy bone. A pathological fracture occurs in diseased or weakened bone with no trauma or with only minor trauma that would not normally break a healthy bone.

Pathological fractures, typically documented as spontaneous fractures, are caused by abnormal weakness of the bone. This may reflect generalized bone fragility caused by many conditions. The pathological fracture may occur at the site of a focal abnormality. It typically presents following minor trauma and may lead to the detection of a previously unsuspected bone abnormality. The facture is characteristically transversely orientated in long bones. The common causes of pathological fracture in the elderly are a secondary deposit from a primary malignancy elsewhere or multiple myeloma of bone. Secondary deposits in bone indicate advanced stages of the disease. A pathological fracture in the vertebrae often represents an exacerbation of a backache. Conditions that weaken a bone and make it susceptible to fracture include:

1. Generalized Disorders in Children

   - Osteogenesis imperfecta

   - Rickets

2. Generalized Disorders in Adults

   - Osteomalacia

   - Osteosclerosis

   - Hyperparathyroidism

3. Generalized Disorders in the Aged

   - Osteoporosis of bone (senile or postmenopausal)

   - Paget's disease of bone

   - Carcinomatosis

   - Multiple Myelomatosis

4. Local Lesions, Benign

   - Solitary bone cyst in children and adolescents

   - Parathyroid lesion (localized)

   - Enchondroma of bone in hands and feet

   - Osteomyelitis

5. Malignant Lesions

   - Secondary deposit in bone from primary lesion in the thyroid, bronchus, breast, kidney, or prostate

   - Primary malignant turmor in bone (eg, Ewing's tumor)

Pathological fractures are coded in category M84.4–. A seventh character is required to indicate the treatment encounter. The pathological fracture is designated as the principal diagnosis when the patient is being treated soley for the pathological fracture. If the reason for treatment is the underlying condition, the condition is coded as the principal diagnosis.

Coding of pathological fractures is discussed in Chapter 10 of this text. Codes for traumatic fractures are located in the Injury and Poisoning Section of ICD-10-CM. Traumatic fractures are discussed in Chapter 11 of this text.

The coder must differentiate between traumatic, accident-induced fractures and spontaneous, pathological fractures (a fracture with or without trauma that would not normally occur in a healthy bone). Always code the pathological fracture to M84.–; this code is based on site and laterality. If the underlying condition of the pathological fracture in known, always code the underlying condition as the secondary diagnosis when treatment is for the pathological fracture. A physician diagnosis of spontaneous fracture is coded in category M84.–, regardless of whether the documentation includes the underlying condition.

Review the following example. Open the ICD-10-CM codebook and, referencing both the Alphabetic Index and the Tabular List, locate the correct diagnosis code(s).

> **EXAMPLE:** *A 62-year-old female with a 3-week history of hip pain is diagnosed with a fracture of the femoral neck on the right side. The problem is further complicated by the fact that the patient has multiple myeloma.*
>
> **Alphabetic Index:**
> *Main term* → *fracture* → *pathological* → *due to neoplastic disease NEC* → *M84.5–*
>
> **Tabular List:**
> *M84.551* → *Pathologic fracture in neoplastic disease right femur*

But wait! The documetation also indicates the patient suffers from multiple myelomas, and this is the underlying condition.

Alphabetic Index:
   Main term ➡ myeloma (multiple) ➡ C90.0–

Tabular List:
   C90.00 ➡ Multiple myeloma not having achieved remission

Correct code(s):
   M84.551, C90.00

CODING TIP When the documentation indicates a spontaneous fracture, code the encounter as a pathological fracture.

CODING TIP When the sole purpose is treatment of the pathological or spontaneous fracture, the patholgic fracture is the first listed diagnosis.

Malunion of a Fracture

The term "malunion" implies that bony healing has occurred, but that the fracture fragments are in poor position. Treatment of a malunion, in general, involves the surgical cutting of the bone (osteotomy), repositioning the bone, and usually the addition of some type of internal fixation with or without bone graft. Malunions are frequently diagnosed during a fracture's healing stages. Many malunions may be left without surgical intervention in hopes that the patient will have no functional problems. Surgery is usually required to reduce functional disability or pain as a result of the poor anatomical position of the bones.

Nonunion of a Fracture

"Nonunion" indicates that healing has not occurred between two fracture parts. Treatment of a nonunion, in general, involves opening the fracture, scraping away the intervening soft tissue (usually scar tissue), and performing a partial debridement of the bone end with repositioning of the bone. Usually, some type of internal fixation and bone grafting is also performed. The treatment of a nonunion is more complicated and difficult to perform than treatment of a malunion.

Because either the malunion or nonunion of a fracture is considered a "late effect" of a fracture, the late effect is referred to as sequelae. Codes may be assigned at any time after the acute injury.

Review the following example. Open the ICD-10-CM codebook and, referencing both the Alphabetic Index and the Tabular List, locate the correct diagnosis code(s).

EXAMPLE: *A 37-year-old patient was previously treated by external fixation for a displaced left tibial fracture. There is now a nonunion of the left proximal tibia, and he is admitted for open reduction of tibia with bone grafting. Approximately 20 grams of cancellous bone were harvested from the iliac crest. The fracture site was exposed and the area of nonunion was osteotomized, cleaned, and repositioned. Interfragmentary compression was applied, and 3 screws and the harvested bone graft were packed into the fracture site.*

Alphabetic Index:
   Fracture ➡ traumatic ➡ tibia (shaft) ➡ comminuted (displaced) ➡ S82.25-

Tabular List:
   S82.25 ➡ Displaced commimited fracture of shaft ➡ left tibia ➡ S82.252 ➡ S82.252S ➡ sequela

Correct code:
   S82.252S Displaced comminuted fracture of left tibia sequela (late effect)

Stress Fractures

Stress fractures usually occur in weight-bearing bones and are caused by repeated minimal stresses, such as overuse or repetitive jarring of the bone. Such fractures can occur following unaccustomed strenuous exercise in patients. Stress fractures commonly occur in the metatarsals of the foot, lumbar spine, upper tibia and fibula, and neck of the femur.

Stress fractures are coded to subclassification M84.3–. Typically, the patient has diffuse pain of a few weeks duration, with no history of any specific injury to the site. The patient may complain of localized tenderness of the site. X-rays may show a hairline crack in the bone and there may be some callus around the site.

Review the following example. Open the ICD-10-CM codebook, and referencing both the Alphabetic Index and the Tabular List, locate the correct diagnosis code(s).

EXAMPLE: *A patient presents to the emergency room with complaint of soreness in the right leg. After a detailed history, the physician discovers that the patient is training for the Boston Marathon and had only run on occasion prior to beginning his training. X-rays are taken, and it is discovered that the patient has a hairline fracture of the right tibia. The physician diagnoses the patient with a stress fracture of the right tibia.*

Alphabetic Index:
  Main term → *Fracture* → *stress* → *tibia* → *M84.36*

Tabular List:
  M84.36 → *Stress fracture of the tibia or fibula* →
  M84.361 → *right* → *M84.361A* → *Stress fracture
  of right tibia, initial encounter*

Correct code:
  M84.361A

CHECKPOINT EXERCISE 8-3

**Using your ICD-10-CM codebook, code the
following:**

1. _____ Osteoarthritis of the neck

2. _____ Systemic lupus erythematosus with
   lung involvement

3. _____ Flat foot, both feet

4. _____ A patient was treated by the orthopedic surgeon for a pathologic fracture
   of the ankle.

5. _____ Disuse osteoporosis

6. _____ Systemic chondromalacia

7. _____ Pyogenic arthritis due to a staph infection. The patient also has Libman-Sacks
   disease with nephritis, which is stable.

8. _____ Cyst of the semilunar cartilage

9. _____ Caplan's syndrome

10. _____ Lumbosacral radiculitis

11. _____ A 46-year-old patient with painful rheu-
    matoid arthritis undergoes an arthrodesis
    of the distal radioulnar joint with removal
    of a 1.5-cm segment of ulnar immediately
    proximal to the distal radioulnar joint.

12. _____ A 23-year-old male who previously
    suffered a metacarpal fracture of the
    left hand, 2nd metacarpal bone, as the
    result of a gunshot wound develops a
    nonunion of the metacarpal.

13. _____ Tenosynovitis

14. _____ A 12-month-old child presents with a
    complex complete syndactyly of the
    long and ring fingers of the right hand.

15. _____ A 12-year-old patient with neuromus-
    cular disease presents with severe hip
    flexion contracture of 110 degrees bilat-
    erally. The contracture has precluded
    the patient from sitting in a wheel chair
    or using braces for erect posture.

Diseases of the Genitourinary System (N00-N99)

Chapter 10 in the Tabular List includes the following
sections:

- Glomerular Diseases (N00-N08)

- Renal Tubulo-Interstitial Diseases (N10-N16)

- Acute Kidney Failure and Chronic Kidney Disease
  (N17-N19)

- Urolithiasis (N20-N23)

- Other Disorders of Kidneys and Ureter (N25-N29)

- Other Disease of the Urinary System (N30-N39)

- Diseases of Male Genital Organs (N40-N53)

- Disorders of Breast (N60-N65)

- Inflammatory Diseases of Female Pelvic Organs
  (N70-N77)

- Noninflammatory Disorders of Female Genital Tract
  (N80-N98)

- Intraoperative and Postprocedural Complications
  and Disorders of Genitourinary System, Not
  Elsewhere Classified (N99)

GLOMERULAR DISEASES

This section excludes hypertensive kidney disease (kidney disease caused by hypertension), which is found
in category I12.–. Some of the diseases coded in this
section include:

- *Nephritis*: inflammation of the kidney.

- *Glomerulonephritis*: a form of nephritis in which the
  lesions involve primarily the glomerulus (bundle of
  capillaries that act as filters in the formation of urine
  in the kidney). Can be acute, subacute, or chronic,
  and the disease is generally bilateral.

- *Nephrotic syndrome*: occurs when damage to glom-
  eruli results in retention of body fluids and loss of
  vital proteins.

- *Nephrosis*: condition in which there are degenerative
  changes in the kidneys without the occurrence of
  inflammation.

- *Renal failure*: decline in kidney efficiency; can
  be acute or chronic. Chronic renal failure is also
  referred to as chronic uremia (toxic condition associated with renal insufficiency and the retention in the
  blood of substances normally excreted by the kidney).

Many of these conditions result from previous infections or other pathology, for example, systemic diseases

such as infectious hepatitis. In these cases, both the Alphabetic Index and the Tabular List instruct the coder to code first the underlying disease.

Review the following example. Open the ICD-10-CM codebook and, referencing both the Alphabetic Index and the Tabular List, locate the correct diagnosis code(s).

> **EXAMPLE:** *A patient is diagnosed with uncontrolled insulin-dependent diabetes mellitus that has resulted in nephrotic syndrome due to the diabetes.*
>
> **Alphabetic Index:**
> Syndrome ➞ Nephrotic (congenital) (see also Nephrosis) ➞ N04.9 ➞ with ➞ diabetic ➞ see diabetes nephrosis ➞ diabetes, diabetic, Type 1 ➞ nephropathy ➞ E10.21
>
> **Correct code:**
> E10.21 Diabetes mellitus with diabetic nephropathy

Note: Diabetes mellitus includes combination codes to identify the type of diabetes mellitus and any associated manifestations.

CODING TIP When a patient has diabetes with chronic kidney disease, there is a combination code to identify the kidney disease and the type of diabetes, which is not coded in the genitourinary chapter but using a diabetes code.

CHRONIC KIDNEY DISEASE

Chronic Kidney Disease (CKD) is classified into category N18, End stage renal disease (ESRD) or chronic kidney disease (CKD), which is the stage of kidney impairment that requires either a regular course of dialysis or kidney transplantation. ESRD occurs from the destruction of normal kidney tissue over a long period of time. Often, there are no symptoms until the kidney has lost more than half of its function. The loss of kidney function in ESRD is usually irreversible and permanent, with the patient most commonly on dialysis.

The term "end stage renal disease" is the technically accurate term for the stage of chronic kidney disease that requires a continuing course of dialysis or kidney transplantation to improve uremic symptoms and to maintain life. The term "chronic kidney disease" alone does not describe this stage of kidney disease completely because many chronic kidney conditions do not require maintenance dialysis or kidney transplant. The stage of kidney disease should be documented in the medical record. The term "end stage" may denote a terminal condition to patients not familiar with this language. "Chronic kidney disease" is the recommended term. Chronic kidney disease often requires

dialysis or transplantation. It develops as a complication of other diseases such as primary hypertension, nephrosis, systemic lupus erythematosus, glomerulonephritis, or polycystic kidney disease, to name a few. Chronic renal failure is coded in category N18.9. There is no further specificity for this condition.

Acute kidney failure (AKF) is coded in category N17.–. AKF is the rapid breakdown of renal (kidney) function that occurs when high levels of uremic toxins (waste products of the body's metabolism) accumulate in the blood. Acute renal failure occurs when the kidneys are unable to excrete (discharge) the daily load of toxins into the urine.

The kidneys filter wastes and excrete fluid by using the bloodstream's own natural pressure. There are numerous potential causes of damage to the kidneys, which include:

- Decreased blood flow may occur when there is extremely low blood pressure caused by trauma, complicated surgery, septic shock, hemorrhage, or burns; associated dehydration; or other severe or complicated illnesses.

- Acute tubular necrosis may occur when tissues aren't getting enough oxygen or when the renal artery is blocked or narrowed.

- Overexposure to metals, solvents, radiographic contrast materials, certain antibiotics, and other medications or substances can cause damage to the kidneys.

- Myoglobinuria (myoglobin in the urine) may be caused by rhabdomyolysis, alcohol abuse, a crush injury, tissue death of muscles from any cause, seizures, and other disorders.

- Direct injury to the kidney.

- Infections such as acute pyelonephritis or septicemia.

- Urinary tract obstruction, such as a narrowing of the urinary tract (stricture), tumors, kidney stones, nephrocalcinosis, or an enlarged prostate with subsequent acute bilateral obstructive uropathy.

- Severe acute nephritic syndrome.

- Disorders of the blood, such as idiopathic thrombocytopenic purpura transfusion reaction, or other hemolytic disorders, malignant hypertension, and disorders resulting from childbirth, such as bleeding placenta or placental previa.

- Autoimmune disorders such as scleroderma.

In young children, hemolytic uremic syndrome is an increasingly common cause of acute renal failure. A toxin-secreting bacterium, *Escherichia coli* (*E coli*), which is found in contaminated undercooked meats, has been implicated as the cause of hemolytic uremic syndrome.

Symptoms include:

- Decreased urine output
- No urine output
- Excessive urination at night
- Edema
- Generalized fluid retention
- Decrease in sensation
- Changes in mental status/mood
- Sluggish movement
- Hand tremor
- Nausea and vomiting
- Seizures
- Prolonged bleeding or bruising
- Flank pain
- Fatigue
- Breath odor
- Breast development in males
- Ear noise/buzzing

Coding Issues

Because there is a relationship with other conditions such as hypertension and diabetes mellitus, there are specific coding rules for both conditions when kidney disease is present.

Hypertensive chronic kidney disease is coded to category I12.–, Hypertensive chronic kidney disease, or to category I13.–, Hypertensive heart and kidney disease when there is a cause and effect. The fifth digit indicates whether the renal failure is a component of the hypertension. See Chapter 7 of this text for the Official Guidelines for reporting hypertensive chronic kidney disease.

Review Table 8.3.

Review the following example. Open the ICD-10-CM codebook and, referencing both the Alphabetic Index and the Tabular List, locate the correct diagnosis code(s).

> **EXAMPLE:** *A 54-year-old hypertensive male with hypertensive chronic kidney disease is in end stage and is now on dialysis. His lifestyle has him frequently eating at restaurants. There are remarkable changes in intake from day to day, and his phosphorus level is rarely controlled. His blood pressure is not well controlled with medication and is malignant.*

> **Alphabetic Index:**
> *Main term → Hypertension → with → stage 5 chronic kidney disease (CKD) or end stage renal disease (ESRD) → I12.0*

> **Tabular List**
> *I12.0 → Hypertensive chronic kidney disease with stage 5 chronic kidney disease or end stage renal diease*

The instructional notes indicate that an additional code is to be used to identify the stage of the chronic kidney disease with N18.5 or N18.6.

TABLE 8.3　　Official Guidelines for Coding and Reporting Chronic Kidney Disease

Chronic kidney disease (CKD)	The ICD-10-CM classifies CKD based on severity. The severity of CKD is designated by stages 1 through 5.
Stages of CKD	Stage 2, code N18.2, equates to mild CKD; stage 3, code N18.3, equates to moderate CKD; and stage 4, code N18.4, equates to severe CKD.
	Code N18.6, End stage renal disease (ESRD), is assigned when the provider has documented ESRD.
	If both a stage of CKD and ESRD are documented, assign code N18.6 only.
CKD and kidney transplant status	Patients who have undergone kidney transplant may still have some form of CKD because the kidney transplant may not fully restore kidney function. Therefore, the presence of CKD alone does not constitute a transplant complication.
	Assign the appropriate N18 code for the patient's stage of CKD and code Z94.0, Kidney transplant status.
	If kidney failure or rejection or other transplant complication is documented, see section I.C.19.g for information on coding complications of a kidney transplant. If the documentation is unclear as to whether the patient has a complication of the transplant, query the provider.
CKD with other conditions	Patients with CKD may also suffer from other serious conditions, most commonly diabetes mellitus or hypertension.
	The sequencing of the CKD code in relationship to codes for other contributing conditions is based on the conventions in the Tabular List.

Source: ICD-10-CM Official Guidelines, Chapter 14, Diseases of Genitourinary System (N00-N99)

Alphabetic Index:
    Failure ➞ kidney ➞ end stage (chronic) N18.6

Tabular List:
    N18.6 ➞ End stage renal disease

You're not finished yet! Because the patient is on dialysis, the instructional note directs the user to report the dialysis status with Z99.2.

Tabular List:
    Z99.2 ➞ Dependence on renal dialysis

Correct code sequencing:
    I12.0, N18.6, Z99.2

Review the following example. Open the ICD-10-CM codebook and code the following patient encounter:

EXAMPLE: *A 64-year-old type 1 IDDM male visits his nephrologist and complains of frequent chest pain and headaches; he is mildly noncompliant with diet. He has occasional problems with his fistula and often requires a longer session for fluid control. He is in stage 5 CKD, nephropathy. The physician evaluates the patient, increases medication dosage, and tells him that he will need dialysis within the next few months.*

In the example above, the coder will code the IDDM as the primary diagnosis and the chronic kidney disease as the secondary diagnosis.

Alphabetic Index:
    Diabetes ➞ Type 1 ➞ with ➞ chronic kidney disease ➞ E10.22

Tabular List:
    E10.22 ➞ Type 1 diabetes mellitus with diabetic chronic kidney disease

There is an instructional note that instructs the coder to use an additional code to identify the stage of the chronic kidney disease.

Alphabetic Index:
    Failure ➞ kidney ➞ chronic ➞ stage 5 ➞ N18.5

Tabular List:
    N18.5 ➞ Chronic kidney disease, stage 5

Correct code sequencing:
    E10.22, N18.5

OTHER DISEASES OF THE URINARY SYSTEM (N30-N39)

Some of the diseases found in this section include the following:

■ Pyelonephritis: inflammation of the kidney pelvis; can be acute or chronic

■ Hydronephrosis: abnormal accumulation of urine in the kidney and renal pelvis due to obstruction

■ Urinary stones (calculi): caused by crystallization of minerals in the urine to form hard, stone-like masses in various locations within the urinary tract, including the kidneys, ureters, and bladder

■ Cystitis: inflammation of the bladder, most commonly caused by *Escherichia coli* (*E coli*), or other gram-negative bacteria such as Proteus, Pseudomonas, *Enterobacter*, and *Klebsiella*. The classic symptoms of cystitis are dysuria (painful urination), urgency, and frequency. Infectious organisms can invade the urinary tract via the urethra. The urethral route is most plaguing to women. In the male, the long penile urethra plus the presence of antibacterial secretions from the prostate discourage this route.

■ Urethritis: inflammation of the urethra

Look for notes that instruct the coder to use an additional code to identify the infectious agent causing inflammation or to identify associated signs and symptoms.

Review the following examples. Open the ICD-10-CM codebook and code the following patient encounter:

EXAMPLE: *A 23-year-old woman is seen by her family doctor for dysuria, urinary frequency, and urgency. She is diagnosed as having acute cystitis due to* Escherichia coli.

Alphabetic Index:
    Cystitis (Main term) ➞ Acute with dysuria ➞ N30.0

Tabular List:
    N30.00 ➞ Acute cystitis without hematuria

The category note instructs the coder to use an additional code to identify the infectious agent (B95-B97).

Tabular List:
    B96.2 ➞ Escherichia coli [E coli] as the cause of diseases classified elsewhere (secondary diagnosis)

Correct code sequencing:
    N30.00, B96.2

EXAMPLE: *A 40-year-old woman has developed a bladder neck obstruction, which has led to postvoid dribbling (inability to control urine flow after urination).*

Alphabetic Index:
    Obstruction (Main term) ➞ Bladder neck (acquired—meaning she developed the condition) ➞ N32.0

Tabular List:
    N32.0 ➞ Bladder neck obstruction

In order to code the encounter completely, we need an additional diagnosis code to identify the patient's postvoid dribbling in addition to the bladder neck obstruction. Can you find the code for postvoid dribbling?

Correct codes:
N32.0 Bladder neck obstruction (first listed diagnosis)

N39.43 Postvoid dribbling (secondary diagnosis)

Correct coding sequence:
N32.0, N39.43

DISEASES OF MALE GENITAL ORGANS (N40-N53)

Diseases of the male genital organs are included in this section because of the anatomic interconnection between the male urinary system and the male reproductive system. Review some of the conditions that are coded in this section prior to coding.

Hyperplasia of the prostate is an enlargement of the prostate, also referred to as hypertrophy. This is usually benign (benign prostatic hypertrophy, or BPH). The most common symptom of prostatic hyperplasia is difficulty initiating and stopping urination. The major complication of prostatic enlargement is obstruction of the urinary tract at the outlet of the bladder. Urinary tract infections frequently occur because of the obstruction. The usual treatment is surgical resection of the gland, and the most common surgical procedure is transurethral resection (TUR) of the excessive prostatic tissue.

CODING TIP Remember that the word "and" in ICD-10-CM means "and/or."

Review the following example. Open the ICD-10-CM codebook and code the following patient encounter:

EXAMPLE: *A 69-year-old male visits his family physician for his 3-month checkup. The physician examines the prostate and notices an enlarged protate during the digital rectal examination. The physician schedules the patient for a biopsy of the prostate to rule out cancer. The physician performs a prostatotomy and removs a fibroadenoma during the encounter. No obstruction is noted. The physician diagnoses the encounter as fibroadenoma of the prostate.*

Alphabetic Index:
Fibroadenoma → prostate → D29.1

Tabular List:
D29.1 → Benign neoplasm of prostate

Correct code:
D29.1

Prostatitis is an inflammation of the prostate that can be acute or chronic and is often associated with considerable pain and discomfort. Orchitis is an inflammation of the testes. Epididymitis is an inflammation of the epididymis (located on the posterior side of each testis and constituting the first part of the excretory duct of each testis).

Review the following example:

EXAMPLE: *A patient is diagnosed with prostatocystitis (inflammation of the prostate and bladder) due to streptococcus.*

Alphabetic Index:
Prostatocystitis (Main term) → N41.3

Tabular List:
N41.3 → Prostatocystitis

There is an instructional note to use an additional code to identify the infectious agent (B95-B97). In this example, the infection is due to streptococcus, but the type is not known.

Tabular List:
B95.5 → Unspecified streptococcus as the cause of diseases classified elsewhere

Correct code sequencing:
N41.3, B95.5

This is an example of a combination code that defines two conditions into one diagnosis code:

- Inflammation of the prostate (N41.9)

- Inflammation of the bladder (N30.9-)

When both of these conditions occur at the same time, there is one code (a combination code) that is used, because these conditions often occur together in males due to of the proximity of the two structures (the prostate sits on either side of the neck of the bladder). When there is a combination code for a diagnostic statement, the index will direct you to that code.

Fibroadenomas of the breast (benign tumors of the breast) are not coded in this section but are coded in Chapter 2 of ICD-10-CM (neoplasms).

DISORDERS OF BREAST (N60-N65)

Although this section of codes would appear to be used to report disorders of the female breast, some of the codes listed in this section apply to both men and women. For example, hypertrophy of breast includes gynecomastia (enlargement of the male breast). Some conditions that are coded from this section include benign mammary dysplasia, which is also referred to as fibrocystic disease, and fibrous masses or cysts, part of a hormonally mediated proliferative condition. Other disorders of the breast include inflammatory disease (eg, abscess, mastitis), hypertrophy, atrophy, and galactocele (milk-filled cyst of the breast caused by a blocked milk duct). This section also includes signs and symptoms in the breast that may require further investigation, including mastodynia (pain in the breast), lump or mass in breast, and nipple discharge.

Review the following example. Open the ICD-10-CM codebook and code the following patient encounter:

> **EXAMPLE:** *A 57-year-old female presents after having a routine mammogram, which shows a 1.5-cm ill-defined mass in the left breast, and an ultrasound, in which the mass is found to be heterogenous and solid. A histologic diagnosis is indicated. In order to more accurately discuss her diagnosis and treatment options, the decision is made, with the patient's consent, to perform an image-guided percutaneous needle core breast biopsy, with imaging guidance. A biopsy is performed and the patient is diagnosed with fibrocystic breast disease.*

> **Alphabetic Index:**
> Fibrocystic ➝ see mathopathy cystic (chronic) (diffuse) ➝ N60.1–

> **Tabular List:**
> N60.1– ➝ Diffuse cystic mastopathy of left breast ➝ N60.12

> **Correct code:**
> N60.12

INFLAMMATORY DISEASE OF FEMALE PELVIC ORGANS (N70-N77)

This section begins with a note to use an additional code(s) for infectious agent, such as staphylococcus or streptococcus. This section excludes inflammatory diseases of the female pelvic organs that are associated with pregnancy, abortion, childbirth, or the puerperium; these are located in Chapter 15 of ICD-10-CM. This section includes acute and chronic inflammatory conditions of the:

- Ovary, fallopian tube, pelvic cellular tissue, and peritoneum

- Uterus, except the cervix

- Cervix, vagina, and vulva

Review the following example. Open the ICD-10-CM codebook and code the following patient encounter:

> **EXAMPLE:** *A 32-year-old female patient complains of swelling and pain around the labial folds. Upon examination, an abscess of the Bartholin's gland (mucus-secreting gland located on each side of the vagina) is found. The*

abscess is incised and drained; a culture is taken of the material drained from the abscess, which shows a staphylococcus infection. The patient is placed on appropriate antibiotic therapy.

> **Alphabetic Index:**
> Abscess (Main term) ➝ Bartholin's gland ➝ N75.1

> **Tabular List:**
> N75.1 ➝ Abscess of Bartholin's gland

Don't forget that there is a note at the beginning of the section instructing the coder to assign an additional code to identify the infectious agent, in this case, staphylococcus.

> **Correct codes:**
> N75.1 Abscess of Bartholin's gland (first listed diagnosis)
>
> B95.8 Staphylococcus (secondary diagnosis)

> **Correct coding sequence:**
> N75.1, B95.8

NONINFLAMMATORY DISORDERS OF FEMALE GENITAL TRACT (N80-N98)

This section includes endometriosis, which is a benign condition in which endometrial material is present outside of the endometrial cavity. Some common sites of endometriosis are the ovaries, uterus, and fallopian tubes.

Genital prolapse is downward displacement or weakness in the walls of the organs of reproduction. This category of codes instructs the coder to use an additional code to identify urinary incontinence associated with the genital prolapse. Some of the conditions included are:

- Cystocele: a hernia of the bladder wall into the vagina causing a soft anterior fullness

- Rectocele: herniation of the terminal rectum into the posterior vagina, causing a collapsible pouch-like fullness

- Enterocele: a vaginal vault hernia containing small intestine, usually in the posterior vagina

Review the following example of multiple coding from this classification. Open the ICD-10-CM codebook and code the following patient encounter:

> **EXAMPLE:** *A 49-year-old woman complains of a sense of heaviness in her pelvis, low backache, dribbling urine even after voiding, and problems with constipation and straining to have a bowel movement. The patient is diagnosed with cystocele with complete uterine prolapse and postvoid dribbling (incontinence of urine).*

Alphabetic Index:
Prolapse → vagina → With prolapse of uterus → Complete → N81.3

Incontinence (main term) → post-void dribbling → N39.43

Tabular List:
N81.3 → Uterovaginal prolapse, complete (first listed diagnosis)

N39.43 → Post-void dribbling (secondary diagnosis)

Correct code sequencing:
N81.3, N39.43

Review this example. Open the ICD-10-CM codebook and code the following patient encounter:

EXAMPLE: A 28-year-old presents with a history of previous episodes of a tender, cystic-feeling mass in the area of the Bartholin's gland and duct. Physical examination confirms that the structure in question is not a hydrocele, Skene's gland, cyst, or solid tumor such as fibroma, fibromyoma, lipoma, or hidrodenoma, but rather a cyst/abscess of the Bartholin's gland and duct. The patient has previously been treated with incision and drainage, marsupialization, and catheter epithelialization, but eitology is not known at this time. The patient is advised that, in cases of symptomatic cysts, refractory to other therapies, excision under anesthesia in the operating room is indicated. Because of this, the patient consents to undergoing an excision of a Bartholin's gland and duct cyst or cyst/abscess.

Alphabetic Index:
Cyst → Bartholin's gland → N75.0

Tabular List:
N75.0 → Cyst of Bartholin's gland

Correct code:
N75.0

Note that in this example, under Category N75–, there is an instructional note to code first the underlying disease. In this example, the underlying disease is not known, therefore, it is not coded.

Review this example. Open the ICD-10-CM codebook and code the following patient encounter:

EXAMPLE: On June 1, 20xx, this 45-year-old female patient presents with pelvic pain and vaginal discharge. The gynecologic exam reveals the external genitalia to be normal anatomically. Cervix appears inflamed, without aceto-white areas. Vagina appears normal. Vaginal discharge is white and watery. Uterus is normal anteverted. The uterus is normal size and shape, tender to movement and movable. Bladder not tender. The physician performs

a Pap and pelvic and sends the specimen to the lab. After receipt of the lab results, the patient is asked to return on June 7, 20xx, for her results. The physician diagnoses the patient with moderate squamous dysplasia.

Alphabetic Index:
Dysplasia → cervix (uteri) → moderate → N87.1

Tabular List:
N87.1 → Moderate cervical dysplasia

Correct code:
N87.1

CHECKPOINT EXERCISE 8-4

Using your ICD-10-CM codebook, code the following:

1. _____ Enlargement of the male breasts bilaterally

2. _____ Chronic pelvic inflammatory disease

3. _____ Intestinouterine fistula

4. _____ Torsion of testis

5. _____ Ovarian cyst

6. _____ Staghorn calculus

7. _____ Impotence of organic origin

8. _____ Endometriosis of ovaries

9. _____ Acute glomerulonephritis due to infectious hepatitis

10. _____ Rupture of bladder (nontraumatic)

11. _____ A 25-year-old who recently delivered vaginally has begun complaining of vaginal pain. An examination reveals a large hematoma in the vaginal canal. The patient is taken to the operating room and the vaginal wall is incised and the hematoma evacuated under anesthesia.

12. _____ A 58-year-old man with left flank pains. Studies demonstrate a left hydronephrosis. The patient elects endoscopic rather than open surgical treatment.

13. _____ A 66-year-old man has a staghorn (branched) calculus filling the entire right renal pelvis and most calyces.

14. _____ Adhesions of the ovaries and fallopian tubes

15. _____ Peripelvic cyst

Test Your Knowledge

Assign codes for the following diagnostic statements.

1. _____ Code a closed treatment of radial and ulnar shaft fractures of the right wrist, with manipulation, initial care performed by the orthopedic surgeon in the emergency room of a local hospital.

2. _____ A juvenile falls and sustains a fracture of the humeral epicondylar, which is reduced anatomically and is percutaneously pinned.

3. _____ Paronychia of right index finger

4. _____ Recurrent dislocation of the right shoulder

5. _____ A 16-year-old female developed a keloid on her right ear 3 weeks after having her ears pierced.

6. _____ Heat rash

7. _____ Two-month-old child with congenital dislocation of both hips

8. _____ Right leg pain that is a late effect of an old tibial stress fracture

9. _____ Laceration of right hand from assault with a knife

10. _____ A 56-year-old female was experiencing severe right knee pain. She went to an orthopedic surgeon for evaluation. After the physician examined the patient and took x-rays of both the right and left knees, the patient was diagnosed with degenerative osteoarthritis of both knees. The physician prescribed a course of medication and physical therapy for the patient.

11. _____ A patient with chronic back pain was referred to the radiology department for chronic low back pain. The radiology report indicated there was no marrow space abnormality, and the conus medullaris is unremarkable. L4-L5: There is a minor diffusely bulging annulus at L4-L5. A small focal disc bulge is seen in far lateral position on the left at L4-L5 within the neural foramen. No definite encroachment on the exiting nerve root at this site is seen. No significant spinal stenosis is identified. L5-S1: There is a diffusely bulging annulus at L5-S1, with a small focal disc bulge centrally at this level. There is minor disc desiccation and disc space narrowing at L5-S1. No significant spinal stenosis is seen at L5-S1. The final diagnosis is minor degenerative disc disease at L4-L5 and L5-S1, as described.

12. _____ A patient is treated by an orthopedic surgeon for osteoarthritis of the right knee. The patient complained of chronic knee pain that worsens at night. The physician prescribed an anti-inflammatory drug to relieve the pain.

13. _____ A 24-year-old patient was seen in the outpatient dermatology clinic at the local hospital. His complaints were moderate itching, which then became severe (pruritus). He also noticed small blisters, redness, and swelling of his lower legs. It was documented that the patient had come in contact with poison ivy. The patient was diagnosed with contact dermatitis due to poison ivy.

14. _____ A 16-month-old patient was seen in the pediatric clinic for a rash on his bottom. He had been taking cephalexin as prescribed. After evaluation, the diagnosis was dermatitis due to an adverse reaction to the cephalexin. A topical cream was prescribed for the patient and cephalexin was discontinued.

15. _____ A patient was seen in the outpatient clinic at the local hospital for treatment of her actinic keratosis 5 lesions of the right arm. Cryosurgery was performed on 5 lesions.

(continued)

Test Your Knowledge *(continued)*

16. _____ Traumatic arthritis following fracture of the left ankle 3 years ago

17. _____ Leg pain from old fracture of femur

18. _____ Foreign body (steel) penetration of the right eyeball and laceration of the periocular area (skin)

19. _____ A patient with difficulty with left shoulder function and deltoid muscle function is in the hospital radiology department for a left shoulder arthrogram to determine if there is a cuff defect. The radiologist diagnosed the patient with rotator cuff syndrome.

20. _____ A patient with a 4.1-cm infected sebaceous cyst on the back and a 2.5-cm infected sebaceous cyst on the neck undergoes surgical excision in the dermatologist's office.

Pregnancy, Childbirth, Puerperium, Conditions Originating in the Perinatal Period, and Congenital Malformations (O00-Q99)

LEARNING OBJECTIVES

- Understand Coding Guidelines for Complications of Pregnancy, Childbirth, and the Puerperium

- Understand Coding Guidelines for the Perinatal Period

- Understand Coding Guidelines for Congenital Malformations, Deformations, and Chromosomal Abnormalities

- Assign ICD-10-CM codes to the highest level of specificity

- Successfully complete checkpoint exercises and test your knowledge exercises

Chapter 15 in the Tabular List includes the following sections:

- Pregnancy with abortive outcome (O00-O08)

- Supervision of high-risk pregnancy (O09)

- Edema, proteinuria, and hypertensive disorders in pregnancy, childbirth, and the puerperium (O10-O16)

- Other maternal disorders predominately related to pregnancy (O20-O29)

- Maternal care related to the fetus and amniotic cavity and possible delivery problems (O30-O48)

- Complications of labor and delivery (O60-O77)

- Encounter for delivery (O80-O82)

- Complications predominately related to the puerperium (O85-O92)

- Other obstetric conditions, not classified elsewhere (O94-O9A)

Chapter 15 includes codes for obstetric (OB) patients. All procedures resulting from conditions located in Chapter 15 are indicated with a procedure code. The first OB code assigned should be based on the reason for the patient encounter. The first assigned diagnosis should be the reason for the encounter. For patient encounters where no delivery occurs, the most significant complication of pregnancy should be sequenced first, if more than one complication occurs.

When delivery occurs, the principal/first listed diagnosis should correspond to the main complication or circumstance of delivery. When cesarean delivery occurs, the principal/first listed diagnosis should correspond to the reason the cesarean delivery was performed, unless the reason is unrelated to the condition resulting in the cesarean delivery. The majority of the codes beginning with category O09 identify a final character indicating the trimester of pregnancy. Time

frames of trimester are provided at the beginning of this chapter. Trimesters are counted from the first day of the last menstrual period.

Trimesters are defined as follows:

- First trimester: less than 14 weeks 0 days

- Second trimester: 14 weeks 0 days to less than 28 weeks 0 days

- Third trimester: 28 weeks 0 days until delivery

Codes for an unspecified trimester should never be reported unless it is impossible to determine the trimester from the documentation in the medical record. The provider's documentation in the medical record based on the number of weeks documented should be used in assigning the appropriate trimester of the pregnancy. Review Table 9.1.

TABLE 9.1   General Rules for Coding Obstetric Cases

Codes from Chapter 15 and sequencing priority	Obstetric cases require codes from Chapter 15, codes in the range O00-O9A, Pregnancy, childbirth, and the puerperium. Chapter 15 codes have sequencing priority over codes from other chapters. Additional codes from other chapters may be used in conjunction with Chapter 15 codes to further specify conditions.
	If the provider documents that the pregnancy is incidental to the encounter, then code Z33.1, Pregnant state, incidental, should be used in place of any Chapter 15 codes. It is the provider's responsibility to state that the condition being treated is not affecting the pregnancy.
Chapter 15 codes used only on the maternal record	Chapter 15 codes are to be used only on the maternal record, never on the record of the newborn.
Final character for trimester	The majority of codes in Chapter 15 have a final character indicating the trimester of pregnancy. The time frames for the trimesters are indicated at the beginning of the chapter. If trimester is not a component of a code, it is because the condition always occurs in a specific trimester or the concept of trimester of pregnancy is not applicable. Certain codes have characters for only certain trimesters because the condition does not occur in all trimesters, but it may occur in more than just one.
	Assignment of the final character for trimester should be based on the provider's documentation of the trimester (or number of weeks) for the current admission/encounter.
	This applies to the assignment of trimester for preexisting conditions as well as those that develop during or are due to the pregnancy.
	The provider's documentation of the number of weeks may be used to assign the appropriate code identifying the trimester.
	Whenever delivery occurs during the current admission and there is an "in childbirth" option for the obstetric complication being coded, the "in childbirth" code should be assigned.
Selection of trimester for inpatient admissions that encompass more than one trimester	In instances when a patient is admitted to a hospital for complications of pregnancy during one trimester and remains in the hospital into a subsequent trimester, the trimester character for the antepartum complication code should be assigned on the basis of the trimester when the complication developed, not the trimester of the discharge. If the condition developed prior to the current admission/encounter or represents a preexisting condition, the trimester character for the trimester at the time of the admission/encounter should be assigned.

(continued)

TABLE 9.1   *(continued)*

Unspecified trimester	Each category that includes codes for trimester has a code for "unspecified trimester." The "unspecified trimester" code should rarely be used, such as when the documentation in the record is insufficient to determine the trimester and it is not possible to obtain clarification.
Fetal extensions	Where applicable, a seventh character is to be assigned for certain categories (O31, O32, O33.3-O33.6, O35, O36, O40, O41, O60.1, O60.2, O64, and O69) to identify the fetus for which the complication code applies.
	Assign seventh character 0:
	• For single gestations
	• When the documentation in the record is insufficient to determine the fetus affected and it is not possible to obtain clarification.
	• When it is not possible to clinically determine which fetus is affected.
Selection of OB principal or first listed diagnosis Routine outpatient prenatal visits	For routine outpatient prenatal visits when no complications are present, a code from category Z34, Encounter for supervision of normal pregnancy, should be used as the first listed diagnosis. These codes should not be used in conjunction with Chapter 15 codes.
Prenatal outpatient visits for high-risk patients	For routine prenatal outpatient visits for patients with high-risk pregnancies, a code from category O09, Supervision of high-risk pregnancy, should be used as the first listed diagnosis. Secondary Chapter 15 codes may be used in conjunction with these codes if appropriate.
Episodes when no delivery occurs	In episodes when no delivery occurs, the principal diagnosis should correspond to the principal complication of the pregnancy that necessitated the encounter. If more than one complication exists, all of which are treated or monitored, any of the complication codes may be sequenced first.
When a delivery occurs	When a delivery occurs, the principal diagnosis should correspond to the main circumstances or complication of the delivery. In cases of cesarean delivery, the selection of the principal diagnosis should be the condition established after study that was responsible for the patient's admission. If the patient was admitted with a condition that resulted in the performance of a cesarean procedure, that condition should be selected as the principal diagnosis. If the reason for the admission/encounter was unrelated to the condition resulting in the cesarean delivery, the condition related to the reason for the admission/encounter should be selected as the principal diagnosis.
Outcome of delivery	A code from category Z37, Outcome of delivery, should be included on every maternal record when a delivery has occurred. These codes are not to be used on subsequent records or on the newborn record.
Preexisting conditions versus conditions due to the pregnancy	Certain categories in Chapter 15 distinguish between conditions of the mother that existed prior to pregnancy (preexisting) and those that are a direct result of pregnancy. When assigning codes from Chapter 15, it is important to assess if a condition was preexisting prior to pregnancy or developed during or due to the pregnancy in order to assign the correct code.
	Categories that do not distinguish between preexisting and pregnancy-related conditions may be used for either. It is acceptable to use codes specifically for the puerperium with codes complicating pregnancy and childbirth if a condition arises postpartum during the delivery encounter.
Preexisting hypertension in pregnancy	Category O10, Preexisting hypertension complicating pregnancy, childbirth, and the puerperium, includes codes for hypertensive heart and hypertensive chronic kidney disease. When assigning one of the O10 codes that include hypertensive heart disease or hypertensive chronic kidney disease, it is necessary to add a secondary code from the appropriate hypertension category to specify the type of heart failure or chronic kidney disease.
	See Section I.C.9, Hypertension.
Fetal conditions affecting the management of the mother Codes from categories O35 and O36	Codes from categories O35, Maternal care for known or suspected fetal abnormality and damage, and O36, Maternal care for other fetal problems, are assigned only when the fetal condition is actually responsible for modifying the management of the mother, that is, by requiring diagnostic studies, additional observation, special care, or termination of pregnancy. The fact that the fetal condition exists does not justify assigning a code from this series to the mother's record.

(continued)

TABLE 9.1   *(continued)*

In utero surgery	In cases when surgery is performed on the fetus, a diagnosis code from category O35, Maternal care for known or suspected fetal abnormality and damage, should be assigned identifying the fetal condition. Assign the appropriate procedure code for the procedure performed.
	No code from Chapter 16, the perinatal codes, should be used on the mother's record to identify fetal conditions. Surgery performed in utero on a fetus is still to be coded as an obstetric encounter.
HIV infection in pregnancy, childbirth, and the puerperium	During pregnancy, childbirth, or the puerperium, a patient admitted because of an HIV-related illness should receive a principal diagnosis from subcategory O98.7–, Human immunodeficiency (HIV) disease complicating pregnancy, childbirth, and the puerperium, followed by the code(s) for the HIV-related illness(es).
	Patients with asymptomatic HIV infection status admitted during pregnancy, childbirth, or the puerperium should receive codes from O98.7– and Z21, Asymptomatic human immunodeficiency virus [HIV] infection status.
Diabetes mellitus in pregnancy	Diabetes mellitus is a significant complicating factor in pregnancy. Pregnant women who are diabetic should be assigned a code from category O24, Diabetes mellitus in pregnancy, childbirth, and the puerperium, first, followed by the appropriate diabetes code(s) (E08-E13) from Chapter 4.
Long-term use of insulin	Code Z79.4, Long-term (current) use of insulin, should also be assigned if the diabetes mellitus is being treated with insulin.
Gestational (pregnancy-induced) diabetes	Gestational (pregnancy-induced) diabetes can occur during the second and third trimester of pregnancy in women who were not diabetic prior to pregnancy. Gestational diabetes can cause complications in the pregnancy similar to those of preexisting diabetes mellitus. It also puts the woman at greater risk of developing diabetes after the pregnancy. Codes for gestational diabetes are in subcategory O24.4, Gestational diabetes mellitus. No other code from category O24, Diabetes mellitus in pregnancy, childbirth, and the puerperium, should be used with a code from O24.4
	The codes under subcategory O24.4 include "diet controlled" and "insulin controlled." If a patient with gestational diabetes is treated with both diet and insulin, only the code for insulin-controlled is required.
	Code Z79.4, Long-term (current) use of insulin, should not be assigned with codes from subcategory O24.4.
	An abnormal glucose tolerance in pregnancy is assigned a code from subcategory O99.81, Abnormal glucose complicating pregnancy, childbirth, and the puerperium.
	Sepsis and septic shock complicating abortion, pregnancy, childbirth and the puerperium. When assigning a Chapter 15 code for sepsis complicating abortion, pregnancy, childbirth, and the puerperium, a code for the specific type of infection should be assigned as an additional diagnosis. If severe sepsis is present, a code from subcategory R65.2, Severe sepsis, and code(s) for associated organ dysfunction(s) should also be assigned as the additional diagnoses.
Puerperal sepsis	Code O85, Puerperal sepsis, should be assigned with a secondary code to identify the causal organism (eg, for a bacterial infection, assign a code from category B95-B96, Bacterial infections in conditions classified elsewhere).
	A code from category A40, Streptococcal sepsis, or A41, Other sepsis, should not be used for puerperal sepsis. If applicable, use additional codes to identify severe sepsis (R65.2–) and any associated acute organ dysfunction.
Alcohol and tobacco use during pregnancy, childbirth, and the puerperium Alcohol use during pregnancy, childbirth, and the puerperium	Codes under subcategory O99.31, Alcohol use complicating pregnancy, childbirth, and the puerperium, should be assigned for any pregnancy case when a mother uses alcohol during the pregnancy or postpartum. A secondary code from category F10, Alcohol-related disorders, should also be assigned to identify manifestations of the alcohol use.
Tobacco use during pregnancy, childbirth, and the puerperium	Codes under subcategory O99.33, Smoking (tobacco) complicating pregnancy, childbirth, and the puerperium, should be assigned for any pregnancy case when a mother uses any type of tobacco product during the pregnancy or postpartum. A secondary code from category F17, Nicotine dependence, or code Z72.0, Tobacco use, should also be assigned to identify the type of nicotine dependence.

(continued)

TABLE 9.1   *(continued)*

Poisoning, toxic effects, adverse effects, and underdosing in a pregnant patient	A code from subcategory O9A.2, Injury, poisoning, and certain other consequences of external causes complicating pregnancy, childbirth, and the puerperium, should be sequenced first, followed by the appropriate poisoning, toxic effect, adverse effect, or underdosing code, and then the additional code(s) that specifies the condition caused by the poisoning, toxic effect, adverse effect, or underdosing.
	See Section I.C.19, Adverse effects, poisoning, underdosing, and toxic effects.
Normal delivery, code O80 Encounter for full-term uncomplicated delivery	Code O80 should be assigned when a woman is admitted for a full-term normal delivery and delivers a single, healthy infant without any complications antepartum, during the delivery, or postpartum during the delivery episode.
	Code O80 is always a principal diagnosis. It is not to be used if any other code from Chapter 15 is needed to describe a current complication of the antenatal, delivery, or perinatal period. Additional codes from other chapters may be used with code O80 if they are not related to or are in any way complicating the pregnancy.
Uncomplicated delivery with resolved antepartum complication	Code O80 may be used if the patient had a complication at some point during the pregnancy, but the complication is not present at the time of the admission for delivery.
Outcome of delivery for O80	Z37.0, Single live birth, is the only outcome of delivery code appropriate for use with O80.
The peripartum and postpartum periods	The postpartum period begins immediately after delivery and continues for 6 weeks following delivery. The peripartum period is defined as the last month of pregnancy to 5 months postpartum.
Peripartum and postpartum complication	A postpartum complication is any complication occurring within the 6-week period.
Pregnancy-related complications after the 6-week period	Chapter 15 codes may also be used to describe pregnancy-related complications after the peripartum or postpartum period if the provider documents that a condition is pregnancy related.
Admission for routine postpartum care following delivery outside hospital	When the mother delivers outside the hospital prior to admission and is admitted for routine postpartum care and no complications are noted, code Z39.0, Encounter for care and examination of mother immediately after delivery, should be assigned as the principal diagnosis.
Pregnancy-associated cardiomyopathy	Pregnancy-associated cardiomyopathy, code O90.3, is unique in that it may be diagnosed in the third trimester of pregnancy but may continue to progress months after delivery. For this reason, it is referred to as peripartum cardiomyopathy. Code O90.3 is only for use when the cardiomyopathy develops as a result of pregnancy in a woman who did not have preexisting heart disease.
Code O94, Sequelae of complication of pregnancy, childbirth, and the puerperium Code O94	Code O94, Sequelae of complication of pregnancy, childbirth, and the puerperium, is for use in those cases when an initial complication of a pregnancy develops a sequela requiring care or treatment at a future date.
After the initial postpartum period	This code may be used at any time after the initial postpartum period.
Sequencing of code O94	This code, like all late effect codes, is to be sequenced following the code describing the sequela of the complication.
Abortions Abortion with liveborn fetus	When an attempted termination of pregnancy results in a liveborn fetus, assign a code from subcategory O60.1, Preterm labor with preterm delivery, and a code from category Z37, Outcome of delivery. The procedure code for the attempted termination of pregnancy should also be assigned.
Conception following an abortion	Subsequent encounters for retained products of conception following a spontaneous abortion or elective termination of pregnancy are assigned the appropriate code from category O03, Spontaneous abortion, or code O07.4, Failed attempted termination of pregnancy without complication, and Z33.2, Encounter for elective termination of pregnancy. This advice is appropriate even when the patient was discharged previously with a discharge diagnosis of complete abortion.
Abuse in a pregnant patient	For suspected or confirmed cases of abuse of a pregnant patient, a code(s) from subcategories O9A.3, Physical abuse complicating pregnancy, childbirth, and the puerperium, O9A.4, Sexual abuse complicating pregnancy, childbirth, and the puerperium, and O9A.5, Psychological abuse complicating pregnancy, childbirth, and the puerperium, should be sequenced first, followed by the appropriate codes (if applicable) to identify any associated current injury due to physical abuse, sexual abuse, and the perpetrator of abuse.
	See Section I.C.19.f, Adult and child abuse, neglect and other maltreatment.

Source: Official ICD-10-CM Guidelines for Coding and Reporting, Chapter 15, Pregnancy, Childbirth, and the Puerperium (O00-O9A)

PREGNANCY INCIDENTAL

Obstetric cases require codes from Chapter 15, Pregnancy, Childbirth, and the Puerperium (code range O00-O9a). If the physician documents that the pregnancy is incidental to the encounter, then code Z33.1, Pregnancy, incidental state, should be used in place of any Chapter 15 codes. The physician should document in the medical record that the condition being treated is not affecting the pregnancy.

Review the following example. Open up the ICD-10-CM codebook, referencing both the Alphabetic Index and the Tabular List, locate the correct code.

> **EXAMPLE:** *An obstetrician sees a pregnant woman at 28 weeks of gestation for persistent pain in her left ear that started 3 weeks ago and has gotten progressively worse. The obstetrician examines the patient, determines that she has acute serous otitis media in both ears, and places her on appropriate medication therapy. The otitis media is not related to her pregnancy.*

Sequence the code for the acute otitis media as the principal diagnosis and use Z33.1, Pregnancy, incidental state, as the secondary diagnosis because the condition being treated is not related to or affecting the pregnancy.

Alphabetic Index:
Otitis ➔ media ➔ acute ➔ serous ➔ see Otitis Media, nonsuppurative, acute, serous ➔ nonsuppurative ➔ serous ➔ acute ➔ H65.0–

Tabular List:
H65.0– ➔ H65.03 ➔ *Acute serous otitis media, bilateral*

Z33.1 ➔ *pregnancy state, incidental (secondary)*

Correct code sequencing:
H65.03, Z33.1

Chapter 15 codes have sequencing priority over codes from other chapters. Additional codes from other chapters may be used in conjunction with Chapter 15 codes to further specify conditions. Chapter 15 codes are to be used only on the maternal record, never on the record of the newborn.

An outcome of delivery code (category Z37) should be included on every maternal record when a delivery has occurred. These codes are not to be used on subsequent records or on the newborn record (Official ICD-10-CM Guidelines).

NORMAL PREGNANCY

Normal pregnancy is coded in Chapter 21 (Factors Influencing Health Status and Contact with Health Services) with category Z34, Encounter for supervision of normal pregnancy. A code from this category is selected for routine obstetric care based on trimester and whether the patient's pregnancy is the first or subsequent pregnancy. Review Figure 9.1, which is an example of code(s) for normal pregnancy. There are exclusions for complications and supervision of high-risk pregnancy as well as pregnancy testing.

FIGURE 9.1   Excerpt from the Tabular List: *Z34*

Z34   Encounter for supervision of normal pregnancy
   EXCLUDES 1   *any complication of pregnancy (O00-O99)*
      encounter for pregnancy test (Z32.0-)
      encounter for supervision of high risk
      pregnancy (O09-)
   Z34.0   Encounter for supervision of normal first pregnancy
      Z34.00   Encounter for supervision of normal first pregnancy, unspecified trimester
      Z34.01   Encounter for supervision of normal first pregnancy, first trimester
      Z34.02   Encounter for supervision of normal first pregnancy, second trimester
      Z34.03   Encounter for supervision of normal first pregnancy, third trimester

Review the following example. Open up the ICD-10-CM codebook, referencing both the Alphabetic Index and the Tabular List, locate the correct code.

> **EXAMPLE:** *This 27-year-old female presents today for an initial obstetrical examination. This is her second pregnancy. She took a home pregnancy test, which was positive. The patient indicates fetal activity is not yet detected (due to early stage of pregnancy). She is approximately 5 weeks pregnant. After a comprehensive history and physical examination, Pap smear is submitted for manual screening. Ordered CBC, blood type, hemoglobin, Rh, and fasting blood glucose. The patient is prescribed prenatal multivitamins and will return in 4 weeks for follow-up.*

Alphabetic Index:
Pregnancy ➔ normal (supervision of) ➔ specified ➔ Z34.8–

Tabular List:
Z34.8– ➔ Z34.81 ➔ *Supervision of other normal pregnancy, first trimester*

Correct code:
Z34.81

PREGNANCY WITH ABORTIVE OUTCOME

An ectopic pregnancy is any pregnancy arising from implantation of the ovum outside the cavity of the uterus. About 98% of ectopic pregnancies are tubal. Other sites of ectopic implantation are the peritoneum or abdominal viscera, the ovary, and the cervix. Peritonitis, salpingitis, abdominal surgery, and pelvic tumors may predispose to abnormally situated pregnancy. Symptoms include amenorrhea; tenderness, soreness, and pain on the affected side; and pallor, weak pulse, and signs of shock or hemorrhage. Hydatidiform mole is a rare condition that is similar to an abortion, except that the placenta undergoes degenerative cystic, edematous changes that make it resemble a bunch of grapes. It is thought to be caused by abnormal postfertilization replication of spermatozoal chromosomes.

Ectopic and abnormal products of conception are classified from O00-O08, which include the following subclassifications:

- Hydatidiform mole O01–

- Other abnormal products of conception O02–

- Spontaneous abortion O03–

- Complications following (induced) termination of pregnancy O04–

- Failed attempted termination of pregnancy O07–

- Complications following ectopic and molar pregnancy O08–

- Supervision of high-risk pregnancy O09–

Review the following example. Open up the ICD-10-CM codebook, referencing both the Alphabetic Index and the Tabular List, locate the correct code.

EXAMPLE: *A patient presents with severe abdominal pain and amenorrhea. It is determined that the patient is suffering from a ruptured intrauterine tubal pregnancy, and she is taken to surgery immediately.*

Alphabetic Index:
Pregnancy → complicated by → ectopic → tubal (with abortion)

(with rupture) → O00.1

Tabular List:
O00.1 → Tubal pregnancy

Correct code:
O00.1

An additional diagnosis code should be used to identify any complication from category (O08) whether the complication occurs during the initial encounter or during a later episode of care.

Now review this example. Open up the ICD-10-CM codebook, referencing both the Alphabetic Index and the Tabular List, locate the correct code.

EXAMPLE: *A patient presents with severe abdominal pain and amenorrhea. It is determined that the patient is suffering from a ruptured intrauterine tubal pregnancy, and she is taken to surgery immediately. The patient goes into septic shock one hour after the surgery.*

Alphabetic Index:
Pregnancy → complicated by → ectopic → tubal (with abortion)

(with rupture) → O00.1

Tabular List:
O00.1 → Tubal pregnancy with rupture

Don't forget to code the complication, which is the septic shock.

O08.3 → Shock following abortion or ectopic and molar pregnancies (secondary diagnosis)

Correct code sequencing:
O00.1, O08.3

ABORTION

An abortion is the interruption or termination of pregnancy before the fetus is considered viable. The different types of abortion include:

- Spontaneous abortion: also called miscarriage; abortion occurring without apparent cause

- Complete: an abortion in which the complete products of conception are expelled

- Incomplete: an abortion in which part of the products of conception are retained in the uterus

- Missed: an abortion in which the fetus dies before completion of the twentieth week of gestation, but the products of conception are retained in the uterus for 8 weeks or longer

- Elective abortion: voluntary termination of a pregnancy for other than medical reasons

- Therapeutic abortion: abortion performed when the pregnancy endangers the mother's mental or physical health or when the fetus has a known condition incompatible with life.

The ICD-10-CM guidelines direct the user to select a code from category O03 or O07 for subsequent encounters for retained products of conception following a spontaneous abortion. If the patient attempts to terminate the pregnancy and it results in a liveborn fetus, a code from category O60.1 is assigned. A code from category Z37 is assigned for a patient with preterm labor and delivery. A failed attempt to terminate the pregnancy is coded as Z33.2 (elective termination of pregnancy) if there are no complications.

Review the following example. Open up the ICD-10-CM codebook, referencing both the Alphabetic Index and the Tabular List, locate the correct code.

EXAMPLE: A 30-year-old patient in her first trimester of gestation suffers an incomplete spontaneous abortion (miscarriage). It is determined that the miscarriage occurred because of numerous uterine fibroids.

Alphabetic Index:
Abortion → *Spontaneous* → *see Abortion (complete) (spontaneous)* → *O03.–*

Tabular List:
O03.– → *spontaneous abortion* → *O03.4* → *Incomplete spontaneous abortion without complication*

Alphabetic Index:
Pregnancy → *Complicated (by)* → *Tumor* → *Uterus* → *O34.1–*

Tabular List:
O34.1 → *Maternal care for benign tumor or corpus uteri, first trimester*

O34.11x0 (secondary diagnosis)

Keep in mind that when reporting the complications of pregnancy, a seventh character is required. Because the correct code has five characters, a dummy placeholder, "x," must be added to the code to code to the highest level of specificity.

Correct code sequencing:
O03.4, O34.11x0

Codes from categories O60-O77, Complications occurring mainly in the course of labor and delivery, are not to be used for complications of abortion. An example is when the complication itself was responsible for an episode of medical care, the abortion or ectopic or molar pregnancy itself having been dealt with at a previous episode.

Review the following example. Open up the ICD-10-CM codebook, referencing both the Alphabetic Index and the Tabular List, to locate the correct code.

EXAMPLE: A 27-year-old woman at 10 weeks of gestation presents with bleeding, abdominal pain, and cramps of sudden onset. The patient is diagnosed as having suffered an incomplete spontaneous abortion (miscarriage) with pelvic peritonitis. She is scheduled for an immediate dilation and curettage to remove the retained products of conception.

Alphabetic Index:
Abortion → *Incomplete (spontaneous)* → *O03.4* → *complicated by (following)* → *pelvic peritonitis* → *O03.0*

Tabular List:
O03.0 → *Genital tract and pelvic infection following incomplete spontaneous abortion*

Correct code:
O03.0

SUPERVISION OF HIGH-RISK PREGNANCY (O09)

Codes in this category are to be used for prenatal care for patients with high-risk pregnancies. An example of a patient who is at high risk is one who is under 16 years of age. Review Figure 9.2, which is an illustration of supervision of high-risk pregnancy due to social problems.

FIGURE 9.2 Excerpt from the Tabular List: *O09.7*

O09.7	Supervision of high risk pregnancy due to social problems	
	O09.70	Supervision of high risk pregnancy due to social problems, unspecified trimester
	O09.71	Supervision of high risk pregnancy due to social problems, first trimester
	O09.72	Supervision of high risk pregnancy due to social problems, second trimester
	O09.73	Supervision of high risk pregnancy due to social problems, third trimester

If a trimester character is not provided for a specific code in the category, it is because the condition always occurs in a specific trimester or the trimester is not applicable, such as postpartum care.

Review the following example. Open up the ICD-10-CM codebook, referencing both the Alphabetic Index and the Tabular List, locate the correct code.

EXAMPLE: A patient with a history of infertility was being seen by a new OB/GYN. The patient presents for pregnancy care after moving to the state. She is in her sixteenth week of pregnancy and has received care from her obstetrician in the other state. She brings her records with her and the physician goes over her history and other information on the care she has already received prior to this visit. Obstetric measurements are taken, and the patient is counseled regarding her remaining care. She is otherwise healthy and will continue taking vitamins and control her diet.

Pregnancy → *supervision* → *of high risk* → *due to infertility* → *O09.0-*

Tabular List:
O09.0- → *Supervision of pregnancy with history of infertility* → *second trimester* → *O09.02*

Complications Mainly Related to Pregnancy (O10-O29)

This section includes some of the following conditions:

- Hemorrhage in early pregnancy
- Preexisting hypertension
- Preeclampsia
- Eclampsia
- Antepartum hemorrhage
- Abruptio placentae
- Placenta previa
- Excessive vomiting in pregnancy
- Early or threatened labor
- Prolonged pregnancy
- Gestational diabetes
- Preexisting diabetes mellitus
- Infections in the genitourinary tract during pregnancy
- Gestational edema
- Venous complications in pregnancy

Many of the code categories include a note to use additional code(s) to identify the condition. When referencing the Alphabetic Index, "pregnancy" should be referenced as the main term, followed by "complicated by."

Review the following example. Open up the ICD-10-CM codebook, referencing both the Alphabetic Index and the Tabular List, locate the correct code.

EXAMPLE: *A patient with gestational diabetes is seen by the obstetrician for her routine visit during her seventh month of pregnancy. The patient is doing well and her gestational diabetes is well controlled with diet. The physician counsels the patient on good prenatal care and continuing to stay on her diet and get fresh air and exercise daily.*

Review Figure 9.3.

FIGURE 9.3   Excerpt from the Tabular List: *O24.–*

O24.4	Gestational diabetes mellitus		
	Diabetes mellitus arising in pregnancy		
	Gestational diabetes mellitus NOS		
	O24.41	Gestational diabetes mellitus in pregnancy	
		O24.410	Gestational diabetes mellitus in pregnancy, diet- controlled
		O24.414	Gestational diabetes mellitus in pregnancy, insulin controlled
		O24.419	Gestational diabetes mellitus in pregnancy, unspecified control
		O24.42	Gestational diabetes mellitus in childbirth
		O24.420	Gestational diabetes mellitus in childbirth, diet controlled
		O24.424	Gestational diabetes mellitus in childbirth, insulin controlled
		O24.429	Gestational diabetes mellitus in childbirth, unspecified control
		O24.43	Gestational diabetes mellitus in the puerperium
		O24.430	Gestational diabetes mellitus in the puerperium, diet controlled
		O24.434	Gestational diabetes mellitus in the puerperium, insulin controlled
		O24.439	Gestational diabetes mellitus in the puerperium, unspecified control

Alphabetic Index:
Pregnancy → *complicated by* → *diabetes, gestational O24.–*

Tabular List:
O24.– → *O24.410 Gestational diabetes mellitus in pregnancy, diet-controlled*

Correct code:
O24.410

When a patient is admitted to the hospital due to complications of pregnancy and remains in the hospital for antepartum, delivery, and postpartum complications, the final character that corresponds to the trimester of the occurrence of the complication should be used. It is also acceptable to use codes indicating different trimesters of pregnancy as well as postpartum care within the same record. When a patient has gestational diabetes and is treated with both diet and insulin, the default is for insulin controlled.

EXAMPLE: *A patient in her third trimester develops moderate preeclampsia that complicates her pregnancy during the antepartum period.*

Alphabetic Index:
   Pregnancy → *complicated by* → *preeclampsia* →
   O14.0–

Tabular List:
   O14.0 → *O14.02* → *Mild to moderate preeclampsia,*
   second trimester

Correct code:
   O14.02

CODING TIP When coding for preexisting diabetes in pregnancy, two codes are required, one to identify the complication of pregnancy O24.-=– (diabetes mellitus in pregnancy) and one to report the diabetes in category E08-E13.

CODING FOR MULTIPLE GESTATIONS (O30)

Multiple gestations are coded using category O30–. An extension is added to codes for multiple gestations indicating which fetus is affected by a particular condition or code. Review Figure 9.4.

FIGURE 9.4   Excerpt from the Tabular List: *O30.1*

O30.1	Triplet pregnancy
	O30.10 Triplet pregnancy, unspecified trimester
	O30.11 Triplet pregnancy, first trimester
	O30.12 Triplet pregnancy, second trimester
	O30.13 Triplet pregnancy, third trimester

One of the following seventh characters is to be assigned to each code under category O31. Seventh character 0 is for single gestations and multiple gestations where the fetus is unspecified. Seventh characters 1 through 9 are for cases of multiple gestations to identify the fetus for which the code applies. The appropriate code from category O30, Multiple gestation, must also be assigned when coding from category O31. Review the character extensions for category O30 and O31:

- 0 not applicable or unspecified

- 1 fetus 1

- 2 fetus 2

- 3 fetus 3

- 4 fetus 4

- 5 fetus

- 9 other fetus

Review Figure 9.5, which is an example of category O31.1 for a patient continuing pregnancy after spontaneous abortion of one (or more) fetus.

FIGURE 9.5   Excerpt from the Tabular List: *O31.3*

O31.3	Continuing pregnancy after elective fetal reduction of one fetus or more
	Continuing pregnancy after selective termination of one fetus or more
	O31.30 Continuing pregnancy after elective fetal reduction of one fetus or more, unspecified trimester
	O31.31 Continuing pregnancy after elective fetal reduction of one fetus or more, first trimester
	O31.32 Continuing pregnancy after elective fetal reduction of one fetus or more, second trimester
	O31.33 Continuing pregnancy after elective fetal reduction of one fetus or more, third trimester

---

EXAMPLE: *A patient in her second trimester of pregnancy with 6 fetuses, underwent surgery to reduce the fetuses to 5 in hopes of survival of the other fetuses.*

Principal/first listed diagnosis:
   O31.321 Continuing pregnancy after elective fetal reduction of one fetus or more, second trimester

Note: The seventh character extension is 1 because only one fetus is reduced.

An ectopic pregnancy, which occurs with an intrauterine pregnancy and is considered a multiple gestation, is coded in category O00. Both the ectopic pregnancy and intrauterine pregnancy should be reported with an extension. Any complication resulting from the ectopic pregnancy (O08) should be reported with the same extension as O00. All codes for intrauterine pregnancy should have the same extension to distinguish them form the ectopic pregnancy codes.

ENCOUNTER FOR DELIVERY (O80-O82)

Code O80 is for use in cases when a woman is admitted for a full-term normal delivery and delivers a single, healthy infant without any complications antepartum, during the delivery, or postpartum during the delivery episode. This code is never used alone and must be accompanied by a delivery code. The first listed diagnosis code should coincide with the primary complication of the pregnancy if one exists. If more than one complication exists, all should be listed and any of the complications can be sequenced first.

Code O80 is used only when the following is documented:

- A full-term, single liveborn infant is delivered

- There are no antepartum or postpartum complications

- The presentation is cephalic, requiring minimal assistance without fetal manipulation or the use of instrumentation

- An episiotomy can be performed

A normal delivery includes the following:

- Spontaneous onset of labor

- Cephalic (head-first) vaginal delivery

- Single, liveborn infant of between 38 and 42 completed weeks of gestation

- No mention of fetal manipulation or instrumentation

- Labor less than 20 hours

Code O80 may be used if the patient had complications at some point during the pregnancy, but the complication is not present at the time of the admission for delivery. This code is always a principal diagnosis. It is not to be used if any other code from Chapter 15 is needed to describe a current complication of the antenatal, delivery, or perinatal period. Additional codes from other chapters may be used with code O80 if they are not related to or are in any way complicating the pregnancy; this must be clearly documented in the medical record. Code Z37.0 is to be used to identify the outcome of delivery for a single liveborn.

Code O82 is reported for a cesarean delivery. This code must not be used as the only diagnosis and must be accompanied by a delivery code. There is also an instructional note to identify the outcome of delivery (Z37).

Codes from category O35, Known or suspected fetal abnormality affecting management of the mother, and category O43, Other fetal and placental problems affecting the management of the mother, are assigned only when the fetal condition is actually responsible for modifying the management of the mother, that is, by requiring diagnostic studies, additional observation, special care, or termination of pregnancy. The fact that the fetal condition exists does not justify assigning a code from this series to the mother's record.

Review the following examples. Open up the ICD-10-CM codebook, referencing both the Alphabetic Index and the Tabular List, locate the correct code. The main term in the following example is "delivery."

EXAMPLE: *A liveborn single infant is delivered to a 29-year-old patient by lower-segment cesarean section because delivery was complicated by obstructed labor due to malpresentation in the hospital.*

Alphabetic Index:
Delivery → complicated by → obstruction → due to → malpresentation → O64.9

Note that this category requires a seventh character extension. Because this code has only 4 characters, dummy placeholders (x) must be added to the code to reach the highest level of specificity.

Tabular List:
O64.9 → Obstructed labor due to malposition and malpresentation → O64.9xx1

Now you must code the cesarean delivery.

Alphabetic Index:
Deliver, cesarean (for) → malposition fetus → O32.9

Tabular List:
O32.9 → O32.9xx1 → Maternal care for malpresentation of fetus, unspecified

Don't forget you must select a code for outcome of delivery.

Alphabetic Index:
Outcome of delivery → Z37

Tabular List:
Z37.0 → Single live birth

Correct code sequencing:
O64.9xx1, O32.9xx1, Z37.0

EXAMPLE: *A 31-year-old woman at 28 weeks gestation is seen for decreased fetal movements during the last week.*

Alphabetic Index:
Pregnancy → complicated by → decreased fetal movement → O36.81–

Tabular List:
O36.81 → Decreased fetal movements → O36.813 → Decreased fetal movement, third trimester

Correct code:
O36.813

OUTCOME OF DELIVERY (Z37)

When coding the outcome of the delivery, code from category Z37, which provides information when a patient delivers in the hospital. If the patient delivers elsewhere, you do not use a code from category Z37. This category is intended to be used as an additional code to identify the outcome of delivery for the mother's record. It is not reported on the newborn record.

Review the following for outcome of delivery in ICD-10-CM:

- Z37.0 Single live birth

- Z37.1 Single still birth

- Z37.2 Twins, both liveborn

- Z37.3 Twins, one liveborn and one stillborn

- Z37.4 Twins, both stillborn

- Z37.5 Other multiple births, all liveborn

- Z37.50 Multiple births, unspecified, all liveborn

- Z37.51 Triplets, all liveborn

- Z37.52 Quadruplets, all liveborn

- Z37.53 Quintuplets, all liveborn

- Z37.54 Sextuplets, all liveborn

- Z37.59 Other multiple births, all liveborn

- Z37.6 Other multiple births, some liveborn

- Z37.60 Multiple births, unspecified, some liveborn

- Z37.61 Triplets, some liveborn

- Z37.62 Quadruplets, some liveborn

- Z37.63 Quintuplets, some liveborn

- Z37.64 Sextuplets, some liveborn

- Z37.69 Other multiple births, some liveborn

- Z37.7 Other multiple births, all stillborn

- Z37.9 Outcome of delivery, unspecified

CODING TIP Outcome of delivery code Z37– is not reported on the infant's record. It is reported only on the mother's record.

Review the following example. Open up the ICD-10-CM codebook, referencing both the Alphabetic Index and the Tabular List, locate the correct code.

EXAMPLE: A 23-year-old female patient delivered in the hospital a healthy male without complication.

Alphabetic Index:
   Normal → delivery → O80
   Outcome of delivery → single → Liveborn →
   Z37.0 → single live birth

Tabular List:
   O80 Encounter for full-term uncomplicated delivery
   Z37.0 Outcome of delivery, single liveborn

Correct codes:
   O80 Normal delivery (first listed diagnosis)
   Z37.0 Outcome of delivery, single liveborn (secondary diagnosis)

CODING TIP Category Z37 is intended for coding the outcome of the delivery and should be coded on the mother's record, not the newborn's record.

HIV IN PREGNANCY

HIV in a pregnant patient is reported with O98.7– when a patient has an HIV infection or HIV-related illness, followed by the appropriate HIV code for the disease. A patient who is HIV positive without any HIV-related system is coded O98.7– along with Z21 for the asymptomatic HIV infection status. Review Figure 9.6.

FIGURE 9.6   Excerpt from the Tabular List: *O98.7*

O98.7   Human immunodeficiency [HIV] disease complicating pregnancy, childbirth and the puerperium
   Use additional code to identify the type of HIV disease:
      Acquired immune deficiency syndrome (AIDS) (B20)
      Asymptomatic HIV status (Z21)
      HIV positive NOS (Z21)
      Symptomatic HIV disease (B20)
   O98.71   Human immunodeficiency [HIV] disease complicating pregnancy
      O98.711   Human immunodeficiency [HIV] disease complicating pregnancy, first trimester
      O98.712   Human immunodeficiency [HIV] disease complicating pregnancy, second trimester
      O98.713   Human immunodeficiency [HIV] disease complicating pregnancy, third trimester
      O98.719   Human immunodeficiency [HIV] disease complicating pregnancy, unspecified trimester
   O98.72   Human immunodeficiency [HIV] disease complicating childbirth
   O98.73   Human immunodeficiency [HIV] disease complicating the puerperium

Review the following example. Open up the ICD-10-CM codebook, referencing both the Alphabetic Index and the Tabular List, locate the correct code.

> **EXAMPLE**: *A patient who is HIV postive is in her second trimester of pregnancy. Her pregnancy is progressing well without complications.*

> **Alphabetic Index:**
> *Pregnancy ➡ complicated by ➡ human immunodeficiency (HIV) disease ➡ 098.7–*

> **Tabular List:**
> *098.712 ➡ Human immunodeficiency [HIV] disease complicating pregnancy, second trimester*

> *Z21 ➡ HIV positive NOS*

Don't forget to code the HIV status as the secondary diagnosis.

> **Correct code sequencing:**
> *098.712, Z21*

COMPLICATIONS OF LABOR AND DELIVERY (060-077)

This section includes codes for:

- Preterm labor
- Failed induction of labor
- Abnormalities of forced of labor
- Obstructed labor
- Long labor
- Trauma to perineum and vulva during delivery
- Postpartum hemorrhage
- Retained placenta or membranes, without hemorrhage
- Complications of the administration of anesthetic or other sedation in labor and delivery

Some of the codes in this classification require additional code(s) to further specify the complication. Review the following example. Open up the ICD-10-CM codebook, referencing both the Alphabetic Index and the Tabular List, locate the correct code.

> **EXAMPLE**: *A 27-year-old patient suffered an atonic hemorrhage 6 hours after delivery.*

> **Alphabetic Index:**
> *Hemorrhage ➡ postpartum following delivery of placenta ➡ 072.–*

> **Tabular List:**
> *072.1 ➡ Other immediate postpartum hemorrhage ➡ postpartum hemorrhage (atonic) NOS*

> **Correct code:**
> *072.1*

The puerperium is the period of 42 days after childbirth and expulsion of the placenta and membrane. The postpartum period begins immediately after delivery and continues for 6 weeks after delivery. A postpartum complication is any complication occurring within the 6-week period. If the physician documents that a condition is pregnancy related, Chapter 15 codes may also be used to describe pregnancy-related complications after the 6-week period. The peripartum period is the last month of pregnancy to 5 months postpartum.

Review the following examples. Open up the ICD-10-CM codebook, referencing both the Alphabetic Index and the Tabular List, locate the correct code.

> **EXAMPLE**: *After delivery, the patient was running a postpartum fever for 4 hours. After the physician examined the patient, the patient was given medication to reduce the fever.*

> **Alphabetic index:**
> *Puerperal ➡ postpartum ➡ fever ➡ (of unknown origin) 086.4*

> **Tabular List:**
> *086.4 ➡ Pyrexia of unknown origin following delivery*

> **Correct code:**
> *086.4*

> **EXAMPLE**: *One day after delivering a single liveborn male, the patient was experiencing sharp pains in her lower extremities. The physician examined the patient and then ordered an ultrasound. The ultrasound revealed postpartum deep vein thrombosis.*

> **Alphabetic Index:**
> *Thrombosis, thrombotic ➡ due to ➡ puerperal, postpartum ➡ 087.–*

> **Tabular List:**
> *087.1 ➡ Deep phlebothrombosis in the puerperium ➡ deep vein thrombosis, postpartum*

> **Correct code:**
> *087.1*

EXAMPLE: *A 34-year-old woman is admitted to a hospital two weeks postpartum with disruption of the perineal wound.*

Alphabetic Index:
   Main term → disruption → wound → episiotomy → O90.1

Tabular List:
   O90.1 → Disruption of perineal obstetric wound

Correct code:
   O90.1

Peripartum cardiomyopathy is a condition that may be present during antepartum care, labor and delivery, or the puerperium. Cardiomyopathy is a serious condition with a mortality rate of 50% within 5 years; it has a high rate of recurrence in subsequent pregnancies. This condition tends to affect women aged 30, pregnancies complicated by preeclampsia, and multiple fetal gestations. This condition typically occurs in the postpartum period. This condition is coded in category O99, Other maternal diseases classifiable elsewhere but complicating pregnancy, childbirth, and the puerperium. There is an instructional note to use an additional code to identify the specific condition.

EXAMPLE: *A 40-year-old female presents to the OB/GYN 5 weeks after delivery of her fifth child via cesarean with complaints of swelling, chest pain, shortness of breath, fatigue, and heart palpitations. The physician performs an EKG, noting poor R-wave progressions, intraventricular condition delay, and ST and T wave changes. He orders a chest x-ray, which reveals cardiomegaly with alveolar edema. The patient is diagnosed with postpartum cardiomyopathy and is admitted to the hospital. A course of medical treatment is prescribed.*

Alphabetic Index:
   Main term → cardiomyopathy → postpartum → O90.3

Tabular List:
   O90.3 → Peripartum cardiomyopathy

Correct code:
   O90.3

When the mother delivers outside the hospital before admission, is admitted for routine postpartum care, and no complications are noted, code Z39.0, Postpartum care and examination immediately after delivery, should be assigned as the principal diagnosis. Code O94, Sequelae of complication of pregnancy, childbirth, and the puerperium, is used in those cases when an initial complication of a pregnancy develops a sequela requiring care or treatment at a future date. This code may be used at any time after the initial postpartum period.

CHECKPOINT EXERCISE 9-1

Assign the correct code(s) for the following diagnostic statements:

1. _____ Rubella in a woman at 4 months gestation

2. _____ Pregnancy, 8 months gestation, complicated by preeclampsia

3. _____ Blighted ovum

4. _____ Vaginal delivery of liveborn single infant with third-degree perineal laceration

5. _____ Delivery of two liveborn twins by cesarean section; labor and delivery complicated by obstructed labor due to locked twins

6. _____ Cesarean delivery due to multiple gestations

7. _____ Intraligamentous pregnancy

8. _____ A patient in her third month of pregnancy experienced persistent hyperemesis.

9. _____ A patient went into cardiac arrest after anesthesia was administered during delivery.

10. _____ A patient developed gestational diabetes during the second trimester of antepartum care.

11. _____ A patient who has had benign hypertension for the past 7 years delivers a single liveborn in the hospital.

12. _____ A patient who delivered a healthy set of twins two weeks ago is suffering postpartum uterine hypertrophy.

13. _____ A tearful new mother visited her OB/GYN complaining of pain at the incision site from her cesarean section 3 weeks ago. After examination, the physician determined that the wound was infected.

14. _____ A 22-year-old primigravida presents to the emergency room at 40-weeks gestation in active labor. The physician has not seen this patient before. While monitoring her in labor, the physician notes acute fetal distress, with fetal maternal hemorrhage necessitating an emergency cesarean delivery, which the physician performs.

15. _____ Postpartum deep phlebothrombosis of her legs.

Review the following example:

> **EXAMPLE:** *A 25-year-old patient is diagnosed with painful scarring due to an old second-degree perineal laceration that she suffered during her last pregnancy two years ago (late effect).*
>
> **Alphabetic Index:**
> *Scar, scarring → Painful L90.5*
>
> *Late → Effects → see Sequelae → Sequelae, pregnancy → 094*
>
> **Tabular List:**
> *L90.5 → Scar conditions and fibrosis of skin*
>
> *094 → Sequelae of complication of pregnancy, childbirth and the puerperium (secondary diagnosis)*

CODING TIP There is an instructional note following category 094 to code first the condition that resulted from the complication of pregnancy.

> **Correct code sequencing:**
> *L90.5, 094*

Certain Conditions Originating in the Newborn (perinatal period) (P00-P96)

Conditions originating in the perinatal period are located in Chapter 16 and include the following categories:

- Newborn affected by maternal factors and by complications of pregnancy, labor, and delivery (P00-P04)

- Disorders related to length of gestation and fetal growth (P05-P08)

- Abnormal findings on neonatal screening (P09)

- Birth trauma (P10-P15)

- Respiratory and cardiovascular disorders specific to the perinatal period (P19-P29)

- Infections specific to the perinatal period (P35-P39)

- Hemorrhagic and hematological disorders of newborn (P50-P61)

- Transitory endocrine and metabolic disorders specific to newborn (P70-P74)

- Digestive system disorders of newborn (P76-P78)

- Conditions involving the integument and temperature regulation of newborn (P80-P83)

- Other problems with newborn (P84)

- Other disorders originating in the perinatal period (P90-P96)

The perinatal period covers birth through the twenty-eighth day. Any clinically significant condition noted on the newborn examination is coded with the most serious condition requiring the most care reported first. A condition is considered clinically significant if it requires:

- Clinical evaluation

- Therapeutic treatment

- Diagnostic procedure

- Extended length of hospital stay

- Increased nursing care or monitoring

- Implications for future health care needs

Codes in Chapter 16 are only used for the newborn or infant and not on the maternal record. Codes in this chapter are also only applicable to liveborn infants. If the condition continues through the life of the child, regardless of the age of the patient, it should be coded. If the condition may be due to the birth process or is community acquired, the default should be the complication at birth code(s) from Chapter 16. These conditions are codes from categories P35-P39 based on the infection or condition. The perinatal period is defined as beginning at birth and lasting through the twenty-eighth day after birth. A code for newborn conditions originating in the perinatal period as well as complications arising during the current episode of care classified in other chapters are assigned only if the diagnoses have been documented by the responsible physician at the time of transfer or discharge as having affected the fetus or newborn.

NEWBORN AFFECTED BY MATERNAL FACTORS AND BY COMPLICATIONS OF PREGNANCY, LABOR, AND DELIVERY (P00-P04)

When a newborn is suspected to have a problem due to the condition of the mother, categories P00-P04 are reported. Diagnosis codes for newborns affected by maternal factors and complications of pregnancy, labor, and delivery are used for these patient encounters. If tests or treatment are performed, codes in this category are used. In addition, if the problem is confirmed, a code for the condition is reported followed by a code from P00-P04. Codes from this category are assigned only when the maternal condition has actually affected the fetus or newborn. The fact that the mother has an associated medical condition or experiences some complication of pregnancy, labor, or delivery does not justify the routine assignment of codes from these categories to the newborn record. The Official ICD-10-CM Guidelines indicate that when a patient has a suspected problem with identified signs and/or symptoms, code the sign or symptom instead of using a code in category P00-P04.

Review the following example. Open up the ICD-10-CM codebook, referencing both the Alphabetic Index and the Tabular List, locate the correct code.

> **EXAMPLE:** *A pregnant woman in her late third trimester sustains a complicated fracture of the skull during a car crash. As a result of her injuries, she goes into labor, and the newborn is delivered in respiratory distress.*

> **Alphabetic Index:**
> *Newborn (affected by)* → *maternal injury* → *P00.5*

> **Tabular List:**
> *P00.5* → *Newborn (suspected to be) affected by maternal injury*

Next we need to specify the fetal condition, respiratory distress.

> **Alphabetic Index:**
> *Distress* → *Respiratory* → → *newborn P22.9*

> **Tabular List:**
> *P22.9* → *Respiratory distress of newborn, unspecified*

> **Correct code sequencing:**
> *P22.9, P00.5*

There is an instructional note under category P00 to indicate that the current condition is coded as the first listed diagnosis. In this example, the respiratory distress is the condition that is coded first followed by the code for the affected injury.

Review this example. Open up the ICD-10-CM codebook, referencing both the Alphabetic Index and the Tabular List, locate the correct code.

> **EXAMPLE:** *A two-day-old baby is suspected to be in withdrawal. The neonate's mother was an active cocaine user up until delivery. The documentation in the medical record indicates the neonate is a "crack baby."*

> **Alphabetic Index:**
> *Crack* → *baby* → *P04.41*

> **Tabular List:**
> *P04.41* → *Newborn (suspected to be) affected by maternal use of cocaine*

> **Correct code:**
> *P04.41*

CODING TIP The perinatal guidelines listed above are the same as the general coding guidelines for "additional diagnoses," except for the final point regarding implications for future health care needs. Codes should be assigned for conditions that have been specified by the provider as having implications for future health care needs. Codes from the perinatal chapter should not be assigned unless the provider has established a definitive diagnosis.

DISORDERS OF NEWBORN RELATED TO LENGTH OF GESTATION AND FETAL GROWTH (P05-P08)

Low birth weight is any newborn weighing less than 2,500 grams or 5 pounds, 8 ounces. Low birth weight can contribute to increased risk for health problems throughout the child's life. Many of these newborns require specialized care in an NICU (newborn intensive care unit). Some problems that are related to low birth weight include:

- Intraventricular hemorrhage (IVH)
- Respiratory distress syndrome (RDS)
- Patent ductus arteriosus (PDA)
- Necrotizing enterocolitis (NEC)
- Retinopathy of prematurity (ROP)

The two main reasons a newborn is born with low birth weight include premature birth and fetal growth restriction. In a premature birth, the baby is born before 37 weeks of pregnancy are completed. A newborn with fetal growth restriction is born at full term but is small for gestation age and underweight. These babies are typically healthy even though they are small. Babies that are both premature and growth restricted are at a higher risk for health problems throughout their lives.

Codes from category P05-P08, Disorders of newborn related to short gestation and low birth weight, are used for a child or adult who was premature or had a low birth weight as a newborn and for whom the condition is affecting the patient's current health status. Review some of the categories in this classification.

- P05.0 Newborn light for gestational age
- P05.1 Newborn small for gestational age
- P07.0 Extremely low birth weigh newborn
- P07.1 Other low birth weight newborn
- P07.2 Extreme immaturity of newborn
- P07.3 Other preterm newborn

- P08 Disorders of newborn related to long gestation and high birth weight

Review Figure 9.7.

FIGURE 9.7   Excerpt from the Tabular List: *P05.1*

P05.1	Newborn small for gestational age
P05.10	Newborn small for gestational age, unspecified weight
P05.11	Newborn small for gestational age, less than 500 grams
P05.12	Newborn small for gestational age, 500-749 grams
P05.13	Newborn small for gestational age, 750-999 grams
P05.14	Newborn small for gestational age, 1000-1249 grams
P05.15	Newborn small for gestational age, 1250-1499 grams
P05.16	Newborn small for gestational age, 1500-1749 grams
P05.17	Newborn small for gestational age, 1750-1999 grams
P05.18	Newborn small for gestational age, 2000-2499 grams

Review this example. Open up the ICD-10-CM codebook, referencing both the Alphabetic Index and the Tabular List, locate the correct code.

EXAMPLE: *An infant is born prematurely at 29 weeks gestation and weighs 710 g. The physician assesses the infant as being extremely immature.*

Alphabetic Index:
Prematurity → birth NEC → see preterm infant, newborn → preterm infant newborn → P07.30 → with gestation of → 28-31 weeks → P07.31

Tabular List:
P07.31 → Other preterm newborn 28-31 completed weeks

Keep in mind that an additional code must be reported to identify the low birth weight of the infant.

P07.02
Extremely low birth weight newborn, 500-749 grams

Correct code sequencing:
P07.02, P07.31

CODING TIP When the documentation in the medical record indicates birth weight and gestational age, both should be coded. Birth weight should be sequenced before the gestational age.

Review Table 9.2.

TABLE 9.2   Official Guidelines for Coding and Reporting for Conditions in the Perinatal Period

Use of Chapter 16 codes	Codes in this chapter are never for use on the maternal record. Codes from Chapter 15, the obstetric chapter, are never permitted on the newborn record.
	Chapter 16 codes may be used throughout the life of the patient if the condition is still present.
Principal diagnosis for birth record	When coding the birth episode in a newborn record, assign a code from category Z38, Liveborn infants according to place of birth and type of delivery, as the principal diagnosis.
	A code from category Z38 is assigned only once to a newborn at the time of birth. If a newborn is transferred to another institution, a code from category Z38 should not be used at the receiving hospital.
	A code from category Z38 is used only on the newborn's record, not on the mother's record.
Use of codes from other chapters with codes from Chapter 16	Codes from other chapters may be used with codes from Chapter 16 if the codes from the other chapters provide more specific detail.
	Codes for signs and symptoms may be assigned when a definitive diagnosis has not been established. If the reason for the encounter is a perinatal condition, the code from Chapter 16 should be sequenced first.
Use of Chapter 16 codes after the perinatal period	If a condition originates in the perinatal period and continues throughout the life of the patient, the perinatal code should continue to be used regardless of the patient's age.
Birth process or community-acquired conditions	If a newborn has a condition that may be either due to the birth process or is community acquired and the documentation does not indicate which it is, the default is the birth process and the code from Chapter 16 should be used.
	If the condition is community acquired, a code from Chapter 16 should not be assigned.

(continued)

TABLE 9.2   *(continued)*

Code all clinically significant conditions	All clinically significant conditions noted on routine newborn examination should be coded. A condition is clinically significant if it requires: • clinical evaluation; or • therapeutic treatment; or • diagnostic procedures; or • extended length of hospital stay; or • increased nursing care and/or monitoring; or • has implications for future health care needs **Note:** The perinatal guidelines listed above are the same as the general coding guidelines for "additional diagnoses," except for the final point regarding implications for future health care needs. Codes should be assigned for conditions that have been specified by the provider as having implications for future health care needs.
Observation and evaluation of newborns for suspected conditions not found	Assign a code from categories P00-P04 to identify those instances when a healthy newborn is evaluated for a suspected condition that is determined after study not to be present. Do not use a code from categories P00-P04 when the provider has identified signs or symptoms of a suspected problem; in such cases, code the sign or symptom.
Coding additional perinatal diagnoses Assigning codes for conditions that require treatment	Assign codes for conditions that require treatment or further investigation, prolong the length of stay, or require resource utilization.
Codes for conditions specified as having implications for future health care needs	Assign codes for conditions that have been specified by the provider as having implications for future health care needs. **Note:** This guideline should not be used for adult patients.
Prematurity and fetal growth retardation	Providers utilize different criteria in determining prematurity. A code for prematurity should not be assigned unless it is documented. Assignment of codes in categories P05, Disorders of newborn related to slow fetal growth and fetal malnutrition, and P07, Disorders of newborn related to short gestation and low birth weight, not elsewhere classified, should be based on the recorded birth weight and estimated gestational age. Codes from category P05 should not be assigned with codes from category P07. When both birth weight and gestational age are available, two codes from category P07 should be assigned, with the code for birth weight sequenced before the code for gestational age.
Low birth weight and immaturity status	Codes from category P07, Disorders of newborn related to short gestation and low birth weight, not elsewhere classified, are for use for a child or adult who was premature or had a low birth weight as a newborn and this is affecting the patient's current health status. *See Section I.C.21, Factors influencing health status and contact with health services, Status.*
Bacterial sepsis of newborn	Category P36, Bacterial sepsis of newborn, includes congenital sepsis. If a perinate is documented as having sepsis without documentation of congenital or community acquired, the default is congenital and a code from category P36 should be assigned. If the P36 code includes the causal organism, an additional code from category B95, Streptococcus, staphylococcus, and enterococcus as the cause of diseases classified elsewhere, or B96, Other bacterial agents as the cause of diseases classified elsewhere, should not be assigned. If the P36 code does not include the causal organism, assign an additional code from category B96. If applicable, use additional codes to identify severe sepsis (R65.2–) and any associated acute organ dysfunction.
Stillbirth	Code P95, Stillbirth, is only for use in institutions that maintain separate records for stillbirths. No other code should be used with P95. Code P95 should not be used on the mother's record.

Source: Chapter 16, Official ICD-10-CM Guidelines for Coding Newborn (Perinatal) (P00-P96).

INFECTIONS SPECIFIC TO THE PERINATAL PERIOD (P35-P39)

Categories P35-P39 are used to report infections specific to the perinatal period. According to the Tabular List, when coding for infections specific to the perinatal period, the infections must be acquired before or during the birth, via the umbilicus or 28 days after birth. Conditions excluded from these categories are congenital pneumonia, congenital syphilis, and maternal infectious disease as a cause of mortality or morbidity in fetus or newborn. Fetus or newborn not manifesting the disease, ophthalmia neonatorum due to gonococcus, and other infections not specifically classified in these categories is included.

Review the following example. Open up the ICD-10-CM codebook, referencing both the Alphabetic Index and the Tabular List, locate the correct code.

> **EXAMPLE:** *A newborn was diagnosed with a naval infection due to* Tetanus *bacillus (Tetanus omphalitis) caused by use of accidental nonsterile instruments during delivery.*

Alphabetic Index:
   Omphalitis (congenital) (newborn) ➞ *P38.9* ➞ *tetanus* ➞ *A33*

Tabular List:
   A33 ➞ *Tetanus neonatorum*

Correct code:
   A33

Review this example. Open up the ICD-10-CM codebook, referencing both the Alphabetic Index and the Tabular List, locate the correct code.

> **EXAMPLE:** *A newborn was diagnosed with congenital viral hepatitis by the pediatrician following birth.*

Review Figure 9.8.

FIGURE 9.8   Excerpt from the Tabular List: *P35*

P35 Congenital viral diseases
   INCLUDES infections acquired in utero or during birth
   P35.0 Congenital rubella syndrome
          Congenital rubella pneumonitis
   P35.1 Congenital cytomegalovirus infection
   P35.2 Congenital herpesviral [herpes simplex] infection
   P35.3 Congenital viral hepatitis
   P35.8 Other congenital viral diseases
          Congenital varicella [chickenpox]
   P35.9 Congenital viral disease, unspecified

Alphabetic Index:
   Hepatitis ➞ *congenital* ➞ *P35.3*

Tabular List:
   P35.3 ➞ *Congenital viral hepatitis*

Correct code:
   P35.3

LIVEBORN STATUS (Z38)

When coding the birth of an infant, assign a code from category Z38, according to the type of birth. A code from this series is assigned as a principal diagnosis and is assigned only once to a newborn at the time of birth. This is never reported on the mother's record, only for the newborn on the initial birth record.

Review category Z38 for reporting the type of birth:

- Z38.0 Single liveborn infant, born in hospital
- Z38.00 Single liveborn infant, delivered vaginally
- Z38.01 Single liveborn infant, delivered by cesarean
- Z38.1 Single liveborn infant, born outside hospital
- Z38.2 Single liveborn infant, unspecified as to place of birth
- Z38.3 Twin liveborn infant, born in hospital
- Z38.30 Twin liveborn infant, delivered vaginally
- Z38.31 Twin liveborn infant, delivered by cesarean
- Z38.4 Twin liveborn infant, born outside hospital
- Z38.5 Twin liveborn infant, unspecified as to place of birth
- Z38.6 Other multiple liveborn infant, born in hospital
- Z38.61 Triplet liveborn infant, delivered vaginally
- Z38.62 Triplet liveborn infant, delivered by cesarean
- Z38.63 Quadruplet liveborn infant, delivered vaginally
- Z38.64 Quadruplet liveborn infant, delivered by cesarean
- Z38.65 Quintuplet liveborn infant, delivered vaginally
- Z38.66 Quintuplet liveborn infant, delivered by cesarean
- Z38.68 Other multiple liveborn infant, delivered vaginally
- Z38.69 Other multiple liveborn infant, delivered by cesarean
- Z38.7 Other multiple liveborn infant, born outside hospital
- Z38.8 Other multiple liveborn infant, unspecified as to place of birth

CHECKPOINT EXERCISE 9-2

Select the correct code(s) for the following statements:

1. _____ Fetal alcohol syndrome

2. _____ A newborn suffers unspecified birth injury that requires the child to be hospitalized.

3. _____ Fetal blood loss due to ruptured cord

4. _____ Perinatal jaundice due to congenital obstruction of the bile duct

5. _____ Transitory ileus of newborn

6. _____ Pulmonary immaturity

7. _____ Neonatal diabetes mellitus

8. _____ Neonatal jaundice due to Gilbert's syndrome

9. _____ Hyperthermia in newborn

10. _____ A newborn suffers a fracture from a scalpel wound during birth.

11. _____ A mother brings her 6-week-old newborn to the family physician. The umbilical cord has not yet separated from the umbilicus. After examination, the physician determines there is no infection and orders diagnostic tests.

12. _____ Neonatal hypoglycemia

13. _____ A newborn is diagnosed with vitamin K deficiency.

14. _____ A newborn is diagnosed with jaundice from galactosemia.

15. _____ A new mother brought her 3-week-old infant to the pediatrician with a complaint that the newborn was vomiting excessively and could not keep food down.

Congenital Malformations, Deformations, and Chromosomal Abnormalities (Q00-Q99)

Chapter 17 includes the following categories:

- Congenital malformations of the nervous system (Q00–Q07)

- Congenital malformations of the eye, ear, face, and neck (Q10–Q18)

- Congenital malformations of the circulatory system (Q20–Q28)

- Congenital malformations of the respiratory system (Q30–Q34)

- Cleft lip and cleft palate (Q35–Q37)

- Other congenital malformations of the digestive system (Q38–Q45)

- Congenital malformations of the genital organs (Q50–Q56)

- Congenital malformations of the urinary system (Q60–Q64)

- Congenital malformations and deformations of the musculoskeletal system (Q65–Q79)

- Other congenital malformations (Q80–Q89)

- Chromosomal abnormalities, not elsewhere classified (Q90–Q99)

Chapter 17 of the Tabular List, which describes congenital anomalies, is not subdivided in code sections like some of the other chapters that have been discussed thus far. An anomaly is an abnormality of a structure or organ. The term "congenital" refers to an abnormality with which a person was born.

Examples of congenital anomalies are:

- Spina bifida, the failure of the spinal column to close during fetal development

- Absence of a body structure such as an eye, ear lobe, blood vessel, lung

- Cleft palate, a congenital fissure in the roof of the mouth forming a communicating passageway between mouth and nasal cavities

- Polydactyly, the condition of having more than the usual number of fingers and toes

Congenital anomalies or syndromes may occur as a set of symptoms or multiple malformations. If there is not a code for a syndrome, for every manifestation of that syndrome a code should be reported from any chapter in the classification. It there is a specific code to identify the congenital anomaly or syndrome, additional codes may be assigned to identify manifestations not included in the code for the syndrome.

Review the following Official ICD-10-CM Guidelines for coding in this classification (Q00-Q99; Chapter 17):

- Assign an appropriate code(s) from categories Q00-Q99, Congenital malformations, deformations, and chromosomal abnormalities, when a malformation/deformation or chromosomal abnormality is documented. A malformation/deformation or chromosomal abnormality may be the principal/first listed diagnosis on a record or a secondary diagnosis.

- When a malformation/deformation or chromosomal abnormality does not have a unique code assignment, assign additional code(s) for any manifestations that may be present.

- When the code assignment specifically identifies the malformation/deformation or chromosomal abnormality, manifestations that are an inherent component of the anomaly should not be coded separately. Additional codes should be assigned for manifestations that are not an inherent component.

- Codes from Chapter 17 may be used throughout the life of the patient. If a congenital malformation or deformity has been corrected, a personal history code should be used to identify the history of the malformation or deformity. Although present at birth, malformation/deformation or chromosomal abnormality may not be identified until later in life. Whenever the condition is diagnosed by the physician, it is appropriate to assign a code from codes Q00-Q99.

- For the birth admission, the appropriate code from category Z38, Liveborn infants, according to place of birth and type of delivery, should be sequenced as the principal diagnosis, followed by any congenital anomaly codes, Q00-Q99.

Some anomalies are detected at birth (such as spina bifida or cleft palate), while other anomalies are detected many years later (such as absence of an ovary). Congenital anomalies may occur as a set of symptoms or multiple malformations. A code should be assigned for each presenting manifestation of the syndrome if the syndrome is not specifically indexed in ICD-10-CM (Official ICD-10-CM Guidelines).

Now review this example. Open up the ICD-10-CM codebook, referencing both the Alphabetic Index and the Tabular List, locate the correct code.

EXAMPLE: A child is born with spina bifida of the thoracic region with hydrocephalus.

Alphabetic Index:
   Spina bifida → *with hydrocephalus* → *thoracic* → *Q05.–*

Tabular List:
   Q05.1 → *Thoracic spina bifida with hydrocephalus*

Correct code:
   Q05.6

A distinction in the Alphabetic Index between congenital and acquired conditions are indexed with a nonessential modifier associated with the main term or subterm. Review the following examples that identify acquired versus congenital.

Alphabetic Index
   Deformity → *diaphragm (congenital)* → *Q79.1* → *Acquired* → *J98.6*

   Deformity → *chin* → *acquired M95.2* → *congenital* → *Q18.9*

With these examples, the Alphabetic Index assumes the deformity of the chin is acquired, whereas deformity of the diaphragm is classified as congenital if not otherwise specified in the documentation. Congenital anomalies are classified first by the body system involved. Some are listed under general terms such as "congenital" while others are listed under deformity rather than the specific condition.

CHECKPOINT EXERCISE 9-3

Select the correct code(s) for the following statements:

1. _____ Congenital absence of Eustachian tube

2. _____ Cystic eyeball, congenital

3. _____ A child is born with mitral stenosis and hypoplastic left heart syndrome.

4. _____ Unilateral complete cleft palate with cleft lip

5. _____ Cryptorchidism

6. _____ Aseptic necrosis of bone

7. _____ Primary pulmonary hypertension of newborn

8. _____ Renal agenesis and dysgenesis

9. _____ Anomalies of pancreas

10. _____ Gerbode defect

11. _____ Congenital fusion of labia

12. _____ Congenital macroglossia

13. _____ Septo-optic dysplasia of the brain

14. _____ Sirenomelia syndrome

15. _____ Prolapse of the urachus

Test Your Knowledge

Assign codes for the following diagnostic statements.

1. _____ Two-month-old child with congenital dislocation of hip

2. _____ An 18-month-old who was born with hypospadias presents to the hospital for hypospadias correction.

3. _____ Congenital hypoplasia of the eyelid

4. _____ Congenital aortic stenosis

5. _____ Arteriovenous malformation of the brain

6. _____ Ventricular septal defect

7. _____ Congenital malposition of the digestive organs

8. _____ A 3-month-old patient visited the ear doctor because she is suffering from congenital fusion of the ear ossicles.

9. _____ A 5-year-old male with congenital brain malformation and intractable epilepsy.

10. _____ A preterm infant was delivered at 10:00 a.m. this morning vaginally at 35 weeks gestation with a weight of 2,400 grams. This evening he suffered respiratory arrest. The patient was intubated and mechanical ventilation started.

11. _____ A female patient in her first trimester of pregnancy visits her physician with a complaint of persistent vomiting. The patient states she is nauseated mainly in the evenings before bedtime.

12. _____ Total placenta previa with indications of fetal distress; an emergency cesarean section is done with delivery of a viable male infant

13. _____ Urinary tract infection following a missed abortion

14. _____ A patient suffered acute deep vein thrombosis of the right lower extremity (femoral vein) following delivery of a single liveborn delivered vaginally.

15. _____ The patient had some preterm labor and was treated with nifedipine and was stable on nifedipine and bed rest. The patient felt decreased fetal movement yesterday, presented to the hospital for evaluation this morning. At approximately 1330 hours and on admission, no cardiac activity was noted by the physician. The diagnosis was confirmed with ultrasound, and the patient was admitted with a diagnosis of intrauterine fetal demise at 36 weeks gestation.

16. _____ This is a 28-year-old G7, P5 female at 39-4/7th weeks who presents to Labor and Delivery for induction. She was admitted and started on Pitocin. Her cervix is 3 cm, 50% effaced, and −2 station. Artificial rupture of membrane was performed for clear fluid. She did receive epidural anesthesia. She progressed to complete and pushing. She pushed to approximately one contraction and delivered a liveborn female infant at 2030 hours. Apgars were 8 at 1 minute and 9 at 5 minutes. Placenta was delivered intact with 3-vessel cord. The cervix was visualized. No lacerations were noted. Perineum remained intact. Estimated blood loss 300 mL. Complications were none. Mother and baby remained in the birthing room in good condition.

17. _____ A 30-year-old female patient gave birth to twins via C-section in the hospital operating room. She delivered one female and one male 2 minutes apart.

18. _____ A patient with anti-D antibodies was seen by an OB specialist in her second trimester.

19. _____ A patient was feeling dysphoria one week after delivery of a male newborn.

20. _____ A newborn was being treated in the NICU for bradycardia.

CHAPTER 10

Symptoms, Signs, and Abnormal Clinical and Laboratory Findings

Injury, Poisoning, and Certain Other Consequences of External Causes: and External Causes of Morbidity (R00-Y99)

This ICD-10-CM chapter includes codes for symptoms, signs, abnormal results of clinical or other investigative procedures, and ill-defined conditions. Codes from this chapter are assigned when the recorded diagnosis is not classified elsewhere. If a definitive diagnosis cannot be determined as in ICD-10-CM, a sign/symptom code is reported. If a confirmed diagnosis is documented in the medical record, only the confirmed diagnosis is reported unless the sign/symptom is not related to the definitive diagnosis.

Chapter 18 of the Tabular List includes the following sections:

- Symptoms and signs involving the circulatory and respiratory systems (R00-R09)

- Symptoms and signs involving the digestive system and abdomen (R10-R19)

- Symptoms and signs involving the skin and subcutaneous tissue (R20-R23)

- Symptoms and signs involving the nervous and musculoskeletal systems (R25-R29)

- Symptoms and signs involving the genitourinary system (R30-R39)

- Symptoms and signs involving cognition, perception, emotional state, and behavior (R40-R46)

- Symptoms and signs involving speech and voice (R47-R49)

- General symptoms and signs (R50-R69)

- Abnormal findings on examination of blood, without diagnosis (R70-R79)

- Abnormal findings on examination of urine, without diagnosis (R80-R82)

- Abnormal findings on examination of other body fluids, substances, and tissues, without diagnosis (R83-R89)

- Abnormal findings on diagnostic imaging and in function studies, without diagnosis (R90-R94)

- Abnormal tumor markers (R97)

- Ill-defined and unknown cause of mortality (R99)

Signs and symptoms that point to a specific diagnosis have been assigned to a category in other chapters of the classification. However, many codes in this chapter are combination codes that include the diagnosis and the most common symptoms of that diagnosis. When a combination code is the appropriate code to report, a secondary code is not reported for the symptom.

Two rules apply to use the symptom codes with confirmed diagnoses:

- A symptom code should not be used with a confirmed diagnosis when the symptom is routinely associated with the disease process thus integral to the diagnosis.

- A symptom code should be used in addition to a confirmed diagnosis when the symptom is not always associated with that diagnosis, such as various signs and symptoms associated with complex syndromes. In this circumstance, the definitive diagnosis code should be sequenced before the symptom code.

Because terminology is important to this section, the following is a review of the most important terms:

- Symptom: any subjective evidence of a disease, such as pain or a headache, observed by the patient.

- Sign: objective evidence of disease, such as fever, that can be observed by someone other than the patient.

- Syndrome: refers to a set of symptoms that occur together. For example, irritable bowel syndrome consists of many symptoms that usually occur together.

General Coding Guidelines

Signs and symptoms that point rather definitely to a given diagnosis are assigned to some category within the ICD-10-CM classification. In general, categories R50-R64 include the more ill-defined conditions and symptoms that may point to two or more diseases or to two or more systems of the body. Practically all categories in this group could be designated as "not otherwise specified" or as "unknown etiology" or "transient." The Alphabetic Index should be consulted to determine which symptoms and signs are to be coded here and which should be coded to more specific sections of the ICD-10-CM classification.

CODING TIP In the outpatient setting, do not code "rule out," "possible," "probable," or "suspected" statements as being definitive diagnoses. Instead, code for the signs or symptoms with which the patient presented.

Review Table 10.1.

Use codes from Chapter 18 when:

- No more specific diagnosis can be made after investigation

- Signs and symptoms existing at the time of the initial encounter proved to be transient or a cause could not be determined

- A patient fails to return and all you have is a provisional diagnosis

- A case is referred elsewhere before a definitive diagnosis could be made

- A more precise diagnosis was not available for any other reason

- Certain symptoms that represent important problems in medical care exist and it is desirable to classify them in addition to a known cause

TABLE 10.1 General Rules for Coding Symptoms, Signs, and Abnormal Clinical and Laboratory Findings, Not Elsewhere Classified

Use of symptom codes	Codes that describe symptoms and signs are acceptable for reporting purposes when a related definitive diagnosis has not been established (confirmed) by the provider.
Use of a symptom code with a definitive diagnosis code	Codes for signs and symptoms may be reported in addition to a related definitive diagnosis when the sign or symptom is not routinely associated with that diagnosis, such as the various signs and symptoms associated with complex syndromes. The definitive diagnosis code should be sequenced before the symptom code.
	Signs or symptoms that are associated routinely with a disease process should not be assigned as additional codes, unless otherwise instructed by the classification.
Combination codes that include symptoms	ICD-10-CM contains a number of combination codes that identify both the definitive diagnosis and common symptoms of that diagnosis. When using one of these combination codes, an additional code should not be assigned for the symptom.
Repeated falls	Code R29.6, Repeated falls, is used when a patient has recently fallen and the reason for the fall is being investigated.
	Code Z91.81, History of falling, is used when a patient has fallen in the past and is at risk for future falls. When appropriate, both codes R29.6 and Z91.81 may be assigned together.
Coma scale	The coma scale codes (R40.2-) can be used in conjunction with traumatic brain injury codes and acute cerebrovascular disease or sequelae of cerebrovascular disease codes. These codes are primarily for use by trauma registries, but they may be used in any setting where this information is collected. The coma scale codes should be sequenced after the diagnosis code(s).
	These codes, one from each subcategory, are needed to complete the scale. The seventh character indicates when the scale was recorded. The seventh character should match for all 3 codes.
	At a minimum, report the initial score documented on presentation at your facility. This may be a score from the emergency medicine technician or in the emergency department. If desired, a facility may choose to capture multiple Glasgow coma scale scores.
Functional quadriplegia	Functional quadriplegia (code R53.2) is the lack of ability to use one's limbs or to ambulate due to extreme debility. It is not associated with neurologic deficit or injury, and code R53.2 should not be used for cases of neurologic quadriplegia. It should only be assigned if functional quadriplegia is specifically documented in the medical record.
SIRS due to noninfectious process	The systemic inflammatory response syndrome (SIRS) can develop as a result of certain noninfectious disease processes, such as trauma, malignant neoplasm, or pancreatitis. When SIRS is documented with a noninfectious condition, and no subsequent infection is documented, the code for the underlying condition, such as an injury, should be assigned, followed by code R65.10, Systemic inflammatory response syndrome (SIRS) of noninfectious origin without acute organ dysfunction, or code R65.11, Systemic inflammatory response syndrome (SIRS) of noninfectious origin with acute organ dysfunction. If an associated acute organ dysfunction is documented, the appropriate code(s) for the specific type of organ dysfunction(s) should be assigned in addition to code R65.11. If acute organ dysfunction is documented, but it cannot be determined if the acute organ dysfunction is associated with SIRS or due to another condition (eg, directly due to the trauma), the provider should be queried.
Death NOS	Code R99, Ill-defined and unknown cause of mortality, is only for use in the very limited circumstance when a patient who has already died is brought into an emergency department or other health care facility and is pronounced dead upon arrival. It does not represent the discharge disposition of death.

Source: ICD-10-CM Official Guidelines, Chapte 18 Symptoms, Signs, and Abnormal Clinical and Laboratory Findings, Not Elsewhere Classified

Do not use codes from Chapter 18 when:

- A definitive diagnosis is available, for example, the diagnostic statement says cough due to acute bronchitis. The code for cough is category J40, which is located in Chapter 10 of ICD-10-CM. Because the reason for the cough is acute bronchitis, you would not include the code for the symptom of cough. The only code you would assign would be from category J40.

- The symptom is considered to be an integral part of the disease process, for example, dysuria (painful urination), urinary frequency, and urgency due to urinary tract infection. Dysuria, frequency, and urgency are classic symptoms of a urinary tract infection. Therefore, you would not assign codes for the symptoms. The only code you would assign is N39.0 for the urinary tract infection.

Review the following examples. Open up the ICD-10-CM codebook, referencing both the Alphabetic Index and the Tabular List, locate the correct code.

> **EXAMPLE:** *Mrs. Jones was referred to a cardiologist by her family practitioner with symptoms of generalized fatigue and intermittent chest pain. After an EKG was performed, the cardiologist could not find any abnormalities and ordered a stress test to rule out any cardiac involvement.*

Alphabetic Index:
   Pain ➞ *chest (central)* ➞ *R07.9*

   Fatigue ➞ *general* ➞ *R53.83*

Tabular List:
   R07.89 ➞ *Other chest pain*

   R53.83 ➞ *Other fatigue* ➞ *fatigue*

Correct code sequencing:
   R07.9, R53.83

In this example, either code may be sequenced first. Because the chest pain was the focus of the visit, it makes sense to report the chest pain as the first listed diagnosis.

> **EXAMPLE:** *A patient visited his family physician with symptoms of nausea and vomiting. The symptoms began two days ago. The patient has no other symptoms. The physician examines the patient and prescribes medication to help with the condition.*

Review Figure 10.1.

FIGURE 10.1   Excerpt from the Tabular List: *R11*

R11	Nausea and vomiting
EXCLUDES 1	cyclical vomiting associated with migraine (G43.81-) excessive vomiting in pregnancy (O21.-) hematemesis (K92.0) neonatal hematemesis (P54.0) newborn vomiting (P92.0) psychogenic vomiting (F50.8) vomiting following gastrointestinal surgery (K91.0)
R11.0	Nausea Nausea NOS Nausea without vomiting
R11.1	Vomiting
R11.10	Vomiting, unspecified Vomiting NOS
R11.11	Vomiting without nausea
R11.12	Projectile vomiting
R11.13	Vomiting of fecal matter
R11.14	Bilious vomiting Bilious emesis
R11.2	Nausea with vomiting, unspecified

Alphabetic Index:
   Nausea ➞ *with vomiting* ➞ *R11.2*

Tabular List:
   R11.2

Correct code:
   R11.2

In this example, there is a code combination that describes both conditions.

> **EXAMPLE:** *A patient is seen by a cardiologist with chest pain and shortness of breath on exertion. The physician documents a diagnosis of bradycardia.*

Alphabetic Index:
   Bradycardia (sinoatrial) (sinus) (vagal) ➞ *R00.1*

Tabular List:
   R00.1 ➞ *Bradycardia, unspecified*

Other examples of new ICD-10-CM category codes include the following:

- R13 Aphagia and dysphagia

- R19.0 Intraabdominal and pelvic swelling, mass and lump

- R25 Abnormal involuntary movements

- R31 Hematuria

- R33.0 Drug-induced retention of urine

- R40.2 Coma

- R43 Disturbances of smell and taste

- R50 Fever of other and unknown origin

- R55 Syncope and collapse

- R58 Hemorrhage, not elsewhere classified

- R77 Other abnormalities of plasma proteins

- R78 Findings of drugs and other substances, not normally found in blood

The codes for abnormal findings have been significantly expanded in ICD-10-CM to provide greater specificity. The block titled Abnormal Findings on Examination of Other Body Fluids, Substances, and Tissues, Without Diagnosis includes the following categories:

- R83 Abnormal findings in cerebrospinal fluid

- R84 Abnormal findings in specimens from respiratory organs and thorax

- R85 Abnormal findings in specimens from digestive organs and abdominal cavity

- R86 Abnormal findings in specimens from male genital organs

- R87 Abnormal findings in specimens from female genital organs

- R88 Abnormal findings in other body fluids and substances

- R89 Abnormal findings in specimens from other organs, systems, and tissues

Falling

Codes for other abnormalities of gait and mobility are to be used when the patient tends to fall when attempting to walk and are not to be confused with the External Cause codes for falls:

- R26.81 Unsteadiness on feet

- R26.82 Other abnormalities of gait and mobility

This code category may be used in conjunction with the External Cause codes for falls. The injury code is reported first, followed by the underlying condition and the External Cause code to describe the type of fall.

Glascow Coma Scale

According to the coding guidelines for ICD-10-CM, the Glascow coma scale must be used in conjunction with the codes for traumatic brain injuries or the sequelae of cerebrovascular accidents. With code R40.2–, one code

from each of the 3 subcategories must be assigned to complete the Glascow scale. When more than one coma assessment is performed (multiple coma assessments), the patient's health record should include a report of the initial coma scale performed at the time of admission and a final rating performed at the time of discharge.

Facility policy should determine which scale ratings are to be reported in the health record. An extension must be added to the coma codes to indicate which ratings are to be reported in the final record. Review Figure 10.2.

FIGURE 10.2   Excerpt from the Tabular List: *R40.2–*

R40.2   Coma
        Coma NOS
        Unconsciousness NOS
        Code first any associated:
                coma in fracture of skull (S02.–)
                coma in intracranial injury (S06.–)
The following seventh character extensions are to be added to
        codes R40.21, R40.22, R40.23
        0 unspecified time
        1 in the field [EMT or ambulance]
        2 at arrival to emergency department
        3 at hospital admission
        4 24 hours after hospital admission
Note: A code from each subcategory is required to complete
        the coma scale
R40.2   Coma (continued)
        R40.20   Unspecified coma
        R40.21   Coma scale, eyes open
                  R40.211   Coma scale, eyes open, never
                  R40.212   Coma scale, eyes open, to pain
                  R40.213   Coma scale, eyes open, to sound
                  R40.214   Coma scale, eyes open, spontaneous

        These codes are intended primarily for trauma registry
        and research but may be utilized by all users of the
        classification who wish to collect this information.
        R40.22   Coma scale, best verbal response
                  R40.221   Coma scale, best verbal response, none
                  R40.222   Coma scale, best verbal response,
                            incomprehensible words
                  R40.223   Coma scale, best verbal response,
                            inappropriate words
                  R40.224   Coma scale, best verbal response,
                            confused conversation
                  R40.225   Coma scale, best verbal response,
                            oriented
        R40.23   Coma scale, best motor response
                  R40.231   Coma scale, best motor response,
                            none
                  R40.232   Coma scale, best motor response,
                            extension
                  R40.233   Coma scale, best motor response,
                            abnormal
                  R40.234   Coma scale, best motor response,
                            flexion withdrawal
                  R40.235   Coma scale, best motor response,
                            localizes pain
                  R40.236   Coma scale, best motor response,
                            obeys commands

CODING TIP   For reporting "coma," always reference the comas scale because coding is based on a coma scale.

CHECKPOINT EXERCISE 10-1

Select the correct ICD-10-CM code(s) for the following diagnostic statements:

1. _____ Abnormal thyroid scan

2. _____ Elevated blood pressure reading

3. _____ Nausea and vomiting, suspect viral gastroenteritis

4. _____ Polydipsia and polyuria, rule out adult-onset diabetes mellitus

5. _____ Hepatomegaly

6. _____ Syncope

7. _____ A patient has symptoms of fever and chills.

8. _____ A patient with symptoms of a rapid heart beat sees her family physician.

9. _____ A pulmonologist ordered a pulmonary function test when the patient complained of shortness of breath, which he has been experiencing for the past 3 months.

10. _____ Abnormal percussion of the chest

11. _____ A 45-year-old patient presented to her internist with symptoms of unexplained memory loss and severe headaches. These symptoms began two days ago, and the patient stated she had not suffered any injuries that would attribute to the memory loss.

12. _____ A 14-year-old female was diagnosed with anorexia and entered a rehabilitation facility that specialized in the condition.

13. _____ A patient with a persistent nosebleed saw her internist for treatment. The physician could not find any specific cause of the nosebleed and ordered additional tests.

14. _____ Male stress incontinence

15. _____ A 55-year-old male is seen by his physician concerned about weight gain and lack of energy. Because the patient has a family history of diabetes mellitus, the physician performs a fasting blood test. The physician documents a fasting glucose of 165 mg/dl and orders a second fasting glucose for later in the week. The physician diagnoses the patient with an abnormal fasting glucose.

External Causes of Morbidity (V00-Y99)

Before discussing Chapter 19, which includes injuries and poisonings, it is important to understand the external causes of morbidity because many of the codes related to injuries and poisonings must include the external cause of morbidity.

Chapter 20 of the Tabular List includes the following sections:

- Pedestrian injured in transport accident (V00-V09)

- Pedal cycle rider injured in transport accident (V10-V19)

- Motorcycle rider injured in transport accident (V20-V29)

- Occupant of 3-wheeled motor vehicle injured in transport accident (V30-V39)

- Car occupant injured in transport accident (V40-V49)

- Occupant of pick-up truck or van injured in transport accident (V50-V59)

- Occupant of heavy transport vehicle injured in transport accident (V60-V69)

- Bus occupant injured in transport accident (V70-V79)

- Other land transport accidents (V80-V89)

- Water transport accidents (V90-V94)

- Air and space transport accidents (V95-V97)

- Other and unspecified transport accidents (V98-V99)

- Slipping, tripping, stumbling, and falls (W00-W19)

- Exposure to inanimate mechanical forces (W20-W49)

- Exposure to animate mechanical forces (W50-W64)

- Accidental non-transport drowning and submersion (W65-W74)

- Exposure to electric current, radiation, and extreme ambient air temperature and pressure (W85-W99)

- Exposure to smoke, fire, and flames (X00-X08)

- Contact with heat and hot substances (X10-X19)

- Exposure to forces of nature (X30-X39)

- Accidental exposure to other specified factors (X52-X58)

- Intentional self-harm (X71-X83)

- Assault (X92-Y09)

- Event of undetermined intent (Y21-Y33)

- Legal intervention, operations of war, military operations, and terrorism (Y35-Y38)

- Misadventures to patients during surgical and medical care (Y62-Y69)

- Medical devices associated with adverse incidents in diagnostic and therapeutic use (Y70-Y82)

- Surgical and other medical procedures as the cause of abnormal reaction of the patient, or of later complication, without mention of misadventure at the time of the procedure (Y83-Y84)

- Supplementary factors related to causes of morbidity classified elsewhere (Y90-Y99)

This chapter permits the classification of environmental events and circumstances as the cause of injury and other adverse effects. Where a code from this section is applicable, it is intended that it shall be used secondary to a code from another chapter indicating the nature of the condition. Most often, the condition will be classifiable to Chapter 19, Injury, poisoning, and certain other consequences of external causes (S00-T98). External cause codes may indicate the external causes of injuries, poisonings, and adverse effects of drugs, chemicals, and substances. However, they can also be reported for diseases due to an external source or other health condition that is applicable. These codes for reporting external causes are important in providing data for injury identification and evaluation of injury prevention. For these conditions, codes from Chapter 20 should be used to provide additional information as to the cause of the condition. These codes are never listed as the principal diagnosis or first listed diagnosis.

External cause codes for injuries and other health conditions provide data for research and prevention strategies. An External Cause code can be used with any code in the rages of A00.0-T88.9 and Z00-Z99 when there is a health condition due to an external cause. These codes capture the cause of the injury or health condition. The External Cause codes identify the intent of the circumstance as:

- Unintentional (accidental)

- Intentional self-harm or assault

- Place where the event occurred

- The activity of the patient at the time of the event

Many insurance carriers require External Cause codes for certain patient encounters. It is important to become familiar with the Official Coding Guidelines related to External Cause codes. Guidelines for External Cause codes apply to all settings, including the physician's office, outpatient clinics, emergency departments, and hospitals.

Injuries are a major cause of mortality, morbidity, and disability. These codes capture how the injury or poisoning happened (cause), the intent (unintentional or accidental, or intentional, such as suicide or assault), and the place where the event occurred. Some major categories of External Cause codes includes:

- Transport accidents

- Poisoning and adverse effects of drugs, medicinal substances, and biologicals

- Accidental falls

- Accidents caused by fire and flames

- Accidents due to natural and environmental factors

- Late effects of accidents, assaults, or self-injury

- Assaults or purposely inflicted injury

- Suicide or self-inflicted injury

CODING TIP Assign as many External Cause codes as necessary to explain fully each cause.

GENERAL CODING GUIDELINES

Sequencing of multiple External Cause codes is based on the sequence of events leading to the injury. If only one External Cause code can be recorded, assign the External Cause code that relates to the principal/first listed diagnosis.

Many times External Cause codes are combination codes that identify sequential events that result in an injury, such as a fall that results in striking against an object. The injury may be due to either event or both. The combination External Cause code used should correspond to the sequence of events regardless of which caused the most serious injury. External cause codes for child and adult abuse take sequencing priority over all other External Cause codes.

Activity Codes

Activity codes are reported with Category Y93– as secondary codes to identify the activity at the time of injury. Only use an activity code one time per patient encounter. It should only be reported for the initial encounter for treatment and not used for subsequent care. Always use an activity code along with a place of occurrence code if the information is available in the documentation.

Sequencing Priority

External cause codes have a specific sequencing priority. Review the following:

- Terrorism takes sequencing priority over all other External Cause code (exception child and adult abuse)

- Cataclysmic events take sequencing priority over all other External Cause codes (exception child and adult abuse and terrorism)

- Transport accidents take sequencing priority over all other External Cause codes (exception cataclysmic events, child and adult abuse, and terrorism)

The selection of the appropriate External Cause code is guided by the Index to External Causes, a separate index in the ICD-10-CM, and by the instructional notes in Chapter 20. The code indicated in the index for the main term is verified in the Tabular List of Chapter 20. The conventions and rules for the classification also apply. Make certain all inclusion and exclusion notes in the Tabular List are reviewed before selecting a code.

There are also sections for legal interventions, operations of war, military operations, terrorism, complications of medical and surgical care, and supplemental factors related to causes of morbidity classified elsewhere.

These extensions match the extensions for the non-fracture T codes that have extensions. An External Cause code may be used for every health care encounter for the duration of treatment of an illness or injury.

Different extensions are needed for Y93, Activity code. No extensions are required for categories Y62-Y84, Complications of medical and surgical care.

Place of Occurrence

In ICD-10-CM, codes from category Y92, Place of occurrence of the external cause, are secondary codes for use with other External Cause codes to identify the location of the patient at the time of injury. A place of occurrence code is used only once, at the initial encounter for treatment. A place of occurrence code should be used in conjunction with an activity code, Y93-. Use place of occurrence code Y92.9, Unspecified place or not applicable, if the place is not stated or is not applicable. Place of occurrence codes are not necessary with poisonings, toxic effects, adverse effects, or underdosing codes, and no extensions are used for Y92-.

Sometimes finding an external code in the Alphabetic Index is a challenge because you are looking for the cause or place of the injury.

UNINTENTIONAL (ACCIDENTAL) INJURIES

The default for external cause is unintentional. If there is no documentation in the medical record as to the intent of an injury, it should be assigned an "unintentional intent" External Cause code.

Review the following examples. Open up the ICD-10-CM codebook, referencing both the Alphabetic Index and the Tabular List, locate the correct code.

> **EXAMPLE:** *A woman fell off a horse she was riding and injured her back on her ranch.*

In order to report the codes correctly, the user must first code the condition, followed by how the injury occurred and where.

> **Alphabetic Index:**
> *Injury → lower back → S39.92*

> **Tabular List:**
> *S39.92 → unspecified injury of lower back*

Note that a seventh character is required to identify the encounter. Because this is the initial encounter, the seventh character is A. You will also need to use a dummy placeholder in order to code to the seventh character. The correct code is S39.92xA.

The next step is to report the external cause.

> **Alphabetic Index to External Causes:**
> *Accident → transport → animal → noncollision → V80.02*

> **Tabular List:**
> *V80.02 → Occupant of animal-drawn vehicle injured by fall from or being thrown from animal-drawn vehicle in noncollision accident (requires seventh character) → V80.02xA (initial encounter)*

The last step is to report the place of occurrence.

> **Alphabetic Index to External Causes:**
> *Place of occurrence → ranch → see place of occurrence farm → specified NEC → Y92.79*

> **Tabular List:**
> *Y92.79 → Other farm location as the place of occurrence of the external cause*

> **Correct code sequencing:**
> *S39.92xA, V80.02xA, Y92.79*

EXAMPLE: *While on vacation in Aspen, a patient fell while skiing and suffered a stress fracture of the right femur.*

Alphabetic Index:
  Fracture ➞ *femur* ➞ *stress fracture* ➞ *M84.35–*

Tabular List:
  M84.351A Stress fracture, right femur, initial encounter

Alphabetic Index to External Causes:
  Accident-snow-ski-V00.32–

Tabular List:
  V00.321 ➞ *fall from snow skis*

Alphabetic Index:
  Activity ➞ *skiing (alpine) (downhill)* ➞ *Y93.23*

Tabular List:
  Y93.23 ➞ *Activity, snow (alpine) (downhill) skiing, snow boarding, sledding, tobogganing and snowtubing as the place of occurrence of the external cause*

Correct code sequencing:
  M84.351A, V00.321, Y93.23, Y99.8

When coding the stress fracture, the seventh character, A, identifies the initial treatment. Also, because this was a nonwork or student activity, a status code is required to report the activity (Y99.8).

CODING TIP Keep in mind that the place of occurrence (Y92–) and activity codes (Y93–) are sequenced after the main External Cause code. Regardless of the number of External Cause codes assigned, there should be only one place of occurrence code and one activity code assigned to a record. An External Cause status in category Y99.– should be used to report accidents and falls as an additional diagnosis.

TRANSPORT ACCIDENTS

The type of vehicle the victim is an occupant in is identified in the first two characters because it is seen as the most important factor to identify for prevention purposes. A transport accident is one in which the vehicle involved must be moving or running or in use for transport purposes at the time of the accident. When accidents involving more than one kind of transport are recorded, the following order of precedence should be used:

- Aircraft and spacecraft (V95-V97)
- Watercraft (V90-V94)
- Other modes of transport (V00-V89, V98-V99)

Where transport accident descriptions do not specify the victim as being a vehicle occupant and the victim is described by terms such as crushed, dragged, hit, or run over, classify the victim as a pedestrian.

If no documentation is available as to whether the victim was the driver or occupant of a vehicle, classify the victim as an occupant.

Use additional External Cause codes with a transport accident code to identify:

- The use of a cell phone or other electronic equipment contributing to the accident (Y93.5–)
- Whether an airbag contributed to any injury (W22.1)
- The type of street or road where the accident occurred, if known (Y92.4–)

Review the following example. Open up the ICD-10-CM codebook, referencing both the Alphabetic Index and the Tabular List, locate the correct code.

EXAMPLE: *The driver of a car was injured when he was involved in a head-on collision with another car on a busy highway. He suffered a superficial injury of the chest wall when the seat belt failed. He was hospitalized for observation.*

Alphabetic Index:
  Injury ➞ *thorax, thoracic (wall)* ➞ *S20.90*

Tabular List:
  S20.90 ➞ *✓7th* ➞ *Unspecified superficial injury of unspecified parts of the thorax* ➞ *S20.90xA (initial encounter)*

Alphabetic Index to External Causes:
  Accident, transport ➞ *car* ➞ *driver* ➞ *collision* ➞ *car* ➞ *in traffic* ➞ *V43.52*

Tabular List:
  V43.52xA ➞ *Car driver injured in collision with other type car in traffic accident, initial encounter (requires seventh character)*

Don't forget to report the place of occurrence.

Alphabetic Index to External Causes:
  Place of occurrence ➞ *highway (interstate)* ➞ *Y92.411*

Tabular List:
  Y92.411 ➞ *Interstate highway as the place of occurrence of the external cause*

Activity code from Category Y99:
  Y99.9 Unspecified external cause status

Correct code sequencing:
  S20.90xA, V43.52xA, Y92.411, Y99.9

FALLS

Categories W00-W19, Falls, include the main fall codes in Chapter 20. Review Figure 8.7. These codes are for standard types of falls, such as those due to ice and snow and falling from stairs or off a ladder. There are other fall codes in Chapter 20 for falls associated with other causes, such as:

- Fires
- Watercraft accidents
- Pedestrian
- Conveyance accidents
- Subsequent striking against objects

Review the following example. Open up the ICD-10-CM codebook, referencing both the Alphabetic Index and the Tabular List, locate the correct code.

> **EXAMPLE:** *A 4-year-old male at the local public pool tripped on the concrete and fell into the water, hitting his head on the wall of the pool. This resulted in a contusion of the head. The mother took the child to the emergency room for care.*

Use the guidelines for external causes and the Alphabetic Index and Tabular List to select the correct codes.

Principal/first listed diagnosis:
   S00.93xA → *Contusion of unspecified part of head (illness or injury code) (initial encounter)*

Secondary diagnosis:
   W16.032A → *Fall into swimming pool striking wall causing other injury (initial encounter)*

Tertiary diagnosis:
   Y93.11 → *Swimming*

Additional diagnosis:
   Y92.34 → *Swimming pool (public) as the place of occurrence of the external cause*

   Y99.8 → *Leisure activity*

Correct code sequencing:
   S00.93xA, W16.032A, Y93.014, Y92.34, Y99.8

Did you locate all of the correct diagnosis codes? If yes, congratulations. If you did not locate all the codes, begin with the Alphabetic Index and start again.

ASSAULT

An assault is an intentional infliction of an injury to another person with the intent to injure or harm. Assault codes X92-Y08 identify the external cause of injury. Other codes are available for terrorism, military operations, operations of war, and legal interventions. Assault codes are not used in these circumstances.

These guidelines are provided for the reporting of external causes of morbidity codes so that there is standardization in the process. These codes are secondary codes for use in any health care setting.

Review Table 10.2.

TABLE 10.2   Official ICD-10-CM I External Cause Coding Guidelines

Used with any code in the range of A00.0-T88.9, Z00-Z99	An External Cause code may be used with any code in the range of A00.0-T88.9, Z00-Z99, for classification that is a health condition due to an external cause. Though they are most applicable to injuries, they are also valid for such things as infections or diseases due to an external source and other health conditions, such as a heart attack that occurs during strenuous physical activity.
External cause code used for length of treatment	Assign the External Cause code, with the appropriate seventh character (initial encounter, subsequent encounter or sequela) for each encounter for which the injury or condition is being treated.
Use the full range of External Cause codes	Use the full range of External Cause codes to completely describe the cause, the intent, the place of occurrence, and, if applicable, the activity of the patient at the time of the event, as well as the patient's status, for all injuries and other health conditions due to an external cause.
Assign as many External Cause codes as necessary	Assign as many External Cause codes as necessary to fully explain each cause. If only one external code can be recorded, assign the code most related to the principal diagnosis.
The selection of the appropriate External Cause code	The selection of the appropriate External Cause code is guided by the Alphabetic Index of External Causes and by Inclusion and Exclusion notes in the Tabular List.

(continued)

TABLE 10.2   *(continued)*

External cause code can never be a principal diagnosis	An External Cause code can never be a principal (first listed) diagnosis.
Combination External Cause codes	Certain External Cause codes are combination codes that identify sequential events that result in an injury, such as a fall that results in striking against an object. The injury may be due to either event or both. The combination External Cause code used should correspond to the sequence of events regardless of which caused the most serious injury.
No External Cause code needed in certain circumstances	No External Cause code from Chapter 20 is needed if the external cause and intent are included in a code from another chapter (eg, T36.0x1, Poisoning by penicillins, accidental [unintentional]).
Place of occurrence guideline	Codes from category Y92, Place of occurrence of the external cause, are secondary codes for use after other External Cause codes to identify the location of the patient at the time of injury or other condition.
	A place of occurrence code is used only once, at the initial encounter for treatment. No seventh characters are used for Y92. Only one code from Y92 should be recorded on a medical record. A place of occurrence code should be used in conjunction with an activity code, Y93.
	Do not use place of occurrence code Y92.9 if the place is not stated or is not applicable.
Activity code	Assign a code from category Y93, Activity code, to describe the activity of the patient at the time the injury or other health condition occurred.
	An activity code is used only once, at the initial encounter for treatment. Only one code from Y93 should be recorded on a medical record. An activity code should be used in conjunction with a place of occurrence code, Y92.
	The activity codes are not applicable to poisonings, adverse effects, misadventures, or late effects.
	Do not assign Y93.9, Unspecified activity, if the activity is not stated.
	A code from category Y93 is appropriate for use with external cause and intent codes if identifying the activity provides additional information about the event.
Place of occurrence, activity, and status codes used with other External Cause code	When applicable, place of occurrence, activity, and external cause status codes are sequenced after the main External Cause code(s). Regardless of the number of External Cause codes assigned, there should be only one place of occurrence code, one activity code, and one external cause status code assigned to an encounter.
If the reporting format limits the number of external cause codes	If the reporting format limits the number of External Cause codes that can be used in reporting clinical data, report the code for the cause/intent most related to the principal diagnosis. If the format permits capture of additional External Cause codes, the cause/intent, including medical misadventures, of the additional events should be reported rather than the codes for place, activity, or external status.
Multiple external cause coding guidelines	More than one External Cause code is required to fully describe the external cause of an illness or injury. The assignment of External Cause codes should be sequenced with the following priority:
	If two or more events cause separate injuries, an External Cause code should be assigned for each cause. The first listed External Cause code will be selected in the following order:
	External codes for child and adult abuse take priority over all other External Cause codes.
	See Section I.C.19, Child and adult abuse guidelines.
	External cause codes for terrorism events take priority over all other External Cause codes except child and adult abuse.
	External cause codes for cataclysmic events take priority over all other External Cause codes except child and adult abuse and terrorism.
	External cause codes for transport accidents take priority over all other External Cause codes except cataclysmic events, child and adult abuse, and terrorism.
	Activity and external cause status codes are assigned following all causal (intent) External Cause codes.
	The first listed External Cause code should correspond to the cause of the most serious diagnosis due to an assault, accident, or self-harm, following the order of hierarchy listed above.

(continued)

TABLE 10.2　*(continued)*

Child and adult abuse guideline	Adult and child abuse, neglect, and maltreatment are classified as assault. Any of the assault codes may be used to indicate the external cause of any injury resulting from the confirmed abuse.
	For confirmed cases of abuse, neglect, and maltreatment, when the perpetrator is known, a code from Y07, Perpetrator of maltreatment and neglect, should accompany any other assault codes.
	See Section I.C.19, Adult and child abuse, neglect and other maltreatment h. Unknown or undetermined intent guideline
	If the intent (accident, self-harm, assault) of the cause of an injury or other condition is unknown or unspecified, code the intent as accidental intent. All transport accident categories assume accidental intent.
Use of undetermined intent	External cause codes for events of undetermined intent are only for use if the documentation in the record specifies that the intent cannot be determined.
Late effects of external cause guidelines Late effect External Cause codes	Late effects are reported using the External Cause code with the seventh character extension S, for sequela. These codes should be used with any report of a late effect or sequela resulting from a previous injury.
Late effect External Cause code with a related current injury	A late effect External Cause code should never be used with a related current nature of injury code.
Use of late effect External Cause codes for subsequent visits	Use a late effect External Cause code for subsequent visits when a late effect of the initial injury is being treated. Do not use a late effect External Cause code for subsequent visits for follow-up care (eg, to assess healing, to receive rehabilitative therapy) of the injury when no late effect of the injury has been documented.
Terrorism guidelines Cause of injury identified by the federal government (FBI) as terrorism	When the cause of an injury is identified by the federal government (FBI) as terrorism, the first listed External Cause code should be a code from category Y38, Terrorism. The definition of terrorism employed by the FBI is found at the inclusion note at the beginning of category Y38. Use additional code for place of occurrence (Y92.–). More than one Y38 code may be assigned if the injury is the result of more than one mechanism of terrorism.
Cause of an injury is suspected to be the result of terrorism	When the cause of an injury is suspected to be the result of terrorism, a code from category Y38 should not be assigned. Suspected cases should be classified as assault.
Code Y38.9, Terrorism, secondary effects	Assign code Y38.9, Terrorism, secondary effects, for conditions occurring subsequent to the terrorist event. This code should not be assigned for conditions that are due to the initial terrorist act.
	It is acceptable to assign code Y38.9 with another code from Y38 if there is an injury due to the initial terrorist event and an injury that is a subsequent result of the terrorist event.
External cause status	A code from category Y99, External cause status, should be assigned whenever any other External Cause code is assigned for an encounter, including an activity code, except for the events noted below. Assign a code from category Y99, External cause status, to indicate the work status of the person at the time the event occurred. The status code indicates whether the event occurred during military activity, whether a nonmilitary person was at work, whether an individual including a student or volunteer was involved in a nonwork activity at the time of the causal event.
	A code from Y99, External cause status, should be assigned, when applicable, with other External Cause codes, such as transport accidents and falls. The external cause status codes are not applicable to poisonings, adverse effects, misadventures, or late effects.
	Do not assign a code from category Y99 if no other External Cause codes (cause, activity) are applicable for the encounter.
	An external cause status code is used only once, at the initial encounter for treatment. Only one code from Y99 should be recorded on a medical record.
	Do not assign code Y99.9, Unspecified external cause status, if the status is not stated.

Source: Official ICD-10-CM Guidelines for External Causes

Review the following example. Open up the ICD-10-CM codebook, referencing both the Alphabetic Index and the Tabular List, locate the correct code.

> **EXAMPLE:** *While having breakfast in the kitchen of their apartment, an angry father poured hot coffee on his 4-year-old child who was badly scalded. The child was taken to the emergency room and diagnosed with second-degree burns of the head, neck, and face.*

> **Alphabetic Index:**
> *Burn ➞ head (and face) (and neck) ➞ T20.00*

> **Tabular List:**
> *T20.00 ➞ T20.20 ➞ Burn of second degree of head, face, and neck, unspecified site ➞ T20.20xA (initial encounter)*

As you review the Tabular List it is evident that a seventh character is required to identify the initial encounter.

> **Alphabetic Index to External Causes:**
> *Accident ➞ caused by ➞ hot ➞ see contact hot ➞ liquid ➞ drinks ➞ X10.0*

> **Tabular List:**
> *X10.0 ➞ Contact with hot drinks ➞ X10.0xxA (initial encounter)*

Note a seventh character is required in this category as well. Now you need to identify the assault.

> **Alphabetic Index to External Causes:**
> *Assault ➞ scalding-see assault burning ➞ assault by steam, vapors, and hot objects ➞ X98*

> **Tabular List:**
> *X98.2 ➞ Assault by hot fluids ➞ X98.2.xxA (initial encounter)*

A seventh character is also required in this category.

> **Alphabetic Index to External Causes:**
> *Place of occurrence ➞ residence ➞ apartment ➞ kitchen ➞ Y92.030*

> *Activity ➞ Y99 ➞ Y99.9 unspecified External Cause status*

> **Correct code sequencing:**
> *T20.20xA, X10.0xxA, X98.2.xxA, Y92.030, Y99.9*

UNDETERMINED INTENT

The default for injuries when the documentation does not indicate intent is unintentional. Codes from categories Y21-Y33, Events of undetermined intent, are only for use when the documentation in the record specifically states that the intent cannot be determined.

LEGAL INTERVENTIONS

The codes from category Y35, Legal intervention, are used for any injury documented as sustained as a result of an encounter with any law enforcement official, serving in any capacity at the time of the encounter, whether on-duty or off-duty. The sixth character for the legal intervention codes identifies the victim, a law enforcement official, a bystander, or the suspect of a crime.

The seventh character extensions for Y35 are the same as for the majority of categories used to identify the initial, subsequent, or sequelae encounter. Review Figure 10.3.

FIGURE 10.3 Excerpt from the Tabular List: *Y35.02–*

Y35.02 Legal intervention involving injury by handgun
        The appropriate seventh character is to be added to each
            code from category Y35
        A initial encounter
        D subsequent encounter
        S sequela
            Y35.021 Legal intervention involving injury by handgun,
                     law enforcement official injured
            Y35.022 Legal intervention involving injury by handgun,
                     bystander injured
            Y35.023 Legal intervention involving injury by handgun,
                     suspect injured

The condition of the patient should be reported as the principal or first listed diagnosis and the cause (legal intervention) should be reported as a secondary diagnosis.

Review the following example. Open up the ICD-10-CM codebook, referencing both the Alphabetic Index and the Tabular List, locate the correct code.

> **EXAMPLE:** *A man was robbing a convenience store. He was using a handgun. He pulled the gun on the store clerk, and the store clerk armed a silent alarm. The police arrived and shot the suspect in the abdomen. He was taken to the hospital, and the physician determined the bullet penetrated into the peritoneal cavity. The suspect was taken to surgery immediately.*

Alphabetic Index:
Wound open → abdomen, abdominal → with penetration into the peritoneal cavity → S31.609

Tabular List:
S31.609A → Unspecified open wound of abdominal wall, unspecified quadrant with penetration into peritoneal cavity (initial encounter)

Secondary diagnosis:
Y35.023A (initial encounter) → Legal intervention involving injury by handgun, suspect injured (what occurred)

Tertiary diagnosis:
Place of occurrence → Store → Y92.512 → Supermarket, store or market as the place of occurrence of the external cause

Status → Y99.8 → other External Cause status

Correct code sequencing:
S31.609A, Y35.023A, Y92.512, Y99.8

OPERATIONS OF WAR/ MILITARY OPERATIONS

Category Y36, Operations of war, is limited to classifying injuries sustained during a time of declared war and that are directly due to the war. Y37, Military operations, is for use to classify injuries to military and civilian personnel that occur during peacetime on military property or during routine military exercises or operations. The extensions for Y36 and Y37 are the same as for the majority of categories for the initial encounter (a), subsequent encounter (d), and sequelae (q).

Review the following examples. Open up the ICD-10-CM codebook, referencing both the Alphabetic Index and the Tabular List, locate the correct code.

> **EXAMPLE:** *While on active duty in Baghdad, a 26-year-old Marine was admitted to the hospital in a foreign country while fighting a war. The patient was in a building when terrorists threw a gasoline bomb through a window in the barracks while he was sleeping on the military base. The blast threw him into the wall. He suffered multiple unstable closed fractures of the pelvis with disruption of the pelvic circle and second-degree burns on the right forearm and right calf.*

Alphabetic Index:
Fracture → pelvic circle → see disruption pelvic ring → disruption → pelvic ring → unstable → S32.811

Tabular List:
S32.811A Multiple fractures of pelvis with unstable disruption of pelvic ring (closed fracture)

The seventh character, A, identifies the closed fracture.

Alphabetic Index:
Burn → upper limb → forearm → right → second degree → T22.211

Tabular List:
T22.211 → Burn of second degree of right forearm → T22.211A → initial encounter

Alphabetic Index:
Burn → calf → right → second degree → T24.231

Tabular List:
T24.231 → Burn of second degree of right lower leg → initial encounter → T24.231A

Alphabetic Index to External Causes:
War operations → explosion → bomb → gasoline → Y36.31–

Tabular List:
Y36.31 → War operations involving gasoline bomb → initial encounter → Y36.310A

Place of Occurrence:
Residence → military base → barracks → Y92.133

Tabular List:
Y92.133 → Barracks on military base as the place of

Now we need to locate the code for the activity. Reference the Alphabetic Index to external caused under the main term "activity."

Activity Code:
Y93.84 → sleeping (sleep)

Now we can also add a status code. You will find this in the Alphabetic Index under the main term "status." Because the status is military activity, it will also be referenced.

Status Code:
Y99.1 → Military activity

Correct code sequencing:
T22.211A, T24.231A, Y36.310A, Y92.133, Y93.84, Y99.1

Transport accidents during peacetime involving military vehicles that are off military property are included with the transport accidents, not in Y36 or Y37.

Injury, Poisoning, and Certain Other Consequences of External Causes (S00-T88)

CHECKPOINT EXERCISE 10-2

Select the External Cause code(s) that best describes the following circumstances:

1. _____ Accidental drowning in a swimming pool at local park

2. _____ A conductor falling off of a railway train when trying to board the train

3. _____ Needle stick accident at a hospital

4. _____ Nonvenomous snakebite

5. _____ Bus accident involving loss of control without collision on the highway due to driver falling asleep; patient is a passenger on the bus

6. _____ Accident caused by blow to the head

7. _____ Flooding resulting from a storm surge

8. _____ Accidental drowning due to sinking ship

9. _____ Accidental perforation during a surgical procedure

10. _____ Prolonged exposure to cold while hiking in the mountains

11. _____ Suicide attempt by amphetamine overdose resulting in cardiac arrest

12. _____ An angry man broke the big toe on his right foot when he kicked a metal pole in an outburst of anger.

13. _____ Observation following automobile accident in which the patient suffered a contusion with a brief loss of consciousness. The patient was a passenger in the vehicle.

14. _____ A boy was brought to the emergency room to have a penny removed from his right nostril. His mother explained that he was showing off to his friends and now she can't remove the coin. The child is having a small amount of difficulty breathing because of the obstruction. As a result of his mother's attempts to remove the coin, the child has suffered a bruise around the affected area.

15. _____ While shooting an action film in Montana, an actor suffered a mild concussion without loss of consciousness from a rough landing while jumping a mound of snow in a snowmobile.

Injury, Poisoning, and Certain Other Consequences of External Causes (S00-T88)

Chapter 19 in ICD-10-CM contains the following categories:

- Injuries to the head (S00-S09)
- Injuries to the neck (S10-S19)
- Injuries to the thorax (S20-S29)
- Injuries to the abdomen, lower back, lumbar spine, pelvis, and external genitals (S30-S39)
- Injuries to the shoulder and upper arm (S40-S49)
- Injuries to the elbow and forearm (S50-S59)
- Injuries to the wrist, hand, and fingers (S60-S69)
- Injuries to the hip and thigh (S70-S79)
- Injuries to the knee and lower leg (S80-S89)
- Injuries to the ankle and foot (S90-S99)
- Unspecified multiple injuries (T07)
- Injury of unspecified body region (T14)
- Effects of foreign body entering through natural orifice (T15-T19)
- Burns and corrosions of external body surface, specified by site (T20-T25)
- Burns and corrosions confined to eye and internal organs (T26-T28)
- Burns and corrosions of multiple and unspecified body regions (T30-T32)
- Frostbite (T33-T34)
- Poisoning by, adverse effects of, and underdosing of drugs, medicaments, and biological substances (T36-T50)
- Toxic effects of substances chiefly nonmedicinal as to source (T51-T65)
- Other and unspecified effects of external causes (T66-T78)
- Certain early complications of trauma (T79)
- Complications of surgical and medical care, not elsewhere classified (T80-T88)

Within the injury and poisoning chapter, external cause of morbidity codes are to be used from Chapter 20 of ICD-10-CM to report the cause of injury. The only exception is if the External Cause code is included in a T-section code that does not require an External Cause code.

These External Cause codes are no longer optional when reporting injuries in ICD-10-CM. In this chapter, codes in the S section are related to different types of injuries in a single body area, and the T section covers injuries to unspecified body areas/regions. In addition, poisonings and certain other consequences of external causes are located in Chapter 19 of ICD-10-CM, but birth and obstetric traumas are excluded from this chapter and are located in other chapters.

INJURIES

Injury is one of the United States' most important health problems. According to the National Safety Council, the leading causes of unintentional death are:

- Motor-vehicle accidents
- Falls
- Poisonings
- Drownings
- Fires

FRACTURES

A fracture is a broken bone. ICD-1-0-CM classifies fractures in terms of their complexity. A closed fracture (with or without delayed healing) is a fracture of the bone with no skin wound. Examples of closed fractures include:

- Comminuted
- Depressed
- Elevated
- Fissured
- Greenstick
- Impacted
- Linear
- March
- Simple
- Slipped epiphysis
- Spiral
- Torus (buckle)
- Compression
- Transverse
- Oblique
- Stress

An open fracture (with or without delayed healing) is a fracture of the bone with skin wound. Examples of open fractures include:

- Compound
- Infected
- Missile
- Puncture
- With foreign body

The accurate assignment in selecting the correct diagnosis for fractures depends upon a clear understating of the anatomic sites and extent of the injuries. As stated earlier, fractures are documented as either "open" or "closed." A closed fracture is one in which the skin is intact at the site of fracture. Other terms may be included in the description that also describe closed fractures, but the code assignment remains the same.

Chapter 19 comprises of S and T codes. S codes are used to report traumatic injuries and T codes are used to report burns and corrosions, poisonings, toxic effects, adverse effects, underdosing, complications of medical care, and other such consequences of external causes. Most categories in Chapter 19 have seventh-character extensions that are required for the applicable code. Most categories use these 3 extensions:

- A initial encounter
- D subsequent encounter
- S sequela

Fractures are reported with additional extensions and are unique to each category.

Extension A is used while the patient is receiving active treatment of an injury. All subsequent encounters require extension D to reflect that the patient has received active treatment of the injury and is receiving routine care for the injury during the healing or recovery phase. An injury code with extension D may be used as long as the patient is treated for the entire course of treatment for a specific injury. Even if the patient delays seeking treatment, the first encounter with the provider is considered the initial encounter. However, if another medical professional has treated the patient previously for the same injury, it is coded as a subsequent treatment. If the encounter is unknown, it is reported with extension A for the initial treatment.

Extension S (sequela) is used for complications or conditions that are a direct result of an injury. A good example is scar formation following a burn. The scars would be sequelae of the burn. The ICD-10-CM guidelines direct the user to report the injury code that precipitated the complication and the code for the sequela. The seventh-character S is added to the injury code, not the code for the complication or sequela. Sequencing for injuries in sequela is important. The following rules apply:

- Sequela is sequenced first (complication or the condition as a result of the injury).

- Injury code is sequenced as the secondary diagnosis.

Remember that when reporting aftercare of injuries, the Z aftercare codes are not used. An acute injury code is assigned with the seventh-character D to report the subsequent encounter for care.

Injury codes, or S codes are reported for injuries. The most severe injury is sequenced first. Injury codes are categorized by type of injury and location (site). In some cases, laterality is critical in the code selection. There are instructional notes to indicate whether any other codes will be needed to describe the injury fully. For open wounds, for example, an instructional note provides guidance to the user to code any associated wound infection. For normal healing surgical wounds, a wound code from this chapter is not used.

Codes in this category are divided into body regions:

S00-S09	Head
S10-S19	Neck
S20-S29	Thorax
S30-S39	Abdomen, lower back, lumbar spine, pelvis, and external genitals
S40-S49	Shoulder and upper arm
S50-S59	Elbow and forearm
S60-S69	Wrist and hand
S70-S79	Hip and thigh
S80-S89	Knee and lower leg
S90-S99	Ankle and foot

Within each body section are categories for type of injury specific to the body section. When coding superficial and open wounds, assign codes based on terms documented in the medical record. For example, if a wound is classified as a bite, it would be classified as an open bite. Superficial wounds are not coded with a more severe injury if the wounds are associated with that injury at the same site.

GENERAL CODING GUIDELINES FOR CODING INJURIES

Following are some general coding guidelines:

- The code for the most serious injury, as determined by the physician, is sequenced first.

- Superficial injuries such as abrasions or contusions are not coded when associated with more severe injuries of the same site.

- Assign separate codes for each injury; the exception is when a combination code is available. The code for unspecified multiple injuries (T07) is only assigned when a more specific code is not available.

- For normal healing surgical wounds or to identify a complication of a wound, the traumatic injury codes (S00-T14.9) are not to be used.

- When a primary injury results in minor damage to peripheral nerves or blood vessels, the primary injury is sequenced first using additional code(s) from categories S04 or S15, Injury to nerves and spinal cord or to blood vessels. When the primary injury is to the blood vessels or nerves, the injury should be sequenced first.

- Traumatic fractures with specified sites are coded individually by site and documented in the medical record.

- Fractures that are not specified as "open" or "closed" are coded as *closed*. A fracture that is not indicated as "displaced" or "not displaced" is coded as *displaced*. It is important to query the physician to identify specificity if possible.

- Use caution and select the appropriate seventh-character extension in the classification.

- For subsequent care after the initial care for a fracture and when the patient is receiving treatment for healing and recovery, the active treatment diagnosis should be reported with the seventh-character D for subsequent care (the aftercare Z codes should not be used for aftercare for injuries).

- A complication code should be used when a complication arises during the healing or recovery phase of fracture care.

- A patient with known osteoporosis who suffers a fracture should be reported in category M80, not with the fracture code(s), even if the condition is minor or traumatic.

- Sequencing of fractures depends on the severity of the fracture. The more serious fracture is sequenced first.

Documentation for fracture coding should include:

- Anatomic site
- Laterality
- Fracture status
- Whether displaced or nondisplaced
- Whether open or closed
- Seventh-character extension as required

Review the following examples. Open up the ICD-10-CM codebook, referencing both the Alphabetic Index and the Tabular List, locate the correct code. When referencing the Alphabetic Index, the main term is "fracture." Keep in mind that if you are referencing "osteoporosis" the main term is "fracture" followed by "pathological." For the following example, this is a traumatic fracture.

> **EXAMPLE:** *A patient fell on his left shoulder and displaced the acromial end of the left clavicle. The orthopedic surgeon evaluated the patient and took him to surgery to repair the fracture.*

Alphabetic Index:
   Fracture, traumatic ➡ *clavicle* ➡ *acromial end (displaced)* ➡ *S42.02–*

Tabular List:
   S42.02– Displaced fracture of shaft of left clavicle initial encounter for closed fracture ➡ *left* ➡ *S42.022*

Don't forget, you will need a seventh-character A for the initial encounter.

Review Figure 10.4.

FIGURE 10.4   Excerpt from the Tabular List: *S42.02–, seventh-character extension*

S42.02-
Fracture codes require seventh character to identify if fracture
   is open or closed
The fracture seventh character extensions are:
A Initial encounter for closed fracture
B Initial encounter for open fracture
D Subsequent encounter for fracture with routine healing
G Subsequent encounter for fracture with delayed healing
K Subsequent encounter for fracture with nonunion
P Subsequent encounter for fracture with malunion
S Sequelae

S42.022, Displaced fracture of shaft of left clavicle initial encounter for closed fracture, requires seventh-character A for the initial encounter.

Correct code:
   S42.022A

> **EXAMPLE:** *A patient with a malunion of a stress fracture of the left femur underwent an open reduction and internal fixation. The original injury occurred 6 months ago.*

In this example, the documentation required to code the patient encounter includes:

- Laterality
- Type of encounter (initial, subsequent, sequela)
- Malunion, not union, healing
- Late effect

Alphabetic Index:
   Fracture, traumatic ➡ *femur* ➡ *M84.35–*

Tabular List:
   M84.35– ➡ *Fracture of femur and pelvis* ➡ *left femur* ➡ *M84.352*

Now you will need to select the seventh-character extension for this code. Because the documentation indicates the condition is a malunion, the seventh character is P.

Correct code:
   M84.352P

You're not finished yet. You must code the late effect. Keep in mind that in the Alphabetic Index, a late effect is listed as the main term "sequelae."

Alphabetic Index:
   Sequelae ➡ *fracture* ➡ *code to injury with extension S*

   Fracture ➡ *femur femoral* ➡ *S72.9–*

Tabular List:
   S72.9 ➡ *unspecified fracture of femur* ➡ *left femur* ➡ *S72.92*

As with other chapters in ICD-10-CM, when a seventh character is required and there are not enough characters in the code, a dummy placeholder x must be added.

Correct code:
   S72.92xS (sequela)

Correct code sequencing:
   M84.352P, S72.92xS

CODING TIP The seventh character S identifies sequela.

CODING TIP A late effect is listed in the Alphabetic Index under the main term "sequelae."

> **EXAMPLE:** A patient who was a passenger in a car involved in a head-on collision with another pickup truck on a major interstate was hospitalized for a closed head injury. He lost consciousness for 45 minutes, was transported by ambulance to the hospital, and was admitted as an inpatient to the ICU.
>
> **Alphabetic Index:**
> Injury ➞ head ➞ with loss of consciousness ➞ S06.9
>
> **Tabular List:**
> S06.9 ➞ Unspecified intracranial injury ➞ with loss of consciousness of 31 minutes to 59 minutes ➞ S06.9x2

Now you need to select the seventh-character extension. Because this is the initial encounter, the appropriate seventh character is A.

You will also need an External Cause code and place of occurrence.

> **Alphabetic Index to External Causes:**
> Accident, transport ➞ car ➞ passenger ➞ collision with ➞ pickup truck ➞ V43.63
>
> Place of occurrence ➞ freeway or highway ➞ Y92.411
>
> **Tabular List:**
> V43.63xA ➞ Car passenger injured in collision with pick-up truck in traffic accident (initial encounter)
>
> Y92.411 ➞ Interstate highway as the place of occurrence of the external cause
>
> Don't forget the External Cause status Y99.9 ➞ unspecified
>
> **Correct code sequencing:**
> S06.9x2A, V43.63xA, Y92.411, Y99

For open fractures of the long bone, extensions identify the degree of severity for the open fracture. The fracture extensions are unique to each type of bone and type of fracture. It is necessary to review the fracture extensions carefully before assigning an extension. A fracture code is reported as long as the patient is receiving treatment for the fracture. Review category 32 (Figure 10.5), Fracture of lumbar spine and pelvis, with note of the seventh-character extensions added to this category.

FIGURE 10.5 Excerpt from the Tabular List: *S32*

S32   Fracture of lumbar spine and pelvis
A fracture not identified as displaced or non displaced should be coded to displaced
A fracture not identified as opened or closed should be coded to closed

INCLUDES   fracture of lumbosacral neural arch
fracture of lumbosacral spinous process
fracture of lumbosacral transverse process
fracture of lumbosacral vertebra
fracture of lumbosacral vertebral arch
Codes first any associated spinal cord and spinal nerve injury (S34-)
EXCLUDES 1 transection of abdomen (S38.3)
EXCLUDES 2 fracture of hip NOS (S72.0-)

The appropriate 7th character is to be added to each code from category S32
A initial encounter for closed fracture
B initial encounter for open fracture
D subsequent encounter for fracture with routine healing
G subsequent encounter for fracture with delayed healing
K subsequent encounter for fracture with nonunion
S sequela

> **EXAMPLE:** A patient underwent surgery for a wedge compression fracture (open) of the second lumbar vertebrae.
>
> **Alphabetic Index:**
> Fracture, traumatic ➞ lumbar ➞ wedge compression
>
> **Tabular List:**
> S32.020– ➞ Fracture of second lumbar vertebra ➞ wedge compression fracture ➞ initial encounter, open fracture ➞ B
>
> **Correct code:**
> S32.020B

A seventh-character extension is required for this category. Since the documentation identifies this as an open fracture, the seventh-character extension is B, initial encounter for open fracture.

> **EXAMPLE:** A patient suffered a closed fracture of the condyle medial that is nondisplaced. The patient was taken to surgery for the repair.
>
> **Alphabetic Index:**
> Fracture ➞ humerus ➞ condyle ➞ medial nondisplaced ➞ S42.46–
>
> **Tabular List:**
> S42.46– ➞ Fracture of medial condyle of humerus ➞ Nondisplaced fracture of medial condyle ➞ unspecified humerus ➞ S42.466 ➞ A
>
> **Correct code:**
> S42.466

In this example, the documentation does not indicate whether the right or left humerus is affected. It is advised that the physician be queried for laterality before submitting a claim.

The seventh-character A indicates the fracture is closed.

> **EXAMPLE:** *A patient is diagnosed with a greenstick fracture of the left ulna from a fall from a scaffold while repairing windows on the fourth floor of an office building where he works. The patient was taken to the emergency room where the orthopedic surgeon repaired the fracture.*
>
> **Alphabetic Index:**
> *Fracture* ➡ *shaft* ➡ *greenstick* ➡ *S52.21–*
>
> **Tabular List:**
> *S52.21– Greenstick fracture of shaft of ulna* ➡ *left ulna* ➡ *S52.212*

A seventh character is required. Because a greenstick fracture is a closed fracture, the seventh character is A.

Don't forget to code for the external cause and place of occurrence. See if you can find the correct code(s).

> **First listed diagnosis:**
> *S52.212A Greenstick fracture of shaft of ulna*
>
> **Secondary diagnosis:**
> *W12.xxxA Fall on and from scaffolding*
>
> **Tertiary diagnosis:**
> *Y92.59 Office building as the place of occurrence of the external cause*
>
> **Additional diagnosis:**
> *Y99.0 civilian activity done for income or pay*

CODING TIP   It is important to understand the types of fractures and which fractures are open versus closed.

DISLOCATION

A dislocation is displacement of a bone from its joint. A subluxation is the partial displacement of a bone from its joint. Coding for a dislocation follows some of the same rules as fracture coding. Coding a dislocation requires the following information regarding the site of the fracture: whether the dislocation is open or closed and laterality. A dislocation not indicated as closed or open should be coded as closed. This note is printed in the section notes for dislocation and is not repeated again within the section. It is important to highlight this note in the ICD-10-CM codebook as a reminder of this rule. A dislocation and fracture of the same bone would be coded to the *fracture* site, not to both the dislocation and fracture.

Review the following examples. Open up the ICD-10-CM codebook, referencing both the Alphabetic Index and the Tabular List, locate the correct code.

> **EXAMPLE:** *A 16-year-old male dislocated his right shoulder joint while playing basketball in the school gym.*
>
> **Alphabetic Index:**
> *Dislocation* ➡ *Shoulder (blade) (ligament) (joint) (traumatic)* ➡ *S43.00–*
>
> **Tabular List:**
> *S43.00–* ➡ *Unspecified subluxation and dislocation of shoulder joint* ➡ *right shoulder* ➡ *S43.004A*
>
> **Correct code:**
> *S43.004A (initial encounter)*
>
> **Alphabetic Index to External Causes:**
> *Activity* ➡ *Y93.67*
>
> *Place of occurrence* ➡ *School gymnasium* ➡ *Y92.39*
>
> **Tabular List:**
> *Y93.67* ➡ *Activity, basketball*
>
> *Y92.39* ➡ *Other specified sports and athletic area as the place of occurrence of the external cause*
>
> **External Cause status:**
> *Y99.8* ➡ *Student activity*
>
> **Correct code sequencing:**
> *S43.004A, Y93.67, Y92.39, Y99.8*

> **EXAMPLE:** *A man suffers a closed fracture and dislocation of the mandible.*
>
> **Alphabetic Index:**
> *Fracture* ➡ *Mandible (lower jaw bone) S02.609*
>
> **Tabular List:**
> *S02.609* ➡ *Fracture of mandible, unspecified*
>
> **Correct code:**
> *S02.609A (initial encounter, closed fracture)*

Do not code for the dislocation. As mentioned above, a dislocation and fracture of the same bone are coded to the fracture.

CRUSH INJURIES

Crush injuries are sequenced first followed by any code to indicate the specific injuries associated with the crushing. Review the following example. Open up the ICD-10-CM codebook, referencing both the Alphabetic Index and the Tabular List, locate the correct code.

> **EXAMPLE:** *A patient was treated in the emergency room 3 days ago for a crushing injury to the right hand due to equipment falling on his hand at a construction site. The emergency department physician treated the patient and referred him to a hand surgeon. The hand surgeon evaluated the patient and determined surgery was indicated.*

Alphabetic Index:
   Crush, crushed, crushing ➡ *hand (except fingers alone)* ➡ *S67.2–*

Tabular List:
   S67.2– ➡ crushing injury of hand ➡ right hand ➡ S67.21xA ➡ Initial encounter

Alphabetic Index to External Causes:
   Contact ➡ with ➡ machinery ➡ x17

   Place of occurrence ➡ industrial construction area ➡ Y92.69

Tabular List:
   X17.xxxA ➡ Contact with hot engines, machinery and tools, initial Encounter

   Y92.69 ➡ Other specified industrial and construction area as the place of occurrence of the external cause

Correct code:
   S67.21xA (initial encounter), X17.xxxA, Y92.69, Y99.0

External Cause status:
   Y99.0 ➡ civilian activity done for income or pay

The encounter is reported as S67.21xA, Crushing injury of right hand. The seventh-character extension, A, is applicable because another physician provided treatment for the initial encounter and treatment by the hand surgeon is subsequent. Keep in mind the dummy placeholder x must be used as the sixth character so that a seventh character can be assigned.

CODING TIP Fracture coding requires a seventh-character extension to identify the highest level of specificity. If there are not six characters in the code, do not forget to use the dummy placeholder x.

Review Table 10.3.

SPRAINS AND STRAINS OF JOINTS AND ADJACENT MUSCLES

A sprain is a rupture of supporting ligament fibers in a joint. A strain is overexertion of a muscle. Sprains and strains are coded according to site.

TABLE 10.3   Official Guidelines Coding Guidelines for Reporting Injuries in Chapter 19

Code extensions	Extension A, initial encounter, is used while the patient is receiving active treatment for the injury. Examples of active treatment are surgical treatment, emergency department encounter, and evaluation and treatment by a new physician.
	Extension D, subsequent encounter, is used for encounters after the patient has received active treatment of the injury and is receiving routine care for the injury during the healing or recovery phase. Examples of subsequent care are cast change or removal, removal of external or internal fixation device, medication adjustment, and other aftercare and follow-up visits following injury treatment.
	The aftercare Z codes should not be used for aftercare of an injury. For aftercare of an injury, assign the acute injury code with the seventh-character D (subsequent encounter).
	Extension S, sequela, is used for complications or conditions that arise as a direct result of an injury, such as scar formation after a burn. The scars are sequela of the burn. When using extension S, it is necessary to use both the injury code that precipitated the sequela and the code for the sequela itself. The S is added only to the injury code, not the sequela code. The S extension identifies the injury responsible for the sequela. The specific type of sequela (eg, scar) is sequenced first, followed by the injury code.
Coding of injuries	When coding injuries, assign separate codes for each injury unless a combination code is provided, in which case the combination code is assigned. Code T07, Unspecified multiple injuries, should not be assigned unless information for a more specific code is not available. Traumatic injury codes (S00-T14.9) are not to be used for normal, healing surgical wounds or to identify complications of surgical wounds.
	The code for the most serious injury, as determined by the provider and the focus of treatment, is sequenced first.
Superficial injuries	Superficial injuries such as abrasions and contusions are not coded when associated with more severe injuries of the same site.
Primary injury with damage to nerves/blood vessels	When a primary injury results in minor damage to peripheral nerves or blood vessels, the primary injury is sequenced first with additional code(s) for injuries to nerves and spinal cord (such as category S04) and/or injury to blood vessels (such as category S15). When the primary injury is to the blood vessels or nerves, that injury should be sequenced first.

(continued)

TABLE 10.3   *(continued)*

Coding of traumatic fractures	The principles of multiple coding of injuries should be followed in coding fractures. Fractures of specified sites are coded individually by site in accordance with both the provisions within categories S02, S12, S22, S32, S42, S49, S52, S59, S62, S72, S79, S82, S89, S92 and the level of detail furnished by medical record content.
	A fracture not indicated as open or closed should be coded to closed. A fracture not indicated as being displaced or not displaced should be coded to displaced.
Initial versus subsequent encounter for fractures	Traumatic fractures are coded using the appropriate seventh-character extension for initial encounter (A, B, C) while the patient is receiving active treatment for the fracture. Examples of active treatment are surgical treatment, emergency department encounter, and evaluation and treatment by a new physician. The appropriate seventh character for initial encounter should also be assigned for a patient who delayed seeking treatment for the fracture or nonunion.
	Fractures are coded using the appropriate seventh-character extension for subsequent care for encounters after the patient has completed active treatment of the fracture and is receiving routine care for the fracture during the healing or recovery phase. Examples of fracture aftercare are cast change or removal, removal of external or internal fixation device, medication adjustment, and follow-up visits following fracture treatment.
	Care for complications of surgical treatment for fracture repairs during the healing or recovery phase should be coded with the appropriate complication codes. Care of complications of fractures, such as malunion and nonunion, should be reported with the appropriate seventh-character extensions for subsequent care with nonunion (K, M, N) or subsequent care with malunion (P, Q, R).
	A code from category M80, not a traumatic fracture code, should be used for any patient with known osteoporosis who suffers a fracture, even if the patient had a minor fall or trauma, if that fall or trauma would not usually break a normal, healthy bone.
	See Section I.C.13, Osteoporosis.
	The aftercare Z codes should not be used for aftercare for traumatic fractures. For aftercare of a traumatic fracture, assign the acute fracture code with the appropriate seventh character.
Multiple fractures sequencing	Multiple fractures are sequenced in accordance with the severity of the fracture.

Source: ICD-10-CM Official Guidelines, Chapter 19, Injuries

Review the following example. Open up the ICD-10-CM codebook, referencing both the Alphabetic Index and the Tabular List, locate the correct code.

> **EXAMPLE:** *A young man sprains his right ankle and is treated in the emergency room of the hospital.*

> **Alphabetic Index:**
> Sprain ➡ Ankle ➡ S93.40–

> **Tabular List:**
> S93.40– ➡ *Sprain of unspecified ligament of right ankle* ➡ *S93.401* ➡ *Initial encounter*

> **Correct code:**
> S93.401A

WOUNDS

Identify wounds by site and complexity. Distinguish between open wounds and superficial wounds. Open wounds include animal bites, avulsions, cuts, lacerations, puncture wounds, and traumatic amputations.

In contrast, superficial wounds include abrasions, blisters, insect bites, and removal of a superficial foreign body. Code superficial injuries to ICD-10-CM categories S00 and S01.

To code an open wound, look under the main term "wound, open" in the Alphabetic Index. Wounds with mention of delayed healing, delayed treatment, or presence of foreign body or major infection would warrant a complicated designation.

Review the following example. Open up the ICD-10-CM codebook, referencing both the Alphabetic Index and the Tabular List, locate the correct code.

> **EXAMPLE:** *A man is bitten on the right lower leg by his dog. He waits two weeks before having a physician examine and treat the bite. The physician discovers that the patient has developed a major infection from the bite and treats it appropriately.*

CHECKPOINT EXERCISE 10-3

Select the ICD-10-CM code(s) for the following diagnostic statements:

1. _____ Abrasion and open wound of right upper arm

2. _____ Concussion

3. _____ Foreign body (small bead) in the right auditory canal

4. _____ Infected open wound of the left thigh

5. _____ Hematoma and contusion of the liver

6. _____ Head injury

7. _____ Torus fracture involving the fibula lower end, the left fibula

8. _____ A patient suffered a skull fracture of the frontal bone and was unconscious for 5 hours.

9. _____ Meniscus tear of the right medial meniscus

10. _____ Closed fracture of the right fibula and tibula

11. _____ A 55-year-old male sustains a comminuted calcaneal fracture after falling from a height. To reconstruct the fracture and joint surface, an open reduction of the intraarticular fracture of the calcaneus is performed using plates and screws.

12. _____ A 28-year-old laborer falls from a height, sustaining tarsometatarsal dislocation. He undergoes open reduction with internal fixation.

13. _____ A 27-year-old female sustains a trimalleolar left ankle fracture after falling down an embankment. Open reduction, internal fixation of the medial and/or lateral malleolus is performed.

14. _____ A patient is seen in the hospital's outpatient surgical area with a diagnosis of a displaced comminuted fracture of the lateral condyle, right elbow.

15. _____ Open cervical fracture of the C1-C4 with spinal cord injury

Alphabetic Index:
Bite(s) → Animal → see also bite by site → Leg (lower) → S81.85–

Tabular List:
S81.85– → Open bite of lower leg → right → S81.851A (Initial encounter)

Based on documentation, the infection should also be coded.

Alphabetic Index:
Infection → leg (skin) NOS → L08.9

Tabular List:
L08.9 → Local infection of the skin and subcutaneous tissue, unspecified

Correct code sequencing:
S81.851A, L08.9

SPINAL CORD INJURIES

For each section of spinal cord injury, the code for the highest level of injury for that section of the cord should be used. If a patient has a cord injury at more than one section of the cord, use a code for the highest level of injury for each section. If the patient has a complete lesion of the cord, it is not necessary to use any additional codes for spinal cord injuries below the level of the complete lesion.

Burns and Corrosions (T20-T32)

Burns and corrosions are coded with categories T20-T32. ICD-10-CM distinguishes between burns and corrosions. The burn codes are used to report thermal burns that come from a heat source, such as a fire or hot appliance. The burn codes are also used for burns resulting from electricity and radiation; corrosions are burns due to chemicals.

The depth of burns is classified by degree: first degree, erythema; second degree, blistering; or third degree (full-thickness involvement). All burns are coded with the highest degree of burn sequenced first. Burns of the same local site (T20-T28) but of different degrees should be classified to the subcategory identifying the highest degree recorded in the diagnosis (Official ICD-10-CM Guidelines).

In ICD-10-CM what must be documented and coded is based on the following:

1. Whether it is a burn or corrosion

   a. Burn codes apply to thermal burns (except sunburns that come from a heat source, such as fire or hot appliance). They include electricity and radiation burns. Corrosions are burns due to chemicals. The guidelines are the same for burns and corrosions.

2. Burns are classified by depth (eg, first, second, third degree).

3. Location of burn (site).

4. Laterality in many cases.

5. If third degree or higher total body surface area (TBSA) is reported as the secondary diagnosis with category in addition to code for burn if known.

6. If an infection is present, an additional code is assigned for the infection.

7. An additional code is required for intent and place of occurrence.

8. Burns of the eye and internal organs (T26–T28) are classified by site, not by degree.

9. Separate codes for each burn site should be assigned.

10. Burn and corrosion, body region unspecified, should be use rarely.

GENERAL GUIDELINES

If a burn is a thermal burn, a burn code should be used. If a burn is a chemical burn, a corrosion code should be used. The guidelines for burns and corrosions are the same. Sunburns are not coded in this category.

When coding a burn of the eye (T26-T28), the codes are classified by site, not degree. When coding burns, assign separate codes for each burn site. Each burn or corrosion site is coded by sequencing the highest degree of burn or corrosion when more than one site is affected. Internal burns and corrosions are reported before external burns if they require more extensive treatment or are more severe. Code burns of the same site to the highest degree, using one code even if the burns or corrosions are of different degrees.

Review the following example. Open the ICD-10-CM codebook, referencing both the Alphabetic Index and the Tabular List, locate the correct code.

EXAMPLE: *A man is diagnosed with a second-degree burn on his left ear and first-degree burns on his chin and nose.*

Alphabetic Index:
Burn → Ear → Second degree T20.21

Burn → Chin → First degree T20.13

Burn → Nose → First degree T20.14

Tabular List:
All 3 burns code in the same category T20, Burn and corrosion of the head, face, and neck. Therefore, the most severe is reported as the first listed diagnosis.

T20.21 Second-degree burn of the face, head, and neck (ear) → T20.212 → left ear

Keep in mind that this code requires a seventh-character extension to identify the type of encounter. In this example, the type is the initial encounter, so the seventh character is A.

Correct code:
T20.21xA, T20.13xA, T20.14xA

CODING TOTAL BODY SURFACE AREA (TBSA) FOR BURNS OR CORROSIONS

An additional code is assigned to one of the following categories when coding a third-degree burn:

- T31 Burns classified according to extent of body surface involved

- T32 Corrosions classified according to extent of body surface involved

These codes are used to indicate the total body surface area burned and should be reported when there is mention of a third-degree burn involving 20% or more TBSA (per Official Coding Guidelines). These codes may be reported, however, if the TBSA is less than 20%; the codes and are optional.

Categories T31 and T32 are based on the classic "rule of nines" in estimating body surface involved:

- Head and neck, 9%

- Each arm, 9%

- Each leg, 18%

- Anterior trunk, 18%

- Posterior trunk, 18%

- Genitalia, 1%

Physicians may change these percentage assignments where necessary to accommodate infants and children who have proportionately larger heads than adults and patients who have large buttocks, thighs, or abdomen that involve burns or corrosions.

CODING TIP Burns are classified by site, depth, and degree.

Review Figure 10.6, which is an example of burns and corrosion for a third-degree burn of the hand.

FIGURE 10.6   Excerpt from the Tabular List: *T23*

T23.301	Burn of third degree of right hand, unspecified site
T23.302	Burn of third degree of left hand, unspecified site
T23.309	Burn of third degree of unspecified hand, unspecified site
T23.701	Corrosion of third degree of right hand, unspecified site
T23.702	Corrosion of third degree of left hand, unspecified site
T23.709	Corrosion of third degree of unspecified hand, unspecified site

Review the following examples. Open up the ICD-10-CM codebook, referencing both the Alphabetic Index and the Tabular List, locate the correct code.

EXAMPLE: The patient is a 38-year-old man admitted to our burn center after sustaining significant burns to both hands while trying put out a trash fire in his backyard, which got out of control after he poured gasoline on the blaze. He has very extensive and deep burns to the right hand. Some of these appear to be fourth-degree type burns with obvious exposure into tendon. He underwent burn excision earlier this week with placement of cadaver allograft skin. Quite a bit of this skin did not take because the underlying tissue remains nonviable due to the severe depth of his injury. He returns to our burn center today requiring a repeat operation for re-excision of the burn wounds on his right hand. We anticipate placing split thickness skin graft at this time. We talked to the patient about risks of infection, bleeding, extensive scarring with significant loss of function, and possible need for finger amputation of the right hand.

Here is what we know: The patient suffered a fourth-degree burn to both hands, but we don't know what part of the hand was affected.

Questions that must be asked are: Which hand is affected? What happened to cause the burn? Where did the incident happen? Is this the initial, subsequent, or sequela visit?

In ICD-10-CM, the intent and cause of the burn must be documented according to the instructional notes in the code categories for burns and corrosions.

First listed diagnosis:
   T23.301D → *Burn of third degree of right hand, unspecified site, subsequent encounter*

Second listed diagnoses:
   X04.xxxD → *Exposure to ignition of gasoline, subsequent encounter*

Additional diagnosis:
   Y92.096 → *Yard, private residence as the place of occurrence of the external cause*

   Y99.8 → *Other External Cause status*

When coding this patient encounter for the second diagnosis, there are only 3 characters, X04. Because a seventh character is required to identify the subsequent encounter, the dummy placeholder, x, must be added to the code to reach the highest level of specificity.

EXAMPLE: A fireman suffered a third-degree burn of the scalp with a 2% total body surface area (TBSA), a second-degree burn of the neck, and a third-degree burn of the right forearm involving 4% TBSA while battling a house fire. He was in a family residence containing the fire when the burns occurred. The flames got out of control; he was burned and taken to the hospital emergency department and treated for a burn of third degree of scalp and right forear, and second degree of the neck.

Alphabetic Index:
   Burn → scalp (any part) → third degree → T20.35

   Burn → forearm → right third degree → T22.31

   Burn → neck → second degree → T20.27

   Burn → unspecified site with TBSA → less than 10% → T31.0

   Exposure → fire flames → building or structure → X00.0

   Place of occurrence → residence → house → Y92.019

Tabular List:
   T20.35xA → Burn of third degree of scalp; (any part), initial encounter

   T22.311A → Burn of third degree of right forearm, initial encounter

   T20.27xA → Burn of second degree of neck, initial encounter

   T31.0 → Burns involving less than 10% of TBSA with third degree burns

   X00.0xxA → Exposure to flames in uncontrolled fire in building or structure, initial encounter

   Y92.019 Unspecified place in single family residence (private) house as the place of occurrence as the external cause

   Y99.0 → Civilian activity done for income or pay

Correct code sequencing:
   T20.35A, T22.311A, T20.27xA, T31.0, X00.xxA, Y92.019, Y99.0

Note: Laterality of the forearm is critical in selection of the code as well as the place of occurrence, the TBSA for third-degree burns.

Review Table 10.4.

Nonhealing burns are coded as acute burns. Necrosis of burned skin should be coded as a nonhealed burn. See example below.

TABLE 10.4   Guidelines for Reporting Burns and Corrosions

Coding of burns and corrosions	The ICD-10-CM makes a distinction between burns and corrosions. The burn codes are for thermal burns, except sunburns, that come from a heat source, such as a fire or hot appliance. The burn codes are also for burns resulting from electricity and radiation. Corrosions are burns due to chemicals. The guidelines are the same for burns and corrosions.
	Current burns (T20-T25) are classified by depth, extent, and agent (x code). Burns are classified by depth as first degree (erythema), second degree (blistering), and third degree (full-thickness involvement). Burns of the eye and internal organs (T26-T28) are classified by site, but not by degree.
Sequencing of burn and related-condition codes	Sequence first the code that reflects the highest degree of burn when more than one burn is present.
	When the reason for the admission or encounter is for treatment of external multiple burns, sequence first the code that reflects the burn of the highest degree.
	When a patient has both internal and external burns, the circumstances of admission govern the selection of the principal diagnosis or first listed diagnosis.
	When a patient is admitted for burn injuries and other related conditions such as smoke inhalation and/or respiratory failure, the circumstances of admission govern the selection of the principal or first listed diagnosis.
Burns of the same local site	Classify burns of the same local site (chapter 3 category level, T20-T28) but of different degrees to the subcategory identifying the highest degree recorded in the diagnosis.
Nonhealing burns	Nonhealing burns are coded as acute burns.
	Necrosis of burned skin should be coded as a nonhealed burn.
Infected burn	For any documented infected burn site, use an additional code for the infection.
Assign separate codes for each burn site	When coding burns, assign separate codes for each burn site.
	Category T30, Burn and corrosion, body region unspecified, is extremely vague and should be used rarely.
Burns and corrosions classified according to extent of body surface involved	Assign codes from category T31, Burns classified according to extent of body surface involved, or T32, Corrosions classified according to extent of body surface involved, when the site of the burn is not specified or when there is a need for additional data. It is advisable to use category T31 as additional coding when needed to provide data for evaluating burn mortality, such as that needed by burn units. It is also advisable to use category T31 as an additional code for reporting purposes when there is mention of a third-degree burn involving 20% or more of the body surface.
	Categories T31 and T32 are based on the classic "rule of nines" in estimating body surface involved: head and neck are assigned 9%; each arm, 9%; each leg, 18%; the anterior trunk, 18%; posterior trunk, 18%; and genitalia, 1%. Providers may change these percentage assignments where necessary to accommodate infants and children who have proportionately larger heads than adults and patients who have large buttocks, thighs, or abdomen that involve burns.
Encounters for treatment of late effects of burns	Encounters for the treatment of the late effects of burns or corrosions (ie, scars or joint contractures) should be coded with a burn or corrosion code with the seventh-character S for sequela.
Sequelae with a late effect code and current burn	When appropriate, both a code for a current burn or corrosion with seventh-character extension A or D and a burn or corrosion code with extension S may be assigned on the same record (when both a current burn and sequela of an old burn exist). Burns and corrosions do not heal at the same rate, and a current healing wound may still exist with sequela of a healed burn or corrosion.
Use of an External Cause code with burns and corrosions	An External Cause code should be used with burns and corrosions to identify the source and intent of the burn, as well as the place where it occurred.

Source: Official ICD-10-CM Guidelines, Chapter 19, Burns and Corrosions

EXAMPLE: A woman suffers a third-degree burn on her left thigh (6%) that has subsequently become infected, complicating the treatment of her burn.

Alphabetic Index:
  Burn ➜ Thigh ➜ left ➜ third degree ➜ T24.312

  Burn ➜ unspecified site with TBSA ➜ less than 10% ➜ T31.0

  Infection ➜ skin ➜ L08.9

Tabular List:
  T24.312S ➜ Burn of third degree of left thigh sequela

  T31.0 ➜ Burns involving less than 10% of TBSA with third degree burns

  L08.9 ➜ Local infection of the skin and subcutaneous tissue, unspecified

Correct codes:
  T24.312S, T31.0, L08.9

Using an additional code for the third-degree burn provides additional data for evaluating burns and corrosion mortality that is typically needed by burn units. It is advisable to use a code from category T31, Burns, or T32, Corrosions, as an addition code for reporting purposes when there is mention of a third-degree burn involving 20% or more of the body surface area (per ICD-10-CM Coding Guidelines).

CODING TIP Category T30, Burn and corrosion, body region unspecified, is extremely vague and should be used rarely.

Keep in mind that encounters for the treatment of the late effects of burns or corrosions (ie, scars or joint contractures) should be coded with a burn or corrosion code with the seventh-character S for sequela.

Review the following examples. Open up the ICD-10-CM codebook, referencing both the Alphabetic Index and the Tabular List, locate the correct code.

EXAMPLE: A patient receives a second-degree burn on the right ankle and a third-degree burn on the palm of the left hand when she picks up a saucepan; she dropped the pan and it hit her right ankle. She was cooking in the kitchen in her home.

Alphabetic Index:
  Burn ➜ Ankle ➜ right ➜ second degree T25.211

Tabular List:
  T25.211A ➜ Burn of second degree of right ankle, initial encounter

Alphabetic Index:
  Burn ➜ Palm(s) ➜ left third degree ➜ T23.351

Tabular List:
  T23.352A ➜ Burn of third degree of left palm, initial encounter

Alphabetic Index to External Cause:
  burn ➜ hot ➜ saucepan (glass) (metal) ➜ X15.3

  Place of occurrence ➜ residence ➜ house, single family ➜ kitchen ➜ Y92.010

Tabular List:
  X15.3xxA ➜ Contact with hot saucepan or skillet, initial encounter

  Y92.010 ➜ Kitchen of single-family (private) house as the place of occurrence of the external cause

  Y99.8 ➜ Other External Cause status

Correct codes:
  T24.211A, T24.352A, X15.3xxA, Y92.010, Y99.8

Because we don't have information on the total body surface area (TBSA), it cannot be coded unless the physician is queried.

Poisonings, Toxic Effects, Adverse Effects, and Underdosing (T36-T50)

A poisoning can occur in a variety of ways. It can occur when an error was made in drug prescription or in the administration of the drug by physician, nurse, patient, or other person. If an overdose of a drug was intentionally taken or administered and resulted in drug toxicity, this would be considered a poisoning. If a nonprescribed drug or medicinal agent was taken in combination with a correctly prescribed and properly administered drug, any drug toxicity or reaction resulting from the interaction of the two drugs would be classified as a poisoning.

ICD-10-CM does not provide codes that differentiate between poisonings and adverse effects. The various codes in the block T36-T50, Poisoning by, adverse effects of and underdosing of drugs, medicaments and biological substances, identify the substances that caused the adverse effect. A Table of Drugs and Chemicals is available to assist in coding this category.

A toxic effect is a poisoning due to a toxic substance that has no medicinal use.

CHECKPOINT EXERCISE 10-4

Select the correct ICD-10-CM code(s) for the following diagnostic statements:

1. _____ First-degree burn of the chest wall, third-degree burn of the left forearm, second-degree of left hand (palm)

2. _____ Second- and third-degree burns on the foot while burning trash

3. _____ Second-degree burn on the back (18%) and third-degree burn on the left arm (9%); calculate total body surface area only

4. _____ Burn of the mouth due to ingestion of caustic agent

5. _____ A patient suffering from a third-degree burn on the left forearm was taken to the operating room to remove the arm as a result of the burn.

6. _____ A patient suffered a chemical burn of the cornea and conjunctiva.

7. _____ A patient was taken to the emergency room with a second-degree sunburn due to overexposure.

8. _____ A patient suffered burns on the face, lip, and scalp when a fire started while she was cooking.

9. _____ A firefighter suffered multiple second-degree burns of the hand and wrist when putting out a car fire on the freeway.

10. _____ A 34-year-old female is burned by a cooking oil fire on the right hand. The patient is in extreme pain from her burned hand. The patient is brought to the operating room emergently for debridement and dressing of the burn wound while under general anesthesia. The burn is of the second degree.

11. _____ A 4-year-old child, while playing with his father's aftershave lotion, saturated his body and clothes with the liquid. He subsequently ignited a fireplace starter, burning his clothes. He was found hiding in a closet. He was admitted to the hospital.

12. _____ Evaluation at the community hospital identified a child with full thickness burns of 55% of his body surface area. He was transferred to the regional burn center.

13. _____ A 22-year-old mechanic suffered burns of the neck, shoulder, and arm from a radiator scald injury. The burns involved 10% of the body surface. These burns were deep partial thickness.

14. _____ A patient suffered a second-degree burn of the left lower leg from an exhaust pipe on a motorcycle.

15. _____ A 28-year-old construction worker suffered a chemical burn of the eye.

ADVERSE EFFECT AND UNDERDOSING

An adverse effect is a reaction to a drug that is taken as prescribed and is properly administered. Codes in categories T36-T50 are combination codes that include the substances related to adverse effects, poisonings, toxic effects, and underdosing, as well as the external cause. No additional External Cause code is required for poisonings, toxic effects, adverse effects, and underdosing codes.

The term "underdosing" means taking less of a medication than was prescribed or based on the manufacturer's instruction that results in a negative health consequence.

A noncompliance (Z91.12–, Z91.13–) or failure in dosage during surgical or medical care (Y63.–) code must be used with an underdosing code to indicate intent. Review Figure 10.7 as an example of coding for underdosing.

FIGURE 10.7   Excerpt from the Tabular List: *Z81.2–*

Z91.12   Patient's intentional underdosing of medication regimen
Code first underdosing of medication (T36-T50) with fifth or sixth character
EXCLUDES 1   adverse effect of prescribed drug taken as directed- code to adverse effect poisoning (overdose) -code to poisoning
Z91.120   Patient's intentional underdosing of medication regimen due to financial hardship
Z91.128   Patient's intentional underdosing of medication regimen for other reason

Notice there is an Excludes 1 note to indicate if the patient encounter is an adverse affect, it would not be reported in this category.

Codes related to poisonings and certain other consequences of external causes are located in blocks T07-T88. Category T07, Unspecified multiple injuries, is to be used only when no documentation is available to identify the specific injuries. Code T07 would never be used in an inpatient setting.

Categories T36-T50, Poisoning, adverse effects and underdosing by drugs, medicaments and biological substances, and T51-T65, Toxic effects of substances chiefly nonmedicinal as to source, are the categories for the different classes of drugs and chemical agents that may cause a poisoning, toxic effect, or adverse effect. Review Figure 10.8.

FIGURE 10.8   Excerpt from the Tabular List: *T36.–*

T36   Poisoning by, adverse effect of and underdosing of systemic antibiotics

    T36.0   Poisoning by, adverse effect of and underdosing of penicillins

        T36.0x1   Poisoning by penicillins, accidental (unintentional)

        T36.0x2   Poisoning by penicillins, intentional self-harm

        T36.0x3   Poisoning by penicillins, assault

        T36.0x4   Poisoning by penicillins, undetermined

        T36.0x5   Adverse effect of penicillins

        T36.0x6   Underdosing of penicillins

Code to the accidental poisoning when there is no intent indicated in the documentation. The code for undetermined intent should be used only when specific documentation in the record indicates that the intent could not be determined. There are fifth and sixth characters to identify the circumstances that caused the adverse effect, such as accidental poisoning or adverse effect, intentional self-harm, assault, or undetermined cause.

Poisonings and toxic effects have an associated intent: accidental, intentional self-harm, assault, and undetermined. The final character code in these categories, usually the sixth character, indicates the intent. Review the final characters:

- Accidental
- Intentional (self-harm)
- Assault
- Undetermined

- Adverse effects (categories T36-T50)
- Poisoning by adverse effects of and underdosing of drugs, medicaments and biological substances (T36-T50)

No additional External Cause code is required for poisonings, toxic effects, adverse effects, and underdosing codes (ICD-10-CM Coding Guidelines).

CODING TIP   Never select the final code in the Table of Drugs and Chemicals. Use this table as a reference. Select the final diagnosis code from the Tabular List.

> *EXAMPLE: A patient took an overdose of penicillin, which was prescribed correctly; this resulted in projectile vomiting.*
>
> **Table of Drugs and Chemicals:**
> *Poisoning* ➞ *penicillins, accidental (unintentional)* ➞ *T36.0x1*
>
> **Tabular List:**
> *T36.0x1A* ➞ *Poisoning by penicillins, accidental (unintentional) initial encounter*
>
> **Alphabetic Index:**
> *Vomiting* ➞ *projectile* ➞ *R11.12*
>
> **Tabular List:**
> *R11.12 Projectile vomiting*

Note: A code from categories T36-T65 is sequenced first, followed by the code(s) that specifies the nature of the adverse effect, poisoning, or toxic effect.

> **Correct code sequence:**
> *T36.0x1A, R11.12*

An example of the Table of Drugs and Chemicals in ICD-10-CM is illustrated in Figure 10.9.

FIGURE 10.9   Excerpt from the ICD-10-CM Table of Drugs and Chemicals

Substance	Poisoning, Accidental (Unintentional)	Poisoning, Intentional self-harm	Poisoning, Undetermined	Poisoning Assault	Adverse Effect	Underdosing
Pengitoxin	T46.0x1	T46.0x2	T46.0x3	T46.0x4	T46.0x5	T46.0x6
Penicillamine	T50.6x1	T50.6x2	T50.6x3	T50.6x4	T50.6x5	T50.6x6
Penicillin (any)	**T36.0x1**	T36.0x2	T36.0x3	T36.0x4	T36.0x5	T36.0x6
Penicillinase	T45.3x1	T45.3x2	T45.3x3	T45.3x4	T45.3x4	T45.3x6
Penicilloyl polylysine	T50.8x1	T50.8x2	T50.8x3	T50.8x4	T50.8x5	T50.8x6
Penimepicycline	T36.4x1	T36.4x2	T36.4x3		T36.4x4	
Pentachloroethane	T53.6x1	T53.6x2	T53.6x3	T53.6x4	- - - - -	- - - - -

FIFTH-CHARACTER x PLACEHOLDER

When reviewing Figure 10.9, notice that the fifth-character "x" is part of many of these codes. The fifth-character "x" at many of the codes in categories T36-T65 is a dummy placeholder to allow for possible future expansion. The "x" must remain in the code and no other character should be used in its place. Not all codes in the Table of Drugs and Chemicals will have an "x" as part of the code.

For example, if a patient is poisoned by penicillin by taking an overdose accidently, using the ICD-10-CM Table of Drugs and Chemicals, it is coded in category T36.0x1. If the patient takes the correct prescribed dosage of penicillin and has an adverse reaction, the encounter is still reported using T36.0x1 because in ICD-10-CM both are considered a poisoning. Use caution because a seventh character is required to identify the encounter and it can only be referenced in the Tabular List.

A poisoning is reported using a minimum of two codes:

- The first code, from the Poisoning column of the Table of Drugs and Chemicals, identifies the drug.

- The second code indicates the condition(s) that resulted from the poisoning.

Use the following guidelines to assign codes for poisonings by drugs and medicinal and biological substances (Official ICD-10-CM Guidelines):

- Do not code directly from the Table of Drugs and Chemicals. Always refer back to the Tabular List.

- Use as many codes as necessary to describe completely all drugs or medicinal or biological substances.

- If two or more drugs or medicinal or biological substances are reported, code each individually, unless a combination code is listed in the Table of Drugs and Chemicals.

Review Table 10.5.

TABLE 10.5 Guidelines for Coding Adverse Effects, Poisoning, Underdosing, and Toxic Effects

Adverse effects, poisoning, underdosing, and toxic effects	Codes in categories T36-T65 are combination codes that include the substances related to adverse effects, poisonings, toxic effects, and underdosing, as well as the external cause. No additional External Cause code is required for poisonings, toxic effects, adverse effects, and underdosing codes.
	A code from categories T36-T65 is sequenced first, followed by the code(s) that specifies the nature of the adverse effect, poisoning, or toxic effect. **Note:** This sequencing instruction does not apply to underdosing codes (fifth or sixth character 6, for example, T36.0x6–).
Do not code directly from the Table of Drugs and Chemicals	Do not code directly from the Table of Drugs and Chemicals. Always refer back to the Tabular List.
Use as many codes as necessary to describe	Use as many codes as necessary to describe completely all drugs, medicinal, or biological substances.
If the same code would describe the causative agent	If the same code would describe the causative agent for more than one adverse reaction, poisoning, toxic effect, or underdosing, assign the code only once.
If two or more drugs, medicinal, or biological substances	If two or more drugs, medicinal, or biological substances are reported, code each individually unless a combination code is listed in the Table of Drugs and Chemicals.
The occurrence of drug toxicity is classified in ICD-10-CM as follows: (a) Adverse Effect	Assign the appropriate code for adverse effect (eg, T36.0x5–) when the drug was correctly prescribed and properly administered. Use additional code(s) for all manifestations of adverse effects. Examples of manifestations are tachycardia, delirium, gastrointestinal hemorrhaging, vomiting, hypokalemia, hepatitis, renal failure, and respiratory failure.
(b) Poisoning	When coding a poisoning or reaction to the improper use of a medication (eg, overdose, wrong substance given or taken in error, wrong route of administration), assign the appropriate code from categories T36-T50. Poisoning codes have an associated intent: accidental, intentional self-harm, assault, and undetermined. Use additional code(s) for all manifestations of poisonings.
	If there is also a diagnosis of abuse or dependence on the substance, the abuse or dependence is an additional code.
	Examples of poisoning include:
	(i) Error was made in drug prescription: Errors made in drug prescription or in the administration of the drug by provider, nurse, patient, or other person.
	(ii) Overdose of a drug intentionally taken: If an overdose of a drug was intentionally taken or administered and resulted in drug toxicity, it would be coded as a poisoning.

(continued)

TABLE 10.5   *(continued)*

	(iii) Nonprescribed drug taken with correctly prescribed and properly administered drug: If a nonprescribed drug or medicinal agent was taken in combination with a correctly prescribed and properly administered drug, any drug toxicity or other reaction resulting from the interaction of the two drugs would be classified as a poisoning.
	(iv) Interaction of drug(s) and alcohol: When a reaction results from the interaction of a drug(s) and alcohol, this would be classified as poisoning.
	See Section I.C.4, If poisoning is the result of insulin pump malfunctions.
(c) Underdosing	Underdosing refers to taking less of a medication than is prescribed by a provider or a manufacturer's instruction. For underdosing, assign the code from categories T36-T50 (fifth or sixth character 6).
	Codes for underdosing should never be assigned as principal or first listed codes. If a patient has a relapse or exacerbation of the medical condition for which the drug is prescribed because of the reduction in dose, then the medical condition itself should be coded.
	Noncompliance (Z91.12–, Z91.13–) or complication of care (Y63.61, Y63.8-Y63.9) codes are to be used with an underdosing code to indicate intent, if known.
(d) Toxic Effects	When a harmful substance is ingested or comes in contact with a person, this is classified as a toxic effect. The toxic effect codes are in categories T51-T65.
	Toxic effect codes have an associated intent: accidental, intentional self-harm, assault, and undetermined.

Source: ICD-10-CM Official Guidelines, Chapter 19, Poisonings, Toxic Effects, Adverse Effects, and Underdosing

SEQUENCING OF POISONINGS, TOXIC EFFECTS, ADVERSE EFFECTS, AND UNDERDOSING

When sequencing a poisoning, the following applies:

- First from category T36-50

- The code(s) that specifies the nature of the poisoning, toxic effect, or adverse effect is reported secondarily (patient's condition)

Review the following examples. Open up the ICD-10-CM codebook, referencing both the Table of Drugs and Chemicals and the Tabular List, locate the correct code.

EXAMPLE: A 3-year-old accidentally ingests some Motrin (ibuprofen) and procainamide capsules, which results in acute gastritis.

> Locate "Ibuprofen" in the Table of Drugs and Chemicals. Under "Ibuprofen," find the poisoning code (first column) (T39.311).

Tabular List:
> T39.311A ➜ Poisoning by propionic acid derivatives, accidental (unintentional) initial encounter

Poisoning code 2:
> Procainamide

> Table of Drugs and Chemicals: Locate "Procainamide" in the Table of Drugs and Chemicals Under "Procainamide," find the poisoning code (first column) (T46.2x1)

Tabular List:
> T46.2x1 ➜ Poisoning by other antidysrhythmic drugs, accidental (unintentional) initial encounter

Manifestation/Condition:
> Acute gastritis

Alphabetic Index:
> Gastritis ➜ Acute K29.00

Tabular List:
> K29.00 ➜ Acute gastritis without bleeding

Correct code sequencing:
> T46.2x1A, K29.00

EXAMPLE: A patient develops a cardiac arrhythmia after taking Librium with vodka (alcohol grain beverage).

Poisoning code 1:
> Librium

> Locate "Librium" in the Table of Drugs and Chemicals Under "Librium," find the poisoning code (first column) (T42.4x1)

Tabular List:
> T42.4x1A ➜ Poisoning by benzodiazepines, accidental (unintentional), initial encounter

Poisoning code 2:
> Alcohol (grain, beverage)

Section 2 Index:
> Locate "alcohol, grain, beverage" in the Table of Drugs and Chemicals Under "alcohol, grain, beverage," find the poisoning code (first column) (T51.0x1)

Tabular List:
T51.0x1A → *Toxic effect of ethanol, accidental (unintentional), initial encounter*

Manifestation/Condition:
Cardiac arrhythmia

Alphabetic Index:
Arrhythmia (auricle) (cardiac) (juvenile) I49.9

Tabular List:
I49.9 → Cardiac arrhythmia, unspecified

Correct code sequencing:
T42.4x1a, T51.0x1A, I49.9

EXAMPLE: *A patient is diagnosed as having toxic cardiomyopathy that is a late effect of an accidental overdose of Valium one year ago.*

Alphabetic Index:
Cardiomyopathy → Toxic NEC → I42.7

Tabular List:
I42.7 → Cardiomyopathy due to drug and external agent → Code first (T36-T65) to identify cause

Table of Drugs and Chemicals:
Valium-self harm → T42.4x2

Tabular List:
T42.4x2S → Poisoning by benzodiazepines, intentional self-harm, sequela

Correct codes:
T42.4x2S, I42.7

Use caution when reporting late effects because the instructional guidance in the ICD-10-CM should be referenced carefully. When you have a late effect, the seventh character is S for sequela.

POISONINGS, TOXIC EFFECTS, ADVERSE EFFECTS, AND UNDERDOSING IN A PREGNANT PATIENT

Codes from Chapter 15, Pregnancy, childbirth, and the puerperium, are always sequenced first on a medical record. A code from subcategory O9A.22, Injury, poisoning and certain other consequences of external causes complicating pregnancy, childbirth, and the puerperium, should be sequenced first, followed by the appropriate poisoning, toxic effect, adverse effect, or underdosing code and the additional code(s) that specifies the nature of the poisoning, toxic effect, adverse effect, or underdosing.

CODING TIP Use a code from the Undetermined column in the Table of Drugs and Chemicals only when the intent of the poisoning or toxic effect cannot be determined.

OTHER T CODES THAT INCLUDE THE EXTERNAL CAUSE

Certain other T codes are combination codes that include the external cause. For example, the codes in categories T15-T19, Effects of foreign body entering through natural orifice, identify both the foreign body as well as the resulting injury. The intent for these codes is accidental. No secondary External Cause code is needed.

For example, T15 identifies a foreign body on the external eye. Codes from T15-T19 require extension codes to identify whether the visit is the initial encounter, a subsequent encounter, or an encounter to address the sequela of the injury.

Review the following examples. Open up the ICD-10-CM codebook, referencing both the Alphabetic Index and the Tabular List, locate the correct code.

EXAMPLE: *A construction worker was cutting metal, and a metal shaving penetrated the cornea of the right eye. The patient went to an ophthalmologist who removed the foreign body and patched the eye.*

Alphabetic Index:
Foreign body → eye → cornea → T15.01–

Tabular List:
T15.01 → Foreign body in cornea, right eye → initial encounter → T15.01xA

Because this is the initial injury, the seventh-character extension A is reported for the initial encounter.

Correct code:
T15.01xA

But wait, you need to report the accident and, if known, the place of occurrence as additional diagnoses.

Alphabetic Index to External Causes:
Contact → with → metal → NEC → X18

Tabular List:
X18 → Contact with other hot metals → X18.xxxA

When reviewing category X18 → Contact with other hot metals

Note that there is an instructional note to report a seventh character as:

A, initial encounter

D, subsequent encounter

S, sequela

You will also need to report the place of occurrence, which is an industrial and construction area (Y92.69).

Tabular List:

Y92.69 ➝ *Other specified industrial and construction area as the place of occurrence of the external cause*

Y99.0 ➝ *External Cause status* ➝ *Civilian activity done for income or pay*

Correct code sequencing:

T15.01xA, X18.xxxA, Y92.69, Y99.0

EXAMPLE: *A 5-year-old patient was playing in an old refrigerator in the garage of the family home and closed the door, causing asphyxiation. The mother found the child, and the patient was taken to the emergency room.*

Alphabetic Index:

Asphyxiation ➝ due to ➝ being trapped in ➝ refrigerator

Tabular List:

T71.231A ➝ Asphyxiation due to being trapped in a (discarded) refrigerator, accidental (initial encounter)

Note: The sixth-character 1 identifies the asphyxiation as accidental, and the seventh-character A identifies the initial encounter.

Alphabetic Index to External Causes:

Suffocation ➝ (accidental) by external means ➝ T71.–

Place of Occurrence ➝ residence ➝ house, single family home ➝ garage ➝ Y92.015

Correct code sequencing:

T71.231A , Y92.015

Note that the Index references the coder back to category T71, which is used to report a combination code that includes the external cause. But you do need to report the Place of Occurrence.

CHECKPOINT EXERCISE 10-5

Select the correct ICD-10-CM code(s) for the following diagnostic statements:

1. _____ Accidental overdose of digoxin, leading to cardiac arrest

2. _____ Coma due to overdose of Sinequan

3. _____ Electrolyte imbalance due to intentional overdose of furosemide

4. _____ Adverse reaction due to taking a combination of lithium carbonate and Percodan, resulting in respiratory failure

5. _____ Accidental overdose of iron tablets by a 6-year-old, resulting in acute gastritis with hemorrhage

6. _____ A patient was prescribed Tylenol with Codeine and suffered extreme swelling and redness.

7. _____ A patient misread the label on a bottle of Sominex and took an overdose of the medication, which caused nausea and vomiting.

8. _____ A small child suffered seizures after ingesting paint that contained lead and was rushed to the emergency room.

9. _____ A lawn care technician suffered from respiratory distress after inhaling insecticide while spraying.

10. _____ A patient was given the wrong instructions on her prescription for lisinopril, took an overdose, and went into cardiac arrest.

11. _____ A patient suffered from heart palpitations due to adverse reaction to an appetite suppressant.

12. _____ A patient cleaning her bathroom became weak and dizzy after smelling fumes from the Clorox bleach she was using and went to the emergency room.

13. _____ Brachycardia due to inhalation of carbon bisulfide

14. _____ A 19-year-old male took an overdose of Amitriptyline that belonged to his mother, was found unconscious, and rushed to the emergency room.

15. _____ A patient prescribed Coumadin, which became toxic, resulted in gross hematuria. The patient took the drug as prescribed.

Test Your Knowledge

Provide all the applicable ICD-10-CM codes for the following diagnosis statements:

1. _____ A 42-year-old construction worker at an industrial site suffered a fracture of the ribs after a shelf fell on him at work

2. _____ Personal history of cancer of the breast

3. _____ Colostomy status

4. _____ History of allergy to sulfa drugs (sulfonamides)

5. _____ Black eye sustained by a 10-year-old boy after being hit in the face with a swing at a local playground

6. _____ A man falls 20 feet off of a ladder while making home repairs and is found to have a closed fracture of his tibia.

7. _____ Patient was seen in the office for lacerations on the forearm. The patient explained that a dog that had rabies bit her. The physician administered a vaccination and bandaged her arm. He asked that she return for follow-up the next day and to call if she begins to exhibit any unusual symptoms.

8. _____ Encounter for dressing change

9. _____ A young man seen in the emergency department was admitted to the hospital after suffering a concussion. He experienced a brief loss of consciousness of less than 30 minutes after being tackled in a high school football game at a neighboring high school.

10. _____ An elderly woman slipped outside of the post office on a patch of ice and suffered several contusions on the right side of her body.

11. _____ A sky diver suffered a broken wrist when complications occurred while he was jumping from a plane.

12. _____ A fight broke out during the World Series when one of the coaches rushed the mound. The umpire was involved and claimed that when he was kicked he felt something snap in his chest. He was found to have two fractured ribs.

13. _____ Noncompliance with medical treatment

14. _____ A child is seen for vomiting and nausea. At that time, it was discovered that the child had ingested cheese, ice cream, and two glasses of milk the day before. The child's physician determined that the child is allergic to milk and should not have any milk products.

15. _____ A woman was seen in the office for a breast exam. She believes that she has found a lump while performing a self-exam. Her mother died of breast cancer several years before, and this has become a concern of hers.

16. _____ Code a closed treatment of radial and ulnar shaft fractures, with manipulation, initial care performed by the orthopedic surgeon in the emergency room of the local hospital.

17. _____ A juvenile falls and sustains a fracture of the humeral epicondylar, which is reduced anatomically and is percutaneously pinned.

18. _____ A patient was admitted to the burn unit after a truck with paint chemical exploded and he suffered third-degree burns over 55% of his arms, legs, and torso.

19. _____ Painful scarring of the hands due to old third-degree burns

20. _____ Toxic encephalitis due to accidental ingestion of lead dioxide

Factors Influencing Health Status and Contact with Health Services (Z00-Z99)

LEARNING OBJECTIVES

- Understand coding guidelines when using Z codes

- Review categories of Z codes and their use

- Apply correct coding conventions when assigning Z codes

- Assign ICD-10-CM codes to the highest level of specificity

- Successfully complete checkpoint exercises and test your knowledge exercises

Section C21 of the Official ICD-10-CM Guidelines, Classification of Factors Influencing Health Status and Contact with Health Service, provides coding guidelines for reporting Z codes. Z codes, described in ICD-10-CM Chapter 21, Factors Influencing Health Status and Contact with Health Services, are often misunderstood in reporting health care services. These codes are designed for occasions when circumstances other than a disease or injury result in an encounter or are recorded by providers as problems or factors that influence care. If there are signs/symptoms related to a suspected condition or abnormal finding during the examination, codes are reported in categories R70-R94.

Chapter 21 in the Tabular List includes the following sections:

- Persons encountering health services for examination (Z00-Z13)

- Genetic carrier and genetic susceptibility to disease (Z14-Z15)

- Infection and drug-resistant microorganisms (Z16)

- Estrogen receptor status (Z17)

- Retained foreign body fragments (Z18)

- Persons with potential health hazards related to communicable diseases (Z20-Z28)

- Persons encountering health services in circumstances related to reproduction (Z30-Z39)

- Persons encountering health services for specific procedures and health care (Z40-Z53)

- Persons with potential health hazards related to socioeconomic and psychosocial circumstances (Z55-Z65)

- Do not resuscitate (DNR) status (Z66)

- Blood type (Z67)

- Body mass index (BMI) (Z68)

- Persons encountering health services in other circumstances (Z69-Z76)

- Persons with potential health hazards related to family and personal history and certain conditions influencing health status (Z77-Z99)

The Z codes are provided to deal with occasions when circumstances other than a disease or injury classifiable to the other chapters of the ICD-10-CM are recorded as a reason for encounters with a health care provider. Z codes may be used in any health care setting.

There are 4 primary circumstances for the use of Z codes:

- When a person who is not currently sick has a health care encounter for some specific reason

- When a person with a resolving disease or injury or a chronic, long-term condition requiring continuous care has a health care encounter for specific aftercare of that disease or injury

- When circumstances or problems influence a person's health status but are not in themselves a current illness or injury

- For newborns, to indicate birth status

CODING TIP A diagnosis/symptom code, not a Z code, should be used whenever a current, acute condition is being treated or a sign or symptom is being studied. Z codes are for use in both the inpatient and outpatient settings but are generally used more often in the outpatient setting.

Z codes may be used as either principal/first listed codes or as secondary codes, depending on the circumstances of the encounter. Certain Z codes may only be first listed, others only secondary. For example, a screening code may be a first listed code if the reason for the visit is specifically the screening exam. Documentation in the medical record must support the Z code assigned for the patient encounter.

The Z code indicates that a screening exam is planned. Because Z codes are not procedure codes, a corresponding procedure code is required to describe the procedure performed. The listing of the appropriate Z code confirms that the screening was performed.

The screening Z codes/categories are as follows:

- Z11 Encounter for screening for infectious and parasitic diseases

- Z12 Encounter for screening for malignant neoplasms

- Z13 Encounter for screening for other diseases and disorders; Except Z13.9, Encounter for screening, unspecified

- Z36 Encounter for antenatal screening for mother

The following Z codes/categories may only be reported as the principal/first listed diagnosis, except when there are multiple encounters on the same day and the medical records for the encounters are combined:

- Z00 Encounter for general examination without complaint, suspected or reported diagnosis

- Z01 Encounter for other special examination without complaint, suspected or reported diagnosis

- Z02 Encounter for administrative examination

- Z03 Encounter for medical observation for suspected diseases and conditions ruled out

- Z33.2 Encounter for elective termination of pregnancy

- Z31.81 Encounter for male factor infertility in female patient

- Z31.82 Encounter for Rh incompatibility status

- Z31.83 Encounter for assisted reproductive fertibility procedure cycle

- Z31.84 Encounter for fertility preservation procedure

- Z34 Encounter for supervision of normal pregnancy

- Z38 Liveborn infants according to place of birth and type of delivery

- Z39 Encounter for maternal postpartum care and examination

- Z42 Encounter for plastic and reconstructive surgery following medical procedure or healed injury

- Z51.0 Encounter for antineoplastic radiation therapy

- Z51.1– Encounter for antineoplastic chemotherapy and immunotherapy

- Z52 Donors of organs and tissues; Except: Z52.9, Donor of unspecified organ or tissue

- Z76.1 Encounter for health supervision and care of foundling

- Z76.2 Encounter for health supervision and care of other healthy infant and child

- Z99.12 Encounter for respirator (ventilator) dependence during power failure

Review Table 11.1, which lists the main terms typically used for Z codes.

TABLE 11.1 Main Terms for Z Codes

Admission	Follow-up	Test
Aftercare	Health, Healthy	Transplant
Attention to	History (personal)	Unavailability of medical facilities
Boarder	History (family)	Vaccination
Care (of)	Maintenance	
Carrier	Maladjustment	
Checking	Observation	
Contraception	Problem	
Counseling	Procedure (Surgical)	
Dialysis	Prophylactic	
Donor	Replacement	
Encounter	Screening	
Examination	Status	
Fitting of	Supervision (of)	

Classifying Z Codes

The Tabular List for Z codes follows the final chapter of the main classification in the Tabular List. To understand how Z codes are used in the outpatient setting, this section provides a review of the 3 main Z code groupings.

PROBLEM-ORIENTED Z CODES

This group provides codes for conditions or circumstances that could affect the patient in the future but are not a current illness or injury. These codes describe an existing circumstance or problem that may influence future medical care (eg, family history of diabetes).

SERVICE-ORIENTED Z CODES

This group identifies or defines examinations, aftercare, ancillary services, and therapy. Use these Z codes to describe the patient who is not currently ill but seeks medical services for some specific purpose, such as a follow-up visit. These codes can also be used when the patient has no symptoms that can be coded and screening services are provided (eg, screening mammogram for high-risk patient).

FACT-ORIENTED Z CODES

These are V codes that do not describe a problem or a service; they simply state a fact (eg, outcome of delivery or categorizing liveborn infants according to type of birth).

Persons Encountering Health Services for Examinations

General and administration examinations are reported for encounters for routine examinations. The codes from these categories are first listed codes. They are not for use if the examination is for diagnosis of a suspected condition or for treatment purposes. In such cases, a confirmed diagnosis, sign, or symptom code should be used. Codes in the category range from Z00 to Z13. For example, an encounter for well-child check is reported in ICD-10-CM with two potential code options for this classification: Z00.121 and Z00.129.

Review the following example. Open up the ICD-10-CM codebook, referencing both the Alphabetic Index and the Tabular List, locate the correct code.

> **EXAMPLE:** *A 3-year-old female is brought to the doctor by her mother for her routine health well visit. After a detailed history and examination, the physician documents "well visit" without any problems.*

The child is well, and there is not a code that describes circumstances (reason for the encounter). However, a diagnosis with this service must be reported in order to receive reimbursement from a carrier. The solution is to use a Z code for the diagnosis.

> **Alphabetic Index:**
> *Examination → Child (over 28 days old) → Z00.129*
>
> **Tabular List:**
> *Z00.129 → Encounter for routine child health examination without abnormal findings*
>
> **Correct code:**
> *Z00.129*

CODING TIP The terms are Z code indicators, which alert the coder that a Z code will likely be used.

The instructional notes in Z00.10 indicate that if abnormal findings are discovered during the routine examination, the abnormal findings are reported as secondary codes. There is an instructional note that states to use Excludes 1 to report health supervision with Z76.1-Z76.2. Code Z76.1 is for health supervision and care of a foundling, and Z76.2 is reported for other health supervision of a healthy infant and child.

This category is used for:

- Encounter for medical or nursing care or supervision of healthy infant under circumstances such as adverse socioeconomic conditions at home

- Encounter for medical or nursing care or supervision of healthy infant under circumstances such as awaiting foster or adoptive placement

- Encounter for medical or nursing care or supervision of healthy infant under circumstances such as maternal illness

- Encounter for medical or nursing care or supervision of healthy infant under circumstances such as number of children at home preventing or interfering with normal care

Category Z00, Encounter for general examination without complaint, suspected or reported diagnosis, and category Z01, Encounter for other special examination without complaint or suspected or reported diagnosis, include subcategories for general medical examinations, including eye, ear, and dental examinations; general laboratory and radiology examinations; routine child health examinations; as well as encounters for examinations for potential organ donors and controls for participants in clinical trials.

Category Z02, Encounter for administrative examinations, includes codes for such things as pre-employment physicals. The final character of the general health examination codes distinguishes between "without abnormal findings" and "with abnormal findings." For these encounters, if an abnormal condition is discovered, the code for "with abnormal findings" should be used. A secondary code for the specific abnormal finding should be used.

Review the following example. Open up the ICD-10-CM codebook, referencing both the Alphabetic Index and the Tabular List, locate the correct code.

> **EXAMPLE:** *A 30-year-old healthy male went to his internist for a pre-employment examination. The patient had no complaints. The physician counseled the patient on diet and exercise, diagnosed the patient as a healthy male with no significant findings, and cleared him for his new job.*

Alphabetic Index:
   Examination → *pre-employment* → *Z02.1*

Tabular List:
   Z02.1 → *Encounter pre-employment examination*

Correct code:
   Z02.1

Now review Figure 11.1, which is an example of category Z01.3.

FIGURE 11.1   Excerpt from the Tabular List: *Z01.3*

Z01.3 Encounter for examination of blood pressure
Z01.30 Encounter for examination of blood pressure without abnormal findings
Z01.31 Encounter for examination of blood pressure with abnormal findings

The codes for preoperative examination and radiological and imaging examinations that are part of the preprocedural examination are reported with codes Z01.81– to Z01.84. These codes are used for surgical clearance and not when other treatment is provided. Pre-existing and chronic conditions, as long as the examination does not focus on them, may also be assigned with codes from Z00-Z02.

> **EXAMPLE:** *A patient who was scheduled for a hip-knee surgery who has a history of type 1 diabetes mellitus with diabetic polyneuropathy was sent to the cardiologist for preoperative clearance. The patient is doing well on her insulin and diet, and the physician cleared the patient for surgery.*

Alphabetic Index:
   Examination → *preoperative* → *see examination preprocedural* → *other* → *Z01.818*

Tabular List:
   Z01.818 → *Encounter for other preprocedural examination*

You should also report the reason for the preoperative examination or any conditions documented during the patient encounter located in the medical record.

Alphabetic Index:
   Diabetes, diabetic → *type 1* → *with polyneuropathy* → *E10.42*

Tabular List:
   E10.42 → *Type 1 diabetes mellitus with diabetic polyneuropathy*

Correct code sequence:
   Z01.818, E10.42

The preprocedural examination is reported as the first listed diagnosis because the focus of the visit is the preoperative examination and not the patient's condition.

Review the following examples. Open up the ICD-10-CM codebook, referencing both the Alphabetic Index and the Tabular List, locate the correct code.

EXAMPLE: *A patient sees an internist for a complete physical examination prior to entering the army. The physician performs a general multisystem examination, documents the patient is in excellent health, and clears the patient for induction.*

Alphabetic Index:
> *Examination* → *medical* → *admission to* → *armed forces* → *Z02.3*

Tabular List:
> *Z02.3* → *Encounter for examination for recruitment to armed forces*

Correct code:
> *Z02.3*

EXAMPLE: *A teenager presents for a medical examination so that she can be cleared to play on the school soccer team.*

Alphabetic Index:
> *Examination* → *medical (for)* → *sport competition* → *Z02.5*

Tabular List:
> *Z02.5* → *Encounter for examination for participation in sport*

Correct code:
> *Z02.5*

Observation Codes

An observation encounter is one wherein a person without a diagnosis is suspected of having an abnormal condition without signs or symptoms. For example, following an accident or incident, further study, examination, and observation rule out the suspected condition. There are two observation categories in ICD-10-CM. They are:

- Z03- Encounter for medical observation for suspected diseases and conditions

  - Preexisting and chronic conditions may also be assigned with codes from category Z03.-

- Z04- Encounter for observation for other reasons

You may use category Z04.- as long as the observation is not associated with a suspected condition being observed.

  - The Z03-Z04.9 codes are for use in very limited circumstances when a person was observed for a suspected condition that was found not to exist. The fact that the patient may be scheduled for a return encounter following the initial observation encounter does not limit the use of an observation code.

Review the following example. Open up the ICD-10-CM codebook, referencing both the Alphabetic Index and the Tabular List, locate the correct code.

EXAMPLE: *A 6-year-old patient was transported by ambulance to the emergency department following a car accident. The mother was driving on icy roads and the minivan she was driving flipped on its top. After examination, without any significant injuries identified, the physician decided to observe the child for a few hours before releasing the child from the emergency room.*

Alphabetic Index:
> *Examination* → *following* → *accident* → *transport* → *Z04.1*

Tabular List:
> *Z04.1 Encounter for examination and observation following transport Accident*

Correct code:
> *Z04.1*

CODING TIP Do not use an observation code for a patient with any illness, injury, signs, and symptoms. The illness, injury, signs, or symptoms should be coded, with the corresponding external cause code.

Follow-up Codes

The follow-up codes are used to describe encounters for a continuing patient encounter following completed treatment of a disease, condition, or injury. Follow-up care should not be confused with aftercare, which is current treatment for a healing or long-term condition.

A patient who is being followed for a "history (of)" is coded as an encounter for a healed, resolved condition that may still require repeated visits. For instance, a patient who had cancer will require long-term follow-up care, and a history code is reported after the cancer has been eradicated. If the condition is still present or reoccurs, the follow-up visit code should be reported in addition to code for the condition diagnosed during the visit.

Codes used in the category include:

- Z08 Encounter for follow-up examination after completed treatment for malignant neoplasm

- Z09 Encounter for follow-up examination after completed treatment for conditions other than malignant neoplasm

When reporting Z08, it is necessary to assign the appropriate secondary code from category Z85, Personal history of primary and secondary malignant neoplasm. If there is an acquired absence of an organ, it should be reported with category Z90.–. An additional code must be reported in category Z09 to report any history of disease with category Z86-Z87.

Review the following example. Open up the ICD-10-CM codebook, referencing both the Alphabetic Index and the Tabular List, locate the correct code.

> **EXAMPLE:** *A-45 year-old female patient is seen by the oncologist in follow-up after breast cancer two years ago. There is no sign of recurrence.*
>
> **Alphabetic Index:**
> *Examination* ➔ *follow-up (routine) (following)* ➔ *malignant neoplasm* ➔ *Z08*
>
> *History* ➔ *(personal)* ➔ *malignant neoplasm* ➔ *breast* ➔ *Z85.3*
>
> **Tabular List:**
> *Z08* ➔ *Encounter for follow-up examination after completed treatment for malignant neoplasm*
>
> *Z85.3* ➔ *Personal history of malignant neoplasm of breast*
>
> **Correct code sequencing:**
> *Z08, Z85.3*

Screening Codes

Screening is the testing for disease or disease precursors in seemingly healthy individuals so that early detection and treatment can be provided for those who test positive for the disease. The testing of a person to rule out or confirm a suspected diagnosis because the patient has some sign or symptom is a diagnostic test, not a screening. For these cases, the code for the sign or symptom is used to explain the test, not the screening code.

A screening code may be a first listed code if the reason for the encounter is specifically the screening. They may also be used as an additional code(s) if the screening is done during an encounter for other health reasons.

A screening code is not necessary if the screening is inherent to a routine examination, such as a Pap smear done during a routine pelvic examination.

If a condition is discovered during a screening, the screening code should still be used, followed by the code for the condition that is discovered. ICD-10-CM category codes Z11-Z13 are used to report encounters for specific screening examinations.

The screening categories are:

- Z11 Encounter for special screening examination for infectious and parasitic diseases

- Z12 Encounter for special screening for malignant neoplasm

- Z13 Encounter for special screening for other diseases and disorders

Review the following examples. Open up the ICD-10-CM codebook, referencing both the Alphabetic Index and Tabular List, locate the correct code.

> **EXAMPLE:** *A screening mammogram was performed on a 50-year-old woman. The patient does not have a family or personal history of cancer.*
>
> **Alphabetic Index:**
> *Screening* ➔ *neoplasm* ➔ *breast* ➔ *routine mammogram* ➔ *Z12.31*
>
> **Tabular list:**
> *Z12.31* ➔ *Encounter for screening mammogram for malignant neoplasm of breast*
>
> **Correct code:**
> *Z12.31*

> **EXAMPLE:** *A 6-week-old male newborn is being screened for sickle-cell disease. There is a very strong family history, and the pediatrician felt it important to screen the child.*

How do you report these screening services for healthy newborns? Use a Z code to provide the reason for providing this service.

> **Alphabetic Index:**
> *Screening* ➔ *Disease (disorder)* ➔ *Sickle-cell trait* ➔ *Z13.0*
>
> **Tabular List:**
> *Z13.0* ➔ *Encounter for screening for diseases of the blood and blood-forming organs and certain disorders involving the immune mechanism*
>
> **Correct Code:**
> *Z13.0*

CHECKPOINT EXERCISE 11-1

Identify the main term for the following conditions:

Example: Routine general medical <u>examination</u>

1. _____ Observation following an accident at work

2. _____ Family history of asthma

3. _____ Influenza vaccination (prophylactic)

4. _____ Renal dialysis status

5. _____ Screening for cystic fibrosis

6. _____ Well-baby visit

7. _____ General health exam

8. _____ Personal history of prostate cancer

9. _____ Chemotherapy encounter

10. _____ Exposure to tuberculosis

11. _____ Exposure to SARS

12. _____ Insulin pump status

13. _____ Dependence on respirator, status

14. _____ Long-term use of aspirin

15. _____ Genetic susceptibility to malignant neoplasm of the ovary

Status Codes

Status codes indicate that a patient is either a carrier of a disease or has the sequela or residual of a past disease or condition. This includes such things as the use of a prosthetic or mechanical device. A status code is informative because the status may affect any current treatment and its outcome. A status code is distinct from a history code. A history code indicates that the patient no longer has a condition. Codes in this category are used to identify long-term care of drug therapy, to identify a pregnant patient whose condition is incidental to the reason for the patient's visit for treatment, and for a patient who is HIV positive with no symptoms, to name a few. Codes from this category should be added to a patient's record at every encounter. For example, a drug allergy is a chronic and typically life-long condition and should be coded as such. This subcategory includes allergies to foods,

insects, and other nonmedicinal substances, such as latex.

The status Z categories/subcategories codes are:

- Z14 Genetic carrier
- Z15 Genetic susceptibility to disease
- Z16 Infection with drug-resistant microorganism
- Z21 Asymptomatic human immunodeficiency virus (HIV), infection status (HIV) disease

Category Z14 is used to report a person who carries a gene associated with a disease that can be passed to his or her children but do not currently have the disease. Codes in this category include:

- Genetic carrier hemophilia
- Cystic fibrosis

Category Z15 is used to report a confirmed abnormal gene for genetic susceptibility to a disease, including malignant neoplasms. Codes in this category are not reported as the first listed diagnosis, but they are secondary when the active disease or condition is the reason for the patient encounter. The disease is sequenced first, followed by a code from category Z15.–. For genetic counseling, code Z31.5 should be reported as the first listed diagnosis, followed by a code from category Z15.

Persons with Potential Health Hazards Related to Communicable Disease (Z20-Z28)

ICD-10-CM category codes Z20-Z28 are assigned to the records of persons who have been diagnosed as having communicable diseases that pose potential public health hazards. These codes are used for patients who do not have any signs or symptoms of a disease but have been exposed either by close personal contact or where an epidemic has erupted. These codes may be reported as the principal/first listed diagnosis to explain the patient encounter or testing performed or they may be used as a secondary diagnosis to report the potential risk.

Review the following example. Open up the ICD-10-CM codebook, referencing both the Alphabetic Index and the Tabular List, locate the correct code.

EXAMPLE: A-15 year-old female was playing with a puppy at a neighbor's home. It was discovered two days later that the puppy had rabies. The patient was taken to her family physician by her mother to evaluate the situation and determine treatment options.

Alphabetic Index:
   Exposure ➙ *rabies*

Tabular List:
   Z20.3 ➙ *Contact with and (suspected) exposure to rabies*

Correct code:
   Z20.3

Code Z23, Encounter for immunization, is used to indicate that a patient is being seen to receive a pro-phylactic inoculation against a disease. The injection itself must be indicated with a procedure code. This code may be used as a secondary code if the inocula-tion is given as a part of preventive health care, such as a well-baby visit. Instructional notes in the beginning of the category instruct the user to report the routine childhood examination as the first listed diagnosis. Immunizations against many communicable diseases are required in most states for admission to school or for employment.

Review the following example. Open up the ICD-10-CM codebook, referencing both the Alphabetic Index and the Tabular List, locate the correct code.

EXAMPLE: A child presents for routine childhood immuni-zations and is given a measles, mumps, and rubella (MMR) vaccination.

Alphabetic Index:
   Vaccination ➙ *encounter for* ➙ *Z23*

Tabular List:
   Z23 ➙ *Encounter for immunization*

Correct Code:
   Z23

For persons who choose not to receive an immuni-zation for personal or health reasons, a code from category Z28, Immunization not carried out, should be used to identify the reason a required immunization is not given. A fifth character is required to identify the highest level of specificity. Review Figure 11.2, which is an example of immunization not carried out.

FIGURE 11.2   Excerpt from the Tabular List: *Z28.–*

Z28   Immunization not carried out and underimmunization
      status
      Vaccination not carried out
      ✓5th Z28.0   Immunization not carried out because of
                   contraindication
               Z28.01   Immunization not carried out
                        because of acute illness of patient
               Z28.02   Immunization not carried out
                        because of chronic illness or
                        condition of patient
               Z28.03   Immunization not carried out
                        because of immune compromised
                        state of patient
               Z28.04   Immunization not carried out
                        because of patient allergy to vaccine
                        or component
               Z28.09   Immunization not carried out
                        because of other contraindication

Review the following example. Open up the ICD-10-CM codebook, referencing both the Alphabetic Index and the Tabular List, locate the correct code.

EXAMPLE: A patient presents to a health care clinic for care after having unprotected sex with a partner who has a positive HIV test.

Alphabetic Index:
   Exposure ➙ *Human immunodeficiency virus (HIV) Z20.6*

Tabular List:
   Z20.6 Contact and (suspected) exposure to Human Immunodeficiency Virus (HIV)

Correct code:
   Z20.6

Persons Encountering Health Services in Circumstances Related to Reproduction (Z30-Z39)

These codes are used for encounters related to repro-duction and development and include status codes, counseling codes, screenings codes, and pregnancy codes. Z codes for pregnancy are for use when a prob-lem or complication that is included in the Obstetrics chapter exists. These codes are not to be used with any code in the Obstetrics chapter in ICD-10-CM.

The categories/codes related to reproduction include:

- Z30 Encounter for contraceptive management

- Z31 Encounter for procreative management

- Z32 Encounter for pregnancy test and instruction

- (Code Z33.1, Pregnancy state, incidental, is a status code)

- Z33.2 Encounter for elective termination of pregnancy

- Z34 Encounter for supervision of normal pregnancy

- Z36 Encounter for antenatal screening

- Z37 Outcome of delivery

- Z38 Liveborn infant according to place of birth and type of delivery

- Z39 Encounter for maternal postpartum care and examination

Review the following example. Open up the ICD-10-CM codebook, referencing both the Alphabetic Index and the Tabular List, locate the correct code.

> **EXAMPLE:** *A single liveborn delivered by cesarean section in the hospital was diagnosed by the pediatrician right after birth with congenital obstruction of the bile duct. The newborn was moved to the neonatal unit of the hospital for continued care.*
>
> **Alphabetic Index:**
>   *Infant(s)* → *single liveborn* → *cesarean* → *Z38.01*
>
>   *Obstruction* → *bile duct* → *congenital (causing jaundice)* → *Q44.3*
>
> **Tabular List:**
>   *Z38.01* → *Single liveborn infant, delivered by cesarean*
>
>   *Q44.3* → *Congenital stenosis and stricture of bile ducts*
>
> **Correct code sequencing:**
>   *Z38.01, Q44.3*

You will code the liveborn delivery via cesarean as the first listed diagnosis, followed by the patient's condition.

These following encounter codes identify the reason for the visit. Any procedures performed must be identified with a procedure code from the appropriate procedure classification.

- Z33.1 Pregnant state, incidental

- Z79 Long-term (current) drug therapy

- Z88 Allergy status to drugs, medicaments, and biological substances

Review the following example. Open up the ICD-10-CM codebook, referencing both the Alphabetic Index and the Tabular List, locate the correct code.

> **EXAMPLE:** *A 28-year-old patient who is pregnant visited her OB/GYN with complaint of congestion and cough. The physician diagnosed the patient with an acute respiratory infection.*
>
> **Alphabetic Index:**
>   *Infection* → *respiratory* → *acute* → *J22*
>
>   *pregnancy* → *state* → *incidental* → *Z33.1*
>
> **Tabular List:**
>   *J22* → *Unspecified acute lower respiratory infection*
>
>   *Z33.1 Pregnancy state, incidental (secondary diagnosis)*
>
> **Correct code sequencing:**
>   *J22, Z33.1*

Outcome of Delivery

This category is intended for reporting the outcome of delivery for those who are using health care services. This category is to be used in the mother's record, not the newborn record. Codes in this category are generally the first listed diagnosis but may be used as an additional diagnosis if the patient has more than one encounter on one day. The categories are based on the number of births that occur.

Review the following categories:

- Z37.0 Single live birth

- Z37.1 Single stillbirth

- Z37.2 Twins, both liveborn

- Z37.3 Twins, one liveborn and one stillborn

- Z37.4 Twins, both stillborn

- Z37.5– Other multiple births, all liveborn

- Z37.6– Other multiple births, some liveborn

- Z37.7 Other multiple births, all stillborn

- Z37.9 Outcome of delivery, unspecified.

Review the following example. Open up the ICD-10-CM codebook, referencing both the Alphabetic Index and the Tabular List, locate the correct code.

EXAMPLE: *A single liveborn was delivered by cesarean section in the hospital.*

Alphabetic Index:
Outcome → delivery → single liveborn →
cesarean → Z38.01

Tabular List:
Z38.01 → Single liveborn infant, delivered by cesarean

Correct code:
Z38.01

Aftercare

Aftercare visit codes, with such category titles as fitting and adjustment and attention to artificial openings, cover situations when the initial treatment of a disease or injury has been performed and the patient requires continuing care during the healing or recovery phase or for the long-term consequences of an illness. The aftercare Z codes should not be used if treatment is directed at a current disease or injury. The disease or injury code should be used in such cases with the seventh-character D, Subsequent encounter. The exceptions to this rule are radiation therapy, chemotherapy, and immunotherapy for the treatment of neoplasm, as discussed below.

An aftercare code may also be used as a secondary code when some type of aftercare is provided in addition to another reason for an encounter and no diagnosis code is applicable. Certain aftercare codes need a secondary diagnosis code to describe the resolving condition or sequelae. For others, the condition is inherent in the code title. Aftercare codes are not used for mechanical complications or malfunctioning devices.

The aftercare categories are:

- Z43 Encounter for attention to artificial openings
- Z44 Encounter for fitting and adjustment of external prosthetic device
- Z45 Encounter for adjustment and management of implanted device
- Z46 Encounter for fitting and adjustment of other devices
- Z47 Orthopedic aftercare
- Z48 Encounter for other postprocedural aftercare
- Z49 Encounter for care involving renal dialysis
- Z51 Encounter for other aftercare

Review the following example. Open up the ICD-10-CM codebook, referencing both the Alphabetic Index and the Tabular List, locate the correct code.

EXAMPLE: *A patient who recently had a meniscectomy returned to the orthopedic surgeon in follow-up. The patient is doing well and will be released in two weeks to return to work.*

Alphabetic Index:
Aftercare → following surgery → (for) (on) →
orthopedic NEC → Z47.89

Tabular List:
Z47.89 → Other orthopedic aftercare

Correct code:
Z47.89

Encounter for Radiation Therapy and Chemotherapy (Z51.–)

For patients whose encounter is specifically to receive radiation therapy and chemotherapy, codes Z51.0, Encounter for radiotherapy session, and Z51.1, When sequencing, the encounter for chemotherapy or radiation therapy is sequenced first, followed by the condition treated (neoplasm). When a patient is receiving both radiation and chemotherapy during the same encounter, both codes should be used, with either sequenced first.

Review the following example. Open up the ICD-10-CM codebook, referencing both the Alphabetic Index and the Tabular List, locate the correct code.

EXAMPLE: *A patient underwent chemotherapy following an oophorectomy for removal of a malignant tumor of the left ovary.*

Alphabetic Index:
Chemotherapy → (session) (for) → neoplasm →
Z51.11

Neoplasm table → Ovary → C56.–

Tabular List:
Z51.11 → Chemotherapy session for neoplasm
(first listed)

C56.2 → Malignant neoplasm of left ovary

Correct code sequencing:
Z51.11, C56.2

History Codes

There are two types of history (of) codes:

- Personal history

- Family history

Personal history codes indicate a patient's past medical condition that no longer exists but that has the potential for recurrence and, therefore, may require continued monitoring. Personal history codes should be used in conjunction with follow-up codes to explain the condition being followed. Personal history codes are acceptable on any medical record regardless of the reason for the encounter. A personal history or an illness or condition, even if no longer present, is important information that may alter the type of treatment given.

Family history codes are for use when a patient has a family member(s) who has had a particular disease that causes the patient to be at higher risk of also contracting the disease. Family history codes should be used in conjunction with screening codes to explain the need for a test or procedure if a family history of the condition being screened for is applicable.

The history (of) categories/codes are:

- Z80 Family history of primary malignant neoplasm

- Z81 Family history of mental and behavioral disorders

- Z82 Family history of certain disabilities and chronic diseases (leading to disablement)

- Z83 Family history of other specific disorders

- Z84 Family history of other conditions

- Z85 Personal history of primary and secondary malignant neoplasm

- Z86 Personal history of certain other diseases

- Z87 Personal history of other diseases and conditions

- Z91.41 Personal history of adult physical and sexual abuse

- Z91.49 Other personal history of psychological trauma, not elsewhere classified

- Z91.5 Personal history of self-harm

- Z92 Personal history of medical treatment

Review the following example. Open up the ICD-10-CM codebook, referencing both the Alphabetic Index and the Tabular List, locate the correct code.

EXAMPLE: *A patient visits her family physician for evaluation. The patient has a family history of diabetes mellitus but is healthy with no sign of the disease.*

Alphabetic Index:
History of (family) → diabetes mellitus → Z83.3

Tabular list:
Z83.3 → Family history of Diabetes Mellitus

Categories Z89-Z99 are for use only if there is no complication or malfunction of the organ or tissue replaced, of the amputation site, or the equipment on which the patient is dependent. These are always secondary codes.

These code categories include:

- Z89 Acquired absence of limb

- Z90 Acquired absence of organs, not elsewhere classified

- Z91.0 Allergy status, other than to drugs and biological substances

- Z92.2 Personal history of drug therapy

- Z93 Artificial opening status

- Z94 Transplanted organ and tissue status

- Z95 Presence of cardiac and vascular implants and grafts

- Z96 Presence of other functional implants

- Z97 Presence of other devices

- Z98 Other postprocedural states

- Z99 Dependence on enabling machines and devices, not elsewhere classified

Review the following examples. Open up the ICD-10-CM codebook, referencing both the Alphabetic Index and the Tabular List, locate the correct code.

EXAMPLE: *A patient who is diagnosed with acute bilateral otitis externa is also status posttracheostomy that does not require attention or management at this visit.*

Alphabetic Index:
Otitis → externa → H60.0-

Status → tracheostomy → Z93.0

Tabular List:
H60.93 → Unspecified otitis externa, bilateral

Z93.0 → Tracheostomy status

Correct code sequencing:
H60.93, Z93.0

EXAMPLE: *A patient suffering from organic aphonia (R49.1) is attending speech therapy sessions.*

Alphabetic Index:
Therapy ➞ *other specified after care* ➞ *Z51.89*

Tabular List:
Z51.89 ➞ *Encounter for other specified aftercare*

You will also need to report the organic aphonia as the reason for the therapy. The speech therapy is the reason for care, so the therapy is reported as the first listed diagnosis, followed by the condition that precipitated the treatment.

Correct code sequencing:
Z51.89, R49.1

Test Your Knowledge

Using volumes 1 and 2 of ICD-10-CM, find the correct code for the following diagnosis statements:

1. _____ Marital conflict

2. _____ Exercise counseling

3. _____ Tubal ligation status

4. _____ Routine or ritual circumcision

5. _____ Unemployment

6. _____ Fertility testing

7. _____ Problems with learning

8. _____ Viral hepatitis vaccine

9. _____ Observation for suspected malignant neoplasm

10. _____ Preoperative cardiovascular examination

11. _____ Special screening for malignant neoplasm of the cervix

12. _____ Awaiting organ transplant status

13. _____ Measles vaccination

14. _____ Personal history of allergy to penicillin

15. _____ Exposure to *Escherichia coli (E coli)*

16. _____ A patient presents for antepartum care at the end of her seventh month of pregnancy. She has not sought medical care of any type during the pregnancy. Other than insufficient weight gain, the patient does not appear to have any complications or problems.

17. _____ A single live infant is born at a local hospital.

18. _____ A child presents for routine childhood immunizations and is given a measles, mumps, and rubella (MMR) vaccination.

19. _____ Liveborn triplets delivered by cesarean in the hospital

20. _____ A patient was experiencing nausea and vomiting following radiation therapy for treatment of a primary malignant tumor of the parathyroid gland.

CHAPTER 12

Medical Terminology and Anatomy

LEARNING OBJECTIVES

- Understand the importance of medical terminology and anatomy as it relates to diagnosis coding

- Identify the 3 word parts that make up medical terminology

- Recognize common word parts associated with systems of the body

- Define other common diagnostic and procedural medical terminology

Introduction

Every profession has its own "language," and medicine is no different. The language of medicine is more than 2000 years old! Many medical terms used today come from terms used by ancient Greeks and Romans. For example, *pro re nata* (Latin), meaning "when necessary," is currently used in medical prescriptions as the abbreviation *PRN*. A thorough understanding of medical terminology can eliminate many coding errors and help the coder identify the accurate diagnosis code(s).

Since ICD-10-CM is much more specific than ICD-9-CM and contains more clinical detail in the code descriptions, a good understanding of anatomy and medical terminology is needed to code successfully with ICD-10-CM. An understanding of the disease process is also important. This chapter focuses on medical terminology related to the structure and function of the body.

This chapter provides an introduction to the language of medicine for those who have not had a formal medical terminology class. It can also serve as a review for seasoned veterans. The chapter begins by analyzing word structures and then examines the terminology of disease and the anatomy of each body system. Checkpoint exercises, designed to review the terminology just presented, appear throughout the chapter; each section ends with a complete review. The list and outline format conveys the material in a user-friendly and accessible manner. Use your medical dictionary as a reference.

Basic Word Structure

Medical terms are often made up of 3 word parts, as follows:

Prefix / Word Root / Suffix

epi/gastro/cele

The word root is the foundation of the word. To link word roots to other word roots or suffixes, a combining vowel, usually an "o," is used. The word root plus a combining vowel is the combining form:

gastr/o: stomach

cardi/o: heart

derm/o: skin

arthr/o: joint

SUFFIXES

A suffix is a word ending used to further describe or clarify the word root or change the meaning of the word. For example:

-algia: pain

-ectomy: removal or excision

-tomy: incision (cutting) into

-stomy: creating a new opening

-cele: protrusion or hernia

-itis: inflammation

Following are the rules for adding a suffix to a word:

1. If the suffix begins with a vowel, drop the final vowel of the word root and add the suffix.

   stomach pain

   gastro + algia = gastralgia

2. If the suffix begins with a consonant, add it to the complete word root.

   incision into the stomach

   gastro + tomy = gastrotomy

3. In some cases, double the initial consonant before adding the suffix.

   -rhexis: rupture

   rupture of the stomach

   gastro + rhexis = gastrorrhexis

CHECKPOINT EXERCISE 12-1

Write a word that means:

1. removal of the stomach _____

2. inflammation of a joint _____

3. skin pain _____

4. suture of the heart _____

PREFIXES

A prefix is a word beginning used to describe:

amount

proximity

location

See the following examples of prefixes:

ante-: before

post-: after

a-: without

ec-: out from

endo-: within

peri-: around

Using the word parts you just learned, review the following words:

1. Postgastrectomy: after removal of stomach.

   post + gastro + ectomy = postgastrectomy

2. Endocarditis: inflammation within the heart.

   endo + cardio + itis = endocarditis

CHECKPOINT EXERCISE 12-2

Write a word that means:

1. rupture within the heart _____

2. without skin _____

3. inflammation around the stomach _____

4. after incision into a joint _____

MORE SUFFIXES

-centesis: puncture

-pexy: fixation

-al: pertaining to

-ic: referring to

-osis: abnormal condition of

-emia: blood condition

-genic: origin

-logy: study of

CHECKPOINT EXERCISE 12-3

Write a word that means:

1. pertaining to the heart _____

2. fixation of a joint _____

3. abnormal condition of the skin _____

4. study of the stomach _____

MORE PREFIXES

hyper-: above normal, excessive

hypo-: below

multi-: many

bi-: two or both

tri-: three

ab-: from

ad-: to, near

epi-: upon

REVIEW: BASIC WORD STRUCTURE

1. Fill in the blank with the appropriate term:

    a. are word endings _____

    b. are word beginnings _____

    c. are the foundation of words _____

2. Define these word roots:

    a. *cardi/o* _____

    b. *gastr/o* _____

    c. *derm/o* _____

    d. *arthr/o* _____

3. Define these prefixes:

    a. *hyper-* _____

    b. *post-* _____

    c. *endo-* _____

    d. *peri-* _____

4. Define these suffixes:

    a. *-cele* _____

    b. *-logy* _____

    c. *-tomy* _____

    d. *-ectomy* _____

5. Identify and define the word parts of each term:

    a. cardiopexy _____

    b. arthralgia _____

    c. dermatitis _____

    d. cardiocentesis _____

Terms of Disease and Basic Anatomy

DISEASE

1. Disease: "a condition of the body that presents a group of symptoms peculiar to it and that sets the condition apart as abnormal or differing from normal body states."[1] The cause of the disease must be identified in order to cure or treat it.

   word root: *path/o*: disease

   suffix: *-pathy*: disease condition

   word root: *eti/o*: cause

   pathogenic: disease-causing agent: *patho*/disease, *genic*/producing

2. Infection: "a condition in which the body or a part of it is invaded by a pathogenic agent that multiplies and produces effects that are injurious."[1]

3. Inflammation: tissue reaction to injury. The inflamed area undergoes continuous change as the body heals and replaces injured tissue.

4. Diagnosis: problem or nature of disease or injury.

5. Prognosis: probable outcome or estimate of chance of recovery from a disease or injury.

6. Sign: any objective evidence of a disease or injury that can be seen, felt, or measured.

7. Symptom: any subjective change in the body or its function that may indicate disease or injury. These changes are not perceptible to an observer.

8. Syndrome: a set of symptoms that occur together.

9. Acute: a disease that has a rapid onset and is of relatively short duration.

10. Chronic: a disease that has a slow onset and lasts for a long period of time.

11. Localized: restricted to a definite area.

12. Systemic: affects the whole body.

13. Morbid: disease/illness.

14. Moribund: dying condition.

15. Necrosis: death of tissue.

    necrosis: *necr*/dead, *osis*/abnormal condition of

16. Mortality: death.

CHECKPOINT EXERCISE 12-4

Write a word that means:

1. disease condition of the heart _____

2. study of causes _____

3. inflammation within the heart with rapid onset and short duration (two words) _____ _____

4. pain in a joint restricted to a definite area (two words) _____ _____

GROWTH AND DEVELOPMENT TERMS

1. Anomaly: an irregularity; something out of the ordinary.

   Acquired (can develop).

   Congenital (present at birth).

   Hereditary (transmission from parent[s] to offspring).

2. Neoplasm: a growth or tumor.

   word root: *neo*: new

   suffix: *-plasm*: a thing formed

3. Benign: noncancerous.

4. Malignant: deadly or cancerous.

5. Carcinoma: cancerous tumor.

   word root: *carcin/o*: cancer

   suffix: *-oma*: tumor

6. Hyperplasia: increase in number of cells.

   prefix: *hyper-*: above

   suffix: *-plasia*: to form

7. Hypertrophy: increase in size of an organ or structure.

   prefix: *hyper-*: above

   suffix: *-trophy*: growth or nourishment

8. Necrosis: death of tissue.

   word root: *necro*: dead

   suffix: *-osis*: abnormal condition of

9. Ptosis: dropping or drooping of an organ or part.

CHECKPOINT EXERCISE 12-5

Write a word that means:

1. a condition that is present at birth _____

2. something that is considered noncancerous

_____

3. death of tissue _____

4. a growth or tumor _____

MENTAL HEALTH TERMS

Mental health terms can be classified by cause:

1. Organic: lesion in the body causing disturbance.

2. Functional: no identifiable lesion.

The following are some word roots related to mental health:

psycho: mind

phreno: mind

somato: body

phobo: fear

schizo: split

CHECKPOINT EXERCISE 12-6

What do these words mean?

1. psychosomatic _____

2. psychosis _____

3. androphobia _____

4. schizophrenia _____

ANATOMY

The body is a single structure "made up of structural units that build together to form the entire body."[2] The 4 major structural units of the body are the following:

1. Cells: "the smallest structural unit of all living things."[2] All human cells that reproduce do so by the process called mitosis, in which the cell divides to multiply (one cell divides to form two cells).

   word root: *cyt/o*

   suffix: *-cyte*

2. Tissues: "groups of like cells."[2]

   word root: *hist/o*

3. Organs: "structures composed of several kinds of tissues that work together to perform a specific function."[2]

   word root: *cardi/o*: heart (name of organ)

4. Systems: "groups of organs that work together to perform a specific [or similar] function."[2] A system is the largest structural unit in the body. The body is made up of the following 9 systems:

   • Skeletal and muscular system

   • Circulatory system

   • Respiratory system

   • Endocrine system

   • Nervous system (including the senses)

   • Urinary system

   • Digestive system

   • Reproductive system

   • Integumentary (skin) system

"The body may be thought of as a house with four major rooms. The rooms are called cavities. The four body cavities house all of the organs in the body. They are:"[2]

thoracic cavity (lining: pleura)

   word root: *pleur/o*

abdominopelvic cavity (lining: peritoneum)

   word root: *periton/o*

cranial cavity (lining: meninges)

   word root: *mening/o*

spinal cavity (lining: meninges)

   word root: *mening/o*

CHECKPOINT EXERCISE 12-7

Write a word that means:

1. "groups of like cells"[2] _____

2. largest structural unit in the body _____

3. smallest structural unit in the body _____

4. "structures composed of several kinds of tissues that work together to perform a specific function"[2] _____

REVIEW: DISEASE AND BASIC ANATOMY

1. Name the four body cavities and their linings:

a. cavity: _____ lining: _____

b. cavity: _____ lining: _____

c. cavity: _____ lining: _____

d. cavity: _____ lining: _____

2. Define these word roots:

a. *path/o* _____

b. *hist/o* _____

c. *carcin/o* _____

d. *necr/o* _____

3. Define these suffixes:

a. *-cyte* _____

b. *-pathy* _____

c. *-ptosis* _____

d. *-oma* _____

4. Match these words with the correct definition:

a. sign	rapid onset, short duration
b. systemic	slow onset, long duration
c. acute	objective evidence of disease
d. symptom	affects the whole body
e. inflammation	subjective change in the body
f. chronic	restricted to a definite area
g. infection	body invaded by pathogenic agent
h. localized	tissue reaction to injury

Body Systems

The remainder of this chapter will focus on the 9 systems of the body. The final section will address the skin and the senses, the organs of which are classified among various body systems.

SKELETAL AND MUSCULAR SYSTEM

"The skeletal system has six functions:"[2]

1. "Gives support."[2]

2. "Gives shape."[2]

3. "Protects inner organs and structures."[2]

4. "Anchors muscles."[2]

5. "Makes blood cells."[2]

Red blood cells (RBCs).

White blood cells (WBCs).

Platelets.

6. "Stores calcium."[2]

> word root: *osteo, osto*: bone

The adult human body has a total of 206 bones. The place where two or more bones meet is called an articulation or joint.

> word root: *arthro*: joint

CHECKPOINT EXERCISE 12-8

Write a word that means:

1. bone pain _____

2. puncture into sternum _____

3. inflammation of bone and cartilage _____

4. bone tumor _____

The muscular system has 3 functions:

1. Assists in moving the skeleton.

2. Provides warmth.

3. Provides strength.

> word root: *myo*: muscle

Three types of muscle exist:

1. Voluntary or skeletal muscle.

2. Cardiac muscle.

3. Smooth muscle.

The human body has more than 600 muscles, which are attached to bones by tendons.

> word root: *tendo, teno*: tendon

Movement Terms

1. Abduct: to move away from the midline.

2. Adduct: to move toward the midline.

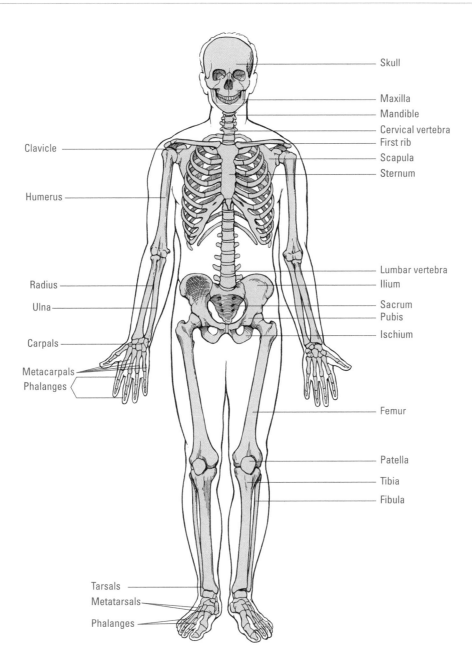

Skull

Maxilla
Mandible
Cervical vertebra
First rib
Scapula
Sternum

Clavicle

Humerus

Lumbar vertebra
Ilium

Radius
Sacrum
Ulna
Pubis

Ischium

Carpals

Metacarpals
Phalanges

Femur

Patella

Tibia
Fibula

Tarsals
Metatarsals

Phalanges

3. Flexion: contraction, to bend a part.

4. Extension: relaxation, to straighten a part.

Position Terms

1. Front vs back.

   anterior/posterior

   ventral/dorsal

2. Top vs bottom (transverse/horizontal).

   superior/inferior

   cephalad/caudal

3. Right vs left (sagittal/vertical).

   lateral (side)

   medial (midline)

4. Face-up vs face-down.

   supine/prone

5. Near attachment vs far from attachment.

   proximal/distal

CHECKPOINT EXERCISE 12-9

Provide the word that means the opposite of these words.

1. anterior vs _____

2. lateral vs _____

3. supine vs _____

4. proximal vs _____

Other Terms

1. Ataxia: loss of muscle coordination and power.

   ataxia: *a*/without, *tax*/order, *ia*/condition

2. Fracture: a broken bone (abbreviation: *fx*).

3. Reduction: to set a broken bone into alignment.

4. Gluteal: of or near the buttocks.

5. Hemiplegia: paralysis of one side of the body.

   hemiplegia: *hemi*/half, *pleg*/paralysis, *ia*/condition of

6. Orthostatic: pertains to an erect position.

   orthostatic: *ortho*/straight, *stat*/stop, stand, *ic*/referring to

7. Paralysis: loss of voluntary motion.

   paralysis: *para*/abnormal, *lysis*/destruction

8. Prosthesis: artificial replacement.

9. Sprain: injury to the ligamentous structure of a joint.

10. Strain: injury to a muscle.

11. Scoliosis: abnormal lateral deviation of the spine.

12. Kyphosis: hunchback.

13. Lordosis: swayback.

More Prefixes

uni-: one

bi-: two or both

mono-: single

anti-: against

inter-: between

dys-: painful or difficult

More Suffixes

-malacia: softening condition

-desis: binding

-genesis: producing

-oid: like

-scopy: examination or visualization of a part with a scope

-scope: instrument used to examine or visualize

CHECKPOINT EXERCISE 12-10

Write a word that means:

1. bone softening _____

2. bone producing _____

3. musclelike _____

4. to examine a joint with a scope _____

REVIEW: SKELETAL AND MUSCULAR SYSTEM

1. Provide the word root for each of these:

   a. bone _____

   b. muscle _____

   c. cartilage _____

   d. wrist bone _____

   e. breast bone _____

2. Match these words with the correct definition:

   a. supine   side

   b. anterior   face-up

   c. lateral   midline

   d. proximal   front

   e. prone   far from attachment

   f. superior   back

   g. medial   face-down

   h. posterior   head; top

   i. inferior   feet; bottom

   j. distal   near attachment

3. Fill in the blanks:

   a. Straightening or stretching a muscle is called _____, while shortening a muscle is called contraction or _____.

   b. Moving a part toward the body is called _____, and moving a part away from the body is called _____.

4. Identify and define the word parts of each term:

   a. osteoarthrotomy _____

   b. osteoid _____

   c. intercostochondritis _____

   d. arthrodesis _____

   e. unilateral _____

   f. arthroscope _____

CIRCULATORY SYSTEM

The circulatory system has 3 functions:

1. "To carry oxygen and nourishment to the body cells."[2]

2. "To exchange oxygen and nourishment for waste products."[2]

3. "To carry the waste products to points of elimination."[2]

Parts of the circulatory system are the heart, the blood vessels, the blood, the lymph and lymph vessels, and the spleen.

The Heart

The heart is a muscular pump.

> word root: *cardi/cardio*

1. Atrium: upper chamber of the heart.

   > word root: *atrio*

2. Ventricle: lower chamber of the heart.

   > word root: *ventriculo*

3. Layers of the heart:

   > *pericardium*: *peri*/around, *cardium*/heart
   >
   > *myocardium*: *myo*/muscle, *cardium*/heart
   >
   > *endocardium*: *endo*/within, *cardium*/heart

4. Systole: contraction phase of heartbeat.

5. Diastole: relaxation phase of heartbeat.

CHECKPOINT EXERCISE 12-11

Write a word that means:

1. disease condition of heart muscle _____

2. repair of the ventricle _____

3. puncture into the heart _____

Blood Vessels

Blood vessels carry blood to and from the heart and body.

> word root: *angio, vaso*

1. Arteries (aorta, large arteries, arteries, arterioles): carry blood away from the heart.

   > word root: *arterio*

2. Veins (vena cava, large veins, veins, venules): carry blood toward the heart.

   > word root: *phlebo, veno*

3. Capillaries: microscopic blood vessels.

   > word root: *capillo*

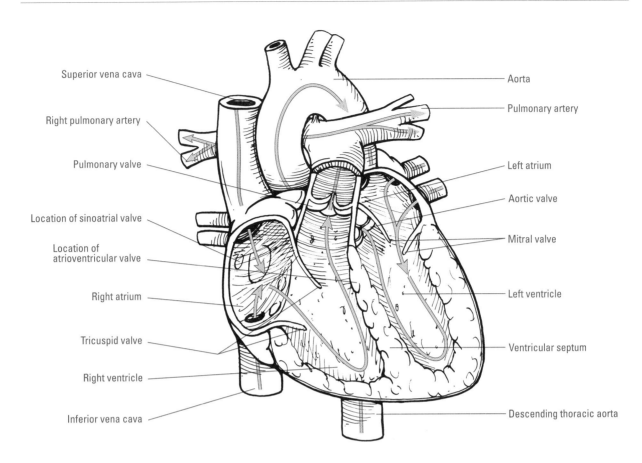

Superior vena cava

Right pulmonary artery

Pulmonary valve

Location of sinoatrial valve

Location of atrioventricular valve

Right atrium

Tricuspid valve

Right ventricle

Inferior vena cava

Aorta

Pulmonary artery

Left atrium

Aortic valve

Mitral valve

Left ventricle

Ventricular septum

Descending thoracic aorta

CHECKPOINT EXERCISE 12-12

Write a word that means:

1. inflammation of a vein _____

2. incision into an artery _____

3. removal of a vein _____

4. relating to the atrium and ventricle _____

Blood

Blood is fluid carried in the blood vessels.

word root: *hemo, hemat, heme*

suffix: *-emia*: blood condition

1. Plasma: liquid portion of blood.

2. Erythrocytes: red blood cells (RBCs).

erythrocyte: erythro/red, cyte/cell

3. Hemoglobin: iron-containing pigment that helps carry oxygen in the blood.

hemoglobin: hemo/blood, globin/pigment

4. Leukocytes: white blood cells (WBCs).

leukocyte: leuko/white, cyte/cell

5. Thrombocytes: platelets; cells that assist in the clotting process.

thrombocyte: thrombo/clot, cyte/cell

CHECKPOINT EXERCISE 12-13

Write a word that means:

1. condition of white blood _____

2. producing red blood cells _____

3. study of blood _____

4. destruction of a clot _____

Lymph, Lymph Vessels, and Spleen

Lymph and lymph vessels work with the circulatory system to return tissue fluid to general circulation, filter out harmful substances, and form some white blood cells.

word root: *lymph*

The spleen is the body's blood bank; it acts as the reservoir of blood in times of emergency and manufactures lymphocytes and monocytes (types of white blood cells).

word root: *spleno*

CHECKPOINT EXERCISE 12-14

Write a word that means:

1. lymph cell _____

2. removal of the spleen _____

3. hernia of the spleen _____

Other Terms

1. Aneurysm: weakening of the wall of an artery.

2. Angina: suffocating chest pain.

3. Arteriosclerosis: hardening of the arteries.

   arteriosclerosis: *arterio*/artery, *scler*/hardening, *osis*/abnormal condition of

4. Atherosclerosis: fatty deposits in the arteries.

   atherosclerosis: *athero*/artery, *scler*/hardening, *osis*/abnormal condition of

5. Thrombus: blood clot.

6. Thrombosis: condition of forming a blood clot.

   thrombosis: *thromb*/clot, *osis*/abnormal condition of

7. Embolus: clot; fat or air bubble that circulates, causing an obstruction.

8. Embolism: state of obstruction caused by an embolus.

9. Electrocardiogram: graphic recording of heart's action potential (abbreviations: *EKG, ECG*).

   electrocardiogram: *electro*/electric, *cardio*/heart, *gram*/record or tracing

10. Infarction: death of tissue due to lack of oxygen.

    myocardial infarction: heart attack

More Prefixes

brady-: slow

tachy-: rapid, fast

intra-: within

dia-: through

in-: not

More Suffixes

-megaly: enlargement

-plasty: repair

-spasm: involuntary contraction

-penia: deficient condition

-ole, -ule: smallness

-emia: blood condition

-ism: state of

-graphy: process of recording

-gram: record or tracing

REVIEW: CIRCULATORY SYSTEM

1. Provide the word root for each of the following:

   a. artery _____

   b. vein _____

   c. spleen _____

   d. blood vessels _____

   e. heart _____

2. Write a word that means:

   a. platelets _____

   b. red blood cells _____

   c. white blood cells _____

   d. heart muscle _____

3. Write a word that means:

   a. microscopic blood vessel _____

   b. white blood cell condition _____

   c. deficient number of platelet cells _____

   d. heart attack _____

   e. contraction phase of the heart cycle _____

   f. relaxation phase of the heart cycle _____

4. Identify and define the word parts of each term:

   a. pericarditis _____

   b. cardioplegia _____

   c. arteriomalacia _____

   d. phleboid _____

   e. splenectomy _____

   f. cardiomegaly _____

   g. tachycardia _____

   h. bradycardia _____

   i. angioplasty _____

   j. hemolysis _____

RESPIRATORY SYSTEM

The respiratory system has 4 functions:

1. "The exchange of gases between the body and its environment."[2]
2. "The production of sound."[2]
3. "The elimination of waste gases and water."[2]
4. "The elimination of excess heat from the body."[2]

Parts of the respiratory system include the following:

1. Nose: warms, moistens, and filters incoming air.

   word root: *rhin/o, nas/o*

2. Pharynx: passageway for both food and air.

   word root: *pharyng/o*

3. Epiglottis: covers entrance to air tube.

   word root: *epiglott/o: epi/*upon, *glotto/*tongue

4. Larynx: beginning of air tube, aids in production of sound.

   word root: *laryng/o*

5. Trachea: passageway for air into the lungs.

   word root: *tracheo*

6. Bronchus: either of the two major branch(es) of the trachea (plural: *bronchi*).

   word root: *broncho*

7. Bronchioles: smaller branches of bronchi that carry air into the alveoli.

   word root: *bronchi/o*

8. Alveoli: air sacs in the lungs, where gas exchange occurs.

   word root: *alveol/o*

9. Lungs: major organ of respiration.

   word root: *pulm/o, pulmon/o*: lungs; *pneum/o*: air

10. Chest: area where the organ of respiration is housed.

    word root: *thorac/o*

11. Diaphragm: major muscle of respiration.

    word root: *phren/o*

12. Ribs: protect and absorb shock to the chest cavity.

    word root: *cost/o*

13. Intercostal muscles: help elevate the ribs during inspiration.

14. Respiratory cycle:

    Inhalation: pulling air into the lungs.

    Exhalation: pulling air out of the lungs.

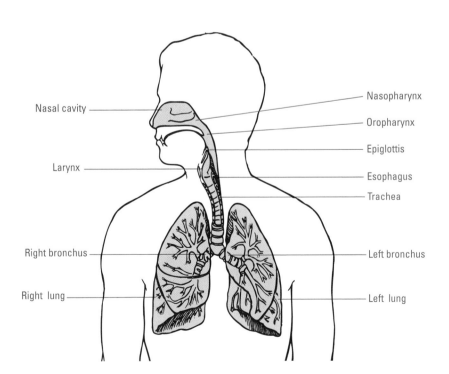

CHECKPOINT EXERCISE 12-15

Write a word that means:

1. inflammation of nose _____

2. creating a new opening in the trachea

   _____

3. removal of the larynx _____

4. involuntary contraction of the bronchus

   _____

Other Word Parts and Terms

1. *-pnea*: suffix that means breathing.

   eupnea: good breathing

   dyspnea: painful or difficult breathing

   orthopnea: straight breathing

   apnea: without breathing

2. Asphyxia: suffocation.

3. Anoxia: deficient oxygen supply to tissues.

   anoxia: *an*/without, *ox*/oxygen, *ia*/condition of

4. Hemoptysis: coughing up blood.

   hemoptysis: *hemo*/blood, *pty*/spittle, *sis*/process or procedure

5. Spirometry: measurement of air capacity of the lungs.

   spirometry: *spiro*/breath, *metry*/to measure (test)

   spirometer: *spiro*/breath, *meter*/to measure (instrument)

6. Cyanosis: bluish discoloration of the skin.

   cyanosis: *cyan*/blue, *osis*/abnormal condition

More Suffixes

-ectasis: dilation

-ary: relating to

-metry: to measure (test)

-meter: to measure (instrument)

CHECKPOINT EXERCISE 12-16

Write a word that means:

1. relating to outside the lungs _____

2. dilation of the bronchi _____

3. pertaining to above the sternum _____

REVIEW: RESPIRATORY SYSTEM

1. Provide the word root for each of these:

   a. trachea _____

   b. lung _____

   c. nose _____

   d. larynx _____

   e. air _____

   f. to breathe _____

2. Write a word that means:

   a. good breathing _____

   b. without breathing _____

   c. condition of being without oxygen

      _____

   d. suffocation _____

   e. coughing up blood _____

3. Identify and define the word parts of each term:

   a. pulmonectomy _____

   b. rhinoplasty _____

   c. pharyngospasm _____

   d. trachealgia _____

   e. thoracolumbar _____

   f. cyanodermia _____

   g. laryngoscope _____

   h. bronchogram _____

   i. laryngoscleroma _____

   j. alveobronchiolitis _____

   k. tracheomalacia _____

   l. pulmonitis _____

ENDOCRINE AND NERVOUS SYSTEMS

The endocrine system and the nervous system control the body's billions of cells, providing a method of communication and integration of function between the cells. The nervous system has a rapid, short-acting response and uses electrical signals.

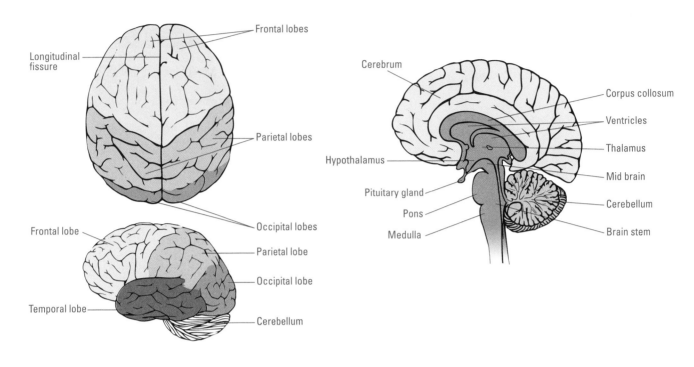

Endocrine System

There are two types of glands in the body:

1. Exocrine glands: secrete substances through ducts.

2. Endocrine glands: secrete substances (hormones) directly into the bloodstream.

The major glands of the endocrine system are the following:

1. Pituitary: "master gland" that secretes a number of hormones that regulate many body processes, such as reproduction and growth.

   word root: *pituitar/o*

2. Thyroid: controls body metabolism and normal growth (produces thyroxine).

   word root: *thyr/o*

3. Parathyroid: maintains normal calcium and phosphorus levels.

   word root: *parathyroid/o*

4. Adrenal: controls chemical balance in the blood and regulates metabolism.

   word root: *adren/o, adrenal/o*

5. Thymus: affects development of the body's immune system.

   word root: *thym/o*

6. Islets of Langerhans (pancreas): regulates body's blood sugar level with the hormone insulin.

   word root: *pancreat/o*

7. Gonads: organs of reproduction:

   Female: ovaries (produce estrogen/progesterone).

   word root: *oophoro*

   Male: testes (produce testosterone).

   word root: *testo, orchio, orchido*

Nervous System

The major parts of the nervous system are the central nervous system (CNS) and the peripheral nervous system (PNS).

Central Nervous System The CNS includes the brain and the spinal cord.

1. Brain: processes sensory information from inside and outside the body to control bodily functions, motor responses, and learning.

   word root: *encephalo*

Cerebrum: center for mental processes.

> word root: *cerebro*

Cerebellum: center of muscular coordination/balance.

> word root: *cerebello*

Hypothalamus: controls hormonal secretion.

> word root: *hypothalamo*

Thalamus: controls sensation and emotion.

> word root: *thalamo*

Brain stem: medulla, pons, and midbrain control vital functions, such as blood pressure, respiration, heartbeat, and diameter of blood vessels.

2. Spinal cord: carries impulses to and from the brain.

> word root: *myelo*

Peripheral Nervous System The PNS includes all the nerves that extend from the CNS to all parts of the body.

> word root: *neuro*: nerve

1. Cranial nerves.

2. Spinal nerves.

3. Autonomic nerves.

> word root: *auto*: self

CHECKPOINT EXERCISE 12-18

What do these words mean?

1. encephalitis _____

2. neuralgia _____

3. cerebrotomy _____

4. autolysis _____

Other Terms

1. Hyperglycemia: increased amount of glucose (sugar) in the blood due to decreased levels of insulin.

> *hyperglycemia*: *hyper*/above, *glyc*/sugar, sweet, *emia*/blood condition

2. Hypothyroidism: decreased activity of the thyroid gland.

> *hypothyroidism*: *hypo*/below, *thyroid*/thyroid, *ism*/state or quality of

3. Aphasia: a loss of ability to speak, write, or comprehend.

> *aphasia*: *a*/without, *phas*/speech, *ia*/condition of

4. Acromegaly: enlargement of the extremities.

> *acromegaly*: *acro*/extremities, *megaly*/enlargement

5. Hydrocephalus: abnormal increase in cerebrospinal fluid around the brain.

6. Syncope: fainting.

7. Vertigo: a sensation of dizziness.

8. Cerebrovascular accident: stroke (abbreviation: CVA).

9. Anesthesia: lack of feeling or sensation.

> *anesthesia*: *an*/without, *esthes*/feeling or sensation, *ia*/condition of

10. Gait: how you walk.

REVIEW: ENDOCRINE AND NERVOUS SYSTEMS

1. Provide the word root for each of the following:

   a. gland _____

   b. brain _____

   c. nerve _____

   d. self _____

   e. head _____

2. Write a word that means:

   a. fainting _____

   b. dizziness _____

   c. condition of lack of feeling or sensation

   _____

   d. stroke _____

   e. headache _____

   f. water on the brain _____

3. Identify and define the word parts of each term:

   a. adenoma _____

   b. thyroiditis _____

   c. cerebellar _____

   d. acroesthesia _____

   e. dysesthesia _____

   f. neurology _____

URINARY SYSTEM

"The urinary system removes wastes from the blood and eliminates them from the body."[2] It is also called the excretory system. The 4 major parts of the urinary system are as follows:

1. Kidneys: major functions include filtration, absorption, and excretion. Wastes are excreted in the form of urine.

    word root: *nephro, reno*; *uro, urino*: urine

2. Ureters: carry urine from kidneys to bladder.

    word root: *uretero*

3. Bladder: muscular storage reservoir for urine.

    word root: *cysto, vesico*

4. Urethra: passageway through which urine is discarded to outside of the body.

    word root: *urethro*

Other Word Parts and Terms

1. *-uria*: suffix that means urine condition.

2. Pyelonephritis: inflammation of the filtration part of the kidneys.

    pyelonephritis: *pyelo*/pelvis, *nephr*/kidney, *itis*/inflammation

3. Calculus: a stone.

    word root: *calc, litho*

4. Ureterolithiasis: presence of stones in the ureter.

    ureterolithiasis: *uretero*/ureter, *lith*/stone, *iasis*/presence of

5. Lithotripsy: procedure to crush stones.

    lithotripsy: *litho*/stone, *tripsy*/crush

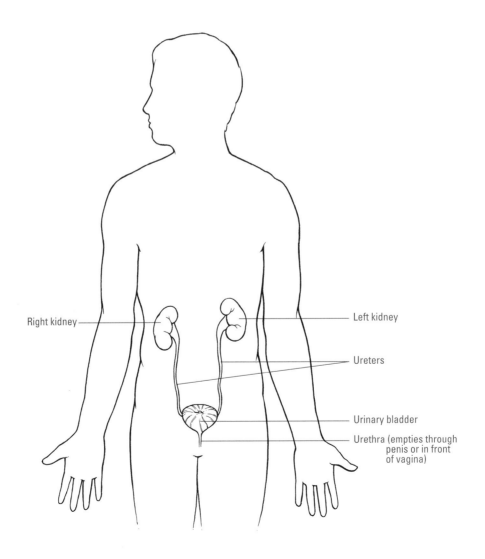

Right kidney

Left kidney

Ureters

Urinary bladder

Urethra (empties through penis or in front of vagina)

CHECKPOINT EXERCISE 12-19

Write a word that means:

1. removal of kidney _____

2. inflammation of the bladder _____

3. incision into the ureter _____

4. pain in the urethra _____

More Prefixes

olig-: few

> *oliguria*: decreased urine: *olig*/few, *uria*/urine condition

poly-: many

> *polyuria*: increased urine: *poly*/many, *uria*/urine condition

py-: pus

> *pyuria*: pus in the urine: *py*/pus, *uria*/urine condition

noct-: night

> *nocturia*: waking at night to urinate: *noct*/night, *uria*/urine condition

dys-: painful or difficult

> *dysuria*: painful urination: *dys*/painful or difficult, *uria*/urine condition

More Suffixes

-uria: urine condition

-rhage, -rhagia: burst forth, hemorrhage

-tripsy: crush

-clasis, -clasia: breaking

-rhaphy: suture

-dynia: pain

-rhea: flow, discharge

-logy: study of

-rhexis: rupture

-ist: specialist

-iasis: presence of

REVIEW: URINARY SYSTEM

1. Provide the word root for each of these:

   a. kidneys _____

   b. bladder _____

   c. urine _____

   d. stone _____

   e. urethra _____

2. Write a word that means:

   a. bedwetting _____

   b. inability to control the flow of urine

   _____

   c. to urinate _____

   d. study of the urinary system _____

   e. painful urine condition _____

3. Define these words:

   a. hematuria _____

   b. vesicorenal _____

   c. nephralgia _____

   d. ureteropyosis _____

   e. urography _____

   f. cystitis _____

   g. urology _____

   h. glycosuria _____

   i. nephradenoma _____

   j. renopathy _____

   k. urinal _____

   l. cystometry _____

   m. ureteroneocystostomy _____

   n. hydronephrosis _____

DIGESTIVE SYSTEM

The digestive system "makes the nourishment taken in during eating available to body cells."[2] It is also called the gastrointestinal (GI) system or alimentary canal:

gastrointestinal: *gastro*/stomach, *intestin*/intestines, *al*/pertaining to

alimentary: *aliment*/nourishment, *ary*/pertaining to

The digestive system has 7 major parts:

1. Mouth: where food is taken into the system.

   word root: *oro, stomo, stomato*

   Tongue.

   word root: *glosso, lingu*

Teeth.

   word root: *denti, dento, odonto*

Salivary glands.

   word root: *sialo*

Cheeks.

   word root: *bucco*

Lips.

   word root: *cheilo, labio*

Gums.

   word root: *gingivo*

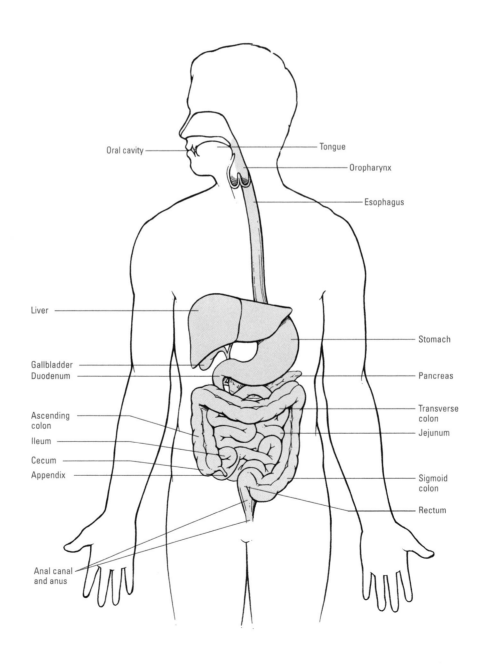

2. Pharynx: passageway for both food and air.

   word root: *pharyngo*

3. Esophagus: carries food from throat to stomach.

   word root: *esophago*

4. Stomach: muscular pouch that serves as reservoir for ingested food.

   word root: *gastro, pepso, pepto*

5. Small intestines: where digestion and absorption are completed.

   word root: *entero*

   Duodenum: first part of the small intestine.

   word root: *duodeno*

   Jejunum: section of the small intestine after the duodenum.

   word root: *jejuno*

   Ileum: last part of the small intestine.

   word root: *ileo*

6. Large intestines: where absorption of water occurs and waste materials pass out of the body in solid form (feces).

   Cecum: pouch connecting the ileum to the large intestine.

   word root: *ceco*

   Appendix: a tube that extends from the cecum.

   word root: *appendo, appendico*

   Colon: the part of the large intestine extending from the cecum to the rectum; includes the ascending, transverse, descending, and sigmoid colon.

   word root: *colo*

   parts of the colon: *ascending, transverse, descending, sigmoid*

   Rectum: final section of the large intestine.

   word root: *recto*

   Anus: opening at the end of the alimentary canal.

   word root: *ano*: anus; *procto*: rectum and anus

7. Accessory organs.

   Pancreas: secretes digestive enzymes including insulin and glucagon.

   word root: *pancreato*

Liver: secretes bile and cleanses the blood.

   word root: *hepa, hepato*

Gallbladder: stores bile from the liver.

   word root: *cholecysto*

Common bile duct: connects the liver and gallbladder to the duodenum.

   word root: *choledocho*

CHECKPOINT EXERCISE 12-20

What do these words mean?

1. gastroenterology _____
2. orolingual _____
3. esophagoenterostomy _____
4. pharyngectomy _____
5. colostomy _____
6. hepatitis _____
7. rectovesical _____
8. hepatosplenomegaly _____

Other Terms

1. Anastomosis: connection between hollow tubes.

2. Cachexia: ill health from malnutrition.

3. Dysphagia: inability to swallow.

   dysphagia: *dys*/painful, difficult, *phag*/eat, *ia*/condition of

4. Edentia: the condition of being without teeth.

   edentia: *e*/without, *dent*/teeth, *ia*/condition of

5. Anorexia: loss of appetite.

6. Peristalsis: a wavelike movement in the digestive organs that propels the contents forward.

7. Jaundice, icterus: yellowish discoloration of the skin and whites of the eyes.

8. Hematemesis: blood in the vomitus.

   hematemesis: *hemat*/blood, *emesis*/vomit

9. Eructation: belching.

10. Flatus: intestinal gas.

REVIEW: DIGESTIVE SYSTEM

1. Provide the word root for each of these:

  a. mouth _____

  b. gums _____

  c. salivary glands _____

  d. liver _____

  e. stomach _____

  f. first part of small intestines

  _____

  g. gallbladder _____

  h. rectum _____

  i. small intestine _____

  j. appendix _____

2. Write a word that means:

  a. chewing _____

  b. elimination of solid wastes

  _____

  c. expulsion of air or gas from the bowel

  _____

  d. hiccup _____

  e. loss of appetite _____

  f. pertaining to the teeth _____

  g. inflammation of the gallbladder

  _____

  h. blood in the vomitus _____

3. What do these words mean?

  a. dentalgia _____

  b. sialoadenitis _____

  c. gastropexy _____

  d. enterorrhaphy _____

  e. colitis _____

  f. rectourethral _____

  g. pancreatolytic _____

  h. hepatocholedochotomy _____

  i. proctosigmoidoscopy _____

  j. esophagogastroplegia _____

REPRODUCTIVE SYSTEM

The primary function of the reproductive system is the continuation of life. The female reproductive system has 5 parts:

1. Uterus: muscular organ that contains the fetus prior to birth.

  word root: *hystero, metro*

2. Fallopian tubes: carry the egg from the ovary to the uterus.

  word root: *salpingo*

3. Ovaries: produces the sex cell (egg) and estrogen/progesterone.

  word root: *oophoro*; *oo*: egg

4. Cervix: the lower portion of the uterus that extends into the vagina.

  word root: *cervico*

5. Vagina: muscular tube that extends from the cervix to the outside of the body.

  word root: *colpo, vagino*

The male reproductive system has 4 parts:

1. Testes (singular: *testis*, *testicle*): produce the sex cell (sperm) and testosterone.

  word root: *testo, orchio, orchido*; *spermato*: sperm

2. Epididymis: a tube at the upper part of each testis; serves as temporary storage area for the sperm.

  word root: *epididymo*

3. Prostate: secretes a fluid that is part of the semen and aids in sperm motility.

  word root: *prostato*

4. Penis: male sex organ that transports sperm into the female vagina.

  word root: *balano*

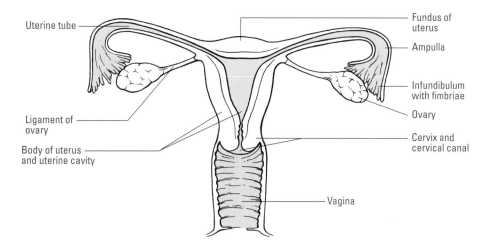

Uterine tube

Fundus of uterus

Ampulla

Infundibulum with fimbriae

Ovary

Ligament of ovary

Body of uterus and uterine cavity

Cervix and cervical canal

Vagina

CHECKPOINT EXERCISE 12-21

What do these words mean?

1. orchiopexy _____

2. oocyte _____

3. salpingoophorectomy _____

4. hysterolith _____

5. endometrium _____

6. vaginitis _____

7. salpingorrhaphy _____

8. prostatectomy _____

9. epididymitis _____

10. balanic _____

4. Lactation: the period of suckling a child.

   word root: *lact, lactat, galac*: milk

   lactation: *lactat*/milk, *ion*/act of

5. Mammary: pertaining to the breast.

   word root: *mammo, masto*: breast

   mammary: *mamm*/breat, *ary*/relating to

6. Primipara: a woman who has given birth to her first child.

   word root: *par, part*: birth

   primipara: *primi*/first, *para*/birth

7. Laparoscopy: abdominal exploration using instruments.

   word root: *laparo*: abdomen

   laparoscopy: *laparo*/abdomen, *scopy*/examine with a scope

Other Terms

1. Amenorrhea: absence or suppression of menstrual flow.

   amenorrhea: *a*/without, *meno*/month, *rhea*/flow

2. Menses: menstrual flow.

3. Ectopic pregnancy: implantation of the fertilized egg cell outside of the uterus.

REVIEW: REPRODUCTIVE SYSTEM

1. Provide the word root for each of these:

    a. vagina _____

    b. uterus _____

    c. ovary _____

    d. prostate _____

    e. testicle _____

    f. fallopian tube _____

    g. egg _____

    h. penis _____

2. Write a word that means:

    a. menstrual flow _____

    b. painful monthly flow _____

    c. inflammation of the breast _____

    d. pregnancy out of place _____

    e. woman who has borne more than one child

    _____

3. What do these words mean?

    a. endometriosis _____

    b. oocyte _____

    c. colpocystotomy _____

    d. prostatectomy _____

    e. vaginocele _____

    f. hysterolith _____

    g. balanoplasty _____

    h. epididymitis _____

    i. hysterocervicotomy _____

    j. laparotomy _____

    k. galactorrhea _____

    l. orchitis _____

    m. mastitis _____

THE SENSES

The "senses" collectively are the faculty by which the nerves and brain respond to physical stimuli. The senses are made up of millions of microscopic-sized sense organs called receptors. These receptors are found in almost every part of the body. This section will review word parts for anatomic and physiologic structures related to sight (eye), hearing (ear), smell (nose), taste (tongue), and touch (skin).

The sense organs can be classified within other major body systems. Skin is a major component of the integumentary system; skin also serves to protect the body and help with temperature and water regulation. The eye and ear are often classified as a part of the nervous system because of the reception of stimuli (light and sound, respectively), while the tongue is classified as part of the gastrointestinal system.

Sight

Sight is provided by specialized receptors located in the eye.

    word root: *op*: vision; *opsy*: to view; *ophthalmo*, *oculo*: eye

Parts of the eye include the following:

1. Conjunctiva: mucous membrane lining the eye.

    word root: *conjunctivo*

2. Eyelid: protective covering over the eye.

    word root: *blepharo*

3. Cornea: clear part of sclera.

    word root: *corne*

4. Tear system (ducts/glands): secretes lubricating fluid.

    word root: *lacrimo*

5. Retina: innermost part of eye, where specialized receptors for sight are located.

    word root: *retino*

Hearing

Hearing is provided by specialized receptors located in the ear.

    word root: *acou, acu*: hear; *oto, aur*: ear

Other word roots pertaining to the ear are as follows:

    tympano, myringo: ear drum

    audio: sound

    phono: voice

    phaso: speech

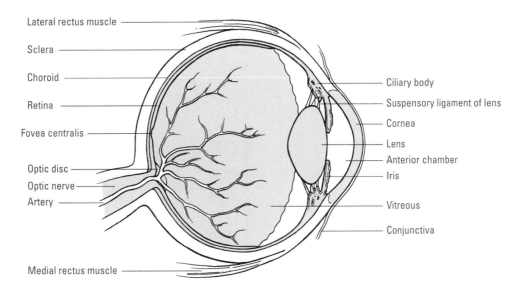

Transverse (horizontal) section of eyeball

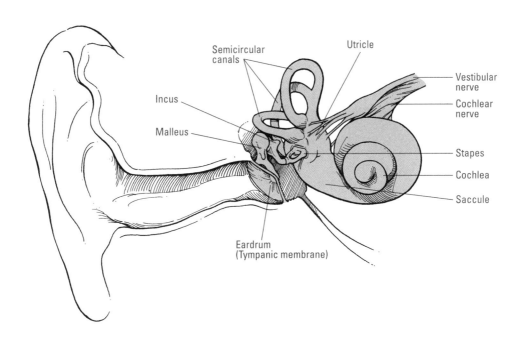

Smell

Smell is provided by specialized receptors located in the nose.

> word root: *olfacto*, *osmo*: smell; *rhino*, *naso*: nose

Taste

Taste is provided by specialized receptors located on the tongue.

> word root: *gusto*, *gustato*: act of tasting; *gloss*: tongue

Touch

Touch is provided by specialized receptors located on the surface of the skin.

> word root: *esthes*: feeling/sensation; *cutaneo*, *dermo*, *dermato*: skin; *onycho*: nail

CHECKPOINT EXERCISE 12-22

What do these words mean?

1. gustation _____

2. autopsy _____

3. ophthalmology _____

4. retinopathy _____

5. lacrimal _____

6. tympanoplasty _____

7. olfactometer _____

8. conjunctivitis _____

9. onychomycosis _____

Other Terms

1. Amblyopia: reduced or dull vision.

   amblyopia: *ambly*/dull, *opia*/vision condition

2. Diplopia: double vision.

   diplopia: *dipl*/double, *opia*/vision condition

3. Photophobia: hypersensitivity to light.

   word root: *photo*: light

   photophobia: *photo*/light, *phob*/fear, *ia*/condition of

4. Epistaxis: nosebleed.

5. Pruritus: itching.

6. Cataract: opacity of the lens of the eye.

7. Urticaria: hives.

8. Cerumen: earwax.

9. Ulcer: break in mucous membrane or skin.

REVIEW: THE SENSES

1. Provide the word root for each of these:

   a. ear _____

   b. eye _____

   c. eyelid _____

   d. sound _____

   e. voice _____

   f. smell _____

   g. taste _____

   h. skin _____

   i. nail _____

   j. feeling or sensation _____

2. Write a word that means:

   a. double vision _____

   b. itching _____

   c. a break in the skin _____

   d. hives _____

   e. earwax _____

   f. opacity of the lens of the eye

   _____

3. What do these words mean?

   a. retinopathy _____

   b. dermatitis _____

   c. otopyosis _____

   d. tympanitis _____

   e. oculist _____

   f. olfactometer _____

   g. otitis media _____

   h. audiometry _____

   i. aphonia _____

Test Your Knowledge

Choose the appropriate letter. Use your medical dictionary.

1. The foundation of a word is the _____.

   a. combining vowel

   b. combining form

   c. word root

   d. prefix

2. The term *proximal* means _____.

   a. nearest the point of attachment

   b. away from the point of attachment

   c. opposite the point of attachment

   d. distal to the point of attachment

3. The medical term for pain in the arm is _____.

   a. brachialis

   b. bradykinesia

   c. brachium

   d. brachialgia

4. The word root *labi* means _____.

   a. mouth

   b. teeth

   c. lip

   d. cheek

5. The inner lining of the heart is the _____.

   a. myocardium

   b. pericardium

   c. septum

   d. endocardium

6. *Appendectomy* means _____.

   a. surgical excision of the appendix

   b. surgical repair of a hernia

   c. surgical excision of the gallbladder

   d. surgical incision into the abdomen

7. The suffix _____ means "the study of."

   a. -logist

   b. -logy

   c. -logo

   d. -logos

(continued)

Test Your Knowledge *(continued)*

8. The _____ plane divides the body into superior and inferior portions.

   a. transverse

   b. frontal

   c. midsagittal

   d. coronal

9. The _____ system consists of the skin and its appendages.

   a. intergumentary

   b. integumentary

   c. cutaneous

   d. subcutaneous

10. The absence of pigment in the skin, hair, and eyes is called _____.

   a. albinism

   b. anhidrosis

   c. acanthosis

   d. alopecia

11. Ankylosis means _____.

   a. a condition of hardening of a joint

   b. a condition of stiffening of a joint

   c. swelling of a joint

   d. any joint disease

12. The word root *chondr* means _____.

   a. cartilage

   b. cancer

   c. clavicle

   d. glue

13. The medical term for fainting is _____.

   a. sciatica

   b. syncope

   c. narcolepsy

   d. palsy

14. The anterior transparent portion of the eyeball is called the _____.

   a. sclera

   b. iris

   c. retina

   d. cornea

(continued)

Test Your Knowledge *(continued)*

15. The combining form *rhino* means _____.

  a. throat

  b. ear

  c. nose

  d. cheek

16. The surgical repair of a fascia is _____.

  a. fascioplasty

  b. faciodesis

  c. fascitis

  d. fasciectomy

17. A condition in which there is an abnormal darkening of muscle tissue is _____.

  a. myoparesis

  b. myorraphy

  c. myorrhexis

  d. myomelanosis

18. The prefix *apo-* means _____.

  a. lack of

  b. away from

  c. separation

  d. toward

19. The term _____ means "lack of appetite."

  a. anorexia

  b. bulimia

  c. emesis

  d. ascites

20. A condition in which the colon is extremely enlarged is _____.

  a. diverticulitis

  b. enteritis

  c. megacolon

  d. microcolon

References

1. *Taber's Cyclopedic Medical Dictionary.* 19th ed. Philadelphia, PA: FA Davis Co; 1999.

2. Rudler-Barnett CS, Suckley LM. *The Last Word in Medical Terminology: A Programmed Text-Workbook.* Boston, MA: Little, Brown, & Co; 1985.

Resources

Ehrlich A. *Medical Terminology for Health Professions.* 4th ed. Albany, NY: Delmar Publishers, Inc; 2006.

Mosby's Medical, Nursing, & Allied Health Dictionary. 5th ed. St Louis, MO: Mosby-Year Book, Inc; 2005.

Rudler-Barnett CS, Suckley LM. *The Last Word in Medical Terminology: A Programmed Text-Workbook.* Boston, MA: Little, Brown, & Co; 1985.

Rice, Jane. *Medical Terminology With Human Anatomy.* Stamford, CT: Appleton and Lange; 2006.

Taber's Cyclopedic Medical Dictionary. 19th ed. Philadelphia, PA: FA Davis Co; 1999.

Glossary

Accident codes—Identify accidental ingestion of drugs for incorrect use in medical or surgical procedures, incorrect administration for ingestion of the drug, or inadvertent or accidental overdose.

Additional Characters Required—A symbol (–) in ICD-10-CM that requires additional characters to be coded to the highest level of specificity.

Adverse effect—A pathologic reaction following the ingestion or exposure to drugs or chemical substance that may result from a cumulative effect of a drug or substance.

AHIMA, American Health Information Management Association—National organization promoting the art and science of medical record management and improving the quality of comprehensive health information and certification.

Alphabetic Index—The alphabetic index of diseases and disorders in the ICD-10-CM.

American Medical Association—The largest US professional association of physicians. Publisher of *Physician's Current Procedural Terminology*®, Fourth Edition (CPT-4).

Brace [ ]—Used in ICD-10-CM to enclose a series of terms, each of which is modified by the statement to the right of the brace.

Carrier—The insurance company or insurer.

Centers for Medicare & Medicaid Services (formerly the Health Care Financing Administration, HCFA)—A governmental department that is part of the Department of Health and Human Services that oversees Medicare and Medicaid.

Certification—Credential issued by a board or association verifying that a person meets a professional standard.

Certified Coding Specialist (CCS)—Inpatient coding certification received after appropriate training and passing a certification examination administered by the American Health Information Management Association.

Certified Coding Specialist-Physician (CCS-P)—Physician-based outpatient coding certification

received after appropriate training and passing a certification examination administered by the American Health Information Management Association.

CMS 1500 claim form—The standard paper insurance claim form used to report outpatient services to insurance carriers.

Coder—A professional who translates documentation, written diagnostics, and procedures into numeric and alphanumeric codes.

Code First Underlying Disease—The note that requires that the underlying disease (etiology) be recorded first and the particular manifestation be recorded second. This note will appear only in the Tabular List.

Coding—Transferring a narrative description of diseases, injuries, and procedures into a numeric designation.

Combination code—Single ICD-10-CM code used to identify etiology and secondary process (manifestation) or complication of a disease.

Comorbidity—An ongoing condition that exists along with the conditions for which the patient is receiving treatment.

Complication—Disease or condition arising during the course of, or as a result of, another disease-modifying medical treatment or outcome.

Conventions—In the diagnostic coding system of the ICD-10-CM, codes are broken down into a 3-character code category or block. Most of these 3-character codes are broken down into 4 to 7 character categories based on the descriptive terms needed to complete the diagnosis and achieve the highest degree of description for coding. It should be noted, however, that not every code will require up to 7 characters to be coded at its highest level of coding. There are a few codes that are at the highest level possible with only the 3-character code.

Current Procedural Terminology® **(CPT 4)**—A medical procedural coding system maintained and published by the American Medical Association (AMA).

Default code—A code listed next to a main term in the ICD-10-CM Index. The default code represents the condition that is most commonly associated with the main term or is the unspecified code for the condition. If a condition is documented in a medical record (eg, appendicitis) without any additional information, such as acute or chronic, the default code should be assigned.

Diagnosis code—The statistical code number assigned by the World Health Organization for a specific diagnosis. This number appears in the *International Classification of Disease*, 10th Revision (ICD-10-CM), distributed by the US Government Printing Office.

Documentation—Chronological detailed recording of pertinent facts and observations about a patient's health recorded in the medical chart and associated reports.

Dummy placeholder—The x used in ICD-10-CM coding as a fifth-character placeholder within certain 6-character codes to allow for future expansion.

External cause codes—ICD-10-CM codes for external causes of injury, poisoning, or other adverse reactions that explain how the injury occurred.

Eponym—Disease or syndrome named after a person.

Encounter form—Routing slip or charge ticket used by a medical practice to record procedures and/or diagnoses for billing purposes.

Modifiers—Subterms that are listed below the main term in alphabetical order and indented two spaces in ICD-10-CM coding.

Etiology—The cause of disease.

Excludes 1—Terms following this word that are to be coded elsewhere are indicated in the notes. This instruction indicates that the code excluded should never be used at the same time as the code above the *Excludes 1* note. An *Excludes 1* is used when two conditions cannot occur together, such as a congenital form versus an acquired form of the same condition. Conditions listed with *Excludes 1* are mutually exclusive.

Excludes 2—Conditions listed with *Excludes 2* are not considered inclusive to a code but may be coexistent. If both conditions are present, both diagnosis codes should be reported.

HCPCS—The Healthcare Common Procedural Coding System used to report outpatient health care services provided to Medicare beneficiaries and other third-party payers.

Department of Health and Human Services (HHS)—A governmental department that develops a system of physician reimbursement and oversees the government programs.

Health insurance—A generic term that applies to all types of insurance indemnifying or reimbursing for medical care costs and lost income arising from illness or injury.

ICD-10-CM codes—The *International Classification of Diseases, 10th Revision, Clinical Modification* (ICD-10-CM), which is a system for classifying diseases and facilitating collection of uniform and comparable health information.

Inpatient—A patient who is admitted to the hospital for a period of time.

Insured—Individual or organization protected by insurance in case of loss under the specific terms of the insurance policy.

Late effect—Inactive residual effect or condition produced after the acute phase of an injury or illness has ended.

Medical necessity—Specific diagnostic requirements for a specific service to indicate medical need.

Not elsewhere classified (NEC)—Terminology used in ICD-10-CM diagnostic coding when the code lacks specific information to code the encounter to a more specific category.

Not otherwise specified (NOS)—Terminology used in ICD-10-CM diagnostic coding when the diagnosis is not specified in the encounter.

Notes—Used to define terms, clarify information, or list choices for additional digits in ICD-10-CM.

Outpatient—A person who encounters health services in a physician's office, hospital clinic, long-term care unit, or the office of other providers of health care services.

Parentheses ( )—Used in ICD-10-CM to enclose supplementary words that may be present or absent in the statement of a disease or procedure without affecting the code number to which it is assigned.

Poisoning—An adverse medical state caused by an overdose of medication, the prescription and use of a medicinal substance prescribed in error, or a drug mistakenly ingested or applied.

Principal/first listed diagnosis—The condition considered to be the major health problem for the patient, always listed and coded first on the claim form.

Provider—A physician or other supplier of medical services or equipment.

See—Directs you to a more specific term in ICD-10-CM under which the correct code can be found.

See Also—Indicates additional information is available in ICD-10-CM that may provide an additional diagnostic code.

See Category—Indicates that you should review the category specified before assigning a code in ICD-10-CM.

Tabular List—The numerical listing of diseases found in ICD-10-CM.

Use Additional Code—A note that appears in categories where you must add further information (by using an additional code) to give a more complete picture of the diagnosis or procedure in ICD-10-CM.

Unspecified nature—A description for a neoplasm when the histology or nature of the tumor has not yet been determined.

ICD-10-CM—The tabular list of diseases in the International Classification of Diseases coding system listed in numerical order by chapter. The alphabetic index lists diseases and etiology.

Z codes—A classification of codes in ICD-10-CM to identify health care encounters for reasons other than illness or injury and to identify patients whose injury or illness is influenced by special circumstances or problems.

Valuable Web Sites and Resource Materials

General Medical

http://www.ncbi.nlm.nih.gov/	Us National Library of Medicine
http://www.webmd.com/	Web MD
http://www.AcronymFinder.com/	Acronym Finder:

Note: (Useful for referencing definitions of acronyms)

http://www.vh.org/	Virtual Hospital

digital library of health information

http://www.adam.com	Health Information Media Products

(Useful for gaining reference materials)

http://www.mtdesk.com	MT Desk

Web site for medical transcriptionists (Useful for referencing medical terminology and reviewing sample chart notes)

WEDI (Workforece for Electronic Data Enterchange) www.wedi.org

Information on ICD-10

Government

http://www.ahcpr.gov	Agency for Healthcare Research and Quality
http://www.access.gpo.gov/cfr	Code of Federal Regulations:

http://www.cms.hhs.gov/ICD-10	Centers for Medicare and Medicaid Services (CMS)-ICD-10 information
http://www.ncvhs.hhs.gov/	National Committee on Vital and Health Statistics
http://www.fda.gov	US Food and Drug Administration
http://www.gpoaccess.gov/cfr/index.html	Federal Register
www.fedworld.gov	Fedworld Information Network/US Department of Commerce
www.access.gpo.gov	US Government Printing Office
www.healthfinder.gov	National Health Information Center/US Department of Health & Human Services
www.jointcommission.org/	Joint Commission on Accreditation of Healthcare Organizations
www.cdc.gov	Centers for Disease Control and Prevention/US Department of Health and Human Services
www.ncqa.org	The National Committee for Quality Assurance
www.oig.hhs.gov/	Office of Inspector General (OIG)
www.ssa.gov	Social Security Online—US Social Security Administration

www.hhs.gov/ocr/hipaa/finalreg.html	Office for Civil Rights—HIPAA/Medical Privacy—National Standards to Protect the Privacy of Personal Health Information

Health Management, Coding, and Training Resources

www.integsoft.com/appeals	Appeal Solutions/Medical Claims Resolution Services (Useful reference: the Appeal Letter, which assists medical providers in appealing denied insurance claims)
www.nlm.nih.gov/	US National Library of Medicine/National Institutes of Health

Professional Organizations and Societies

www.ache.org	American College of Healthcare Executives
www.aclm.org	American College of Legal Medicine
www.acs.org	American College of Surgeons
www.ahima.org	American Health Information Management Association
www.aha.org	American Hospital Association
www.ama-assn.org	American Medical Association
www.hcca-info.org	Health Care Compliance Association
www.hfma.org	Healthcare Financial Management Association
www.physicianswebsites.com	Medical Association of Billers
www.mgma.com	Medical Group Management Association
www.who.org/	World Health Organization
www.ama-assn.org	American Medical Association

Medicolegal

www.nhcaa.org/	National Healthcare Antifraud Association
www.healthlawyers.org	American Health Lawyers Association
www.internets.com/mednets/smedgovt.htm	MedNets Government Searchable Databases
www.mediregs.com/index.html	MediRegs (search engine for managing health care compliance information)

Resource Materials

Centers for Medicare and Medicaid Services; www.cms.hhs.org/ ICD-10

Coding Clinic; American Hospital Association; www.aha.org/

ICD-10-CM Official Guidelines for Coding and Reporting

ICD-10-CM Official Guidelines for Coding and Reporting
2011
Narrative changes appear in bold text
Items <u>underlined</u> have been moved within the guidelines since the 2010 version
Italics are used to indicate revisions to heading changes

The Centers for Medicare and Medicaid Services (CMS) and the National Center for Health Statistics (NCHS), two departments within the U.S. Federal Government's Department of Health and Human Services (DHHS) provide the following guidelines for coding and reporting using the International Classification of Diseases, 10th Revision, Clinical Modification (ICD-10-CM). These guidelines should be used as a companion document to the official version of the ICD-10-CM as published on the NCHS website. The ICD-10-CM is a morbidity classification published by the United States for classifying diagnoses and reason for visits in all health care settings. The ICD-10-CM is based on the ICD-10, the statistical classification of disease published by the World Health Organization (WHO).

These guidelines have been approved by the four organizations that make up the Cooperating Parties for the ICD-10-CM: the American Hospital Association (AHA), the American Health Information Management Association (AHIMA), CMS, and NCHS.

These guidelines are a set of rules that have been developed to accompany and complement the official conventions and instructions provided within the ICD-10-CM itself. The instructions and conventions of the classification take precedence over guidelines. These guidelines are based on the coding and sequencing instructions in **the Tabular List and Alphabetic Index** of ICD-10-CM, but provide additional instruction. Adherence to these guidelines when assigning ICD-10-CM diagnosis codes is required under the Health Insurance Portability and Accountability Act (HIPAA). The diagnosis codes (**Tabular List and Alphabetic Index**) have been adopted under HIPAA for all healthcare settings. A joint effort between the healthcare provider and the coder is essential to achieve complete and accurate documentation, code assignment, and reporting of diagnoses and procedures. These guidelines have been developed to assist both the healthcare provider and the coder in identifying those diagnoses and procedures that are to be reported. The importance of consistent, complete documentation in the medical record cannot be overemphasized. Without such documentation accurate coding cannot be achieved. The entire record should be reviewed to determine the specific reason for the encounter and the conditions treated.

The term encounter is used for all settings, including hospital admissions. In the context of these guidelines, the term provider is used throughout the guidelines to mean physician or any qualified health care practitioner who is legally accountable for establishing the patient's diagnosis. Only this set of guidelines, approved by the Cooperating Parties, is official.

The guidelines are organized into sections. Section I includes the structure and conventions of the classification and general guidelines that apply to the entire classification, and chapter-specific guidelines that correspond to the chapters as they are arranged in the classification. Section II includes guidelines for selection of principal diagnosis for non-outpatient settings. Section III includes guidelines for reporting additional diagnoses in non-outpatient settings. Section IV is for outpatient coding and reporting. It is necessary to review all sections of the guidelines to fully understand all of the rules and instructions needed to code properly.

Section I. Conventions, general coding guidelines and chapter specific guidelines

The conventions, general guidelines and chapter-specific guidelines are applicable to all health care settings unless otherwise indicated. The conventions and instructions of the classification take precedence over guidelines.

A. Conventions for the ICD-10-CM

The conventions for the ICD-10-CM are the general rules for use of the classification independent of the guidelines. These conventions are incorporated within the **Alphabetic Index** and **Tabular List** of the ICD-10-CM as instructional notes.

1. The Alphabetic Index and Tabular List

The ICD-10-CM is divided into the **Alphabetic Index**, an alphabetical list of terms and their corresponding code, and the Tabular List, a chronological list of codes divided into chapters based on body system or condition. **The Alphabetic Index consists of the following parts: the Index of Diseases and Injury, the Index of External Causes of Injury, the Table of Neoplasms and the Table of Drugs and Chemicals.**

See Section I.C2. General guidelines
See Section I.C.19. Adverse effects, poisoning, underdosing and toxic effects

2. Format and Structure:

The ICD-10-CM Tabular List contains categories, subcategories and codes. Characters for categories, subcategories and codes may be either a letter or a number. All categories are 3 characters. A three-character category that has no further subdivision is equivalent to a code. Subcategories are either 4 or 5 characters. Codes may be **3,** 4, 5, 6 or 7 characters. That is, each level of subdivision after a category is a subcategory. The final level of subdivision is a code. Codes that have applicable 7th characters are still referred to as codes, not subcategories. A code that has an applicable 7th character is considered invalid without the 7th character.

The ICD-10-CM uses an indented format for ease in reference.

3. Use of codes for reporting purposes

For reporting purposes only codes are permissible, not categories or subcategories, and any applicable 7th character is required.

4. Placeholder character

The ICD-10-CM utilizes a placeholder character "X". The "X" is used as a placeholder at certain codes to allow for future expansion. An example of this is at the poisoning, adverse effect and underdosing codes, categories T36-T50.

Where a placeholder exists, the X must be used in order for the code to be considered a valid code.

5. **7th Characters**

Certain ICD-10-CM categories have applicable 7th characters. The applicable 7th character is required for all codes within the category, or as the notes in the Tabular List instruct. The 7th character must always be the 7th character in the data field. If a code that requires a 7th character is not 6 characters, a placeholder X must be used to fill in the empty characters.

6. **Abbreviations**

    a.   *Alphabetic* **Index abbreviations**

        NEC   "Not elsewhere classifiable"
                This abbreviation in the **Alphabetic Index** represents "other specified". When a specific code is not available for a condition, the **Alphabetic Index** directs the coder to the "other specified" code in the **Tabular List**.

        NOS   **"Not otherwise specified"**
                This abbreviation is the equivalent of unspecified.

    b.   *Tabular List* **abbreviations**

        NEC   "Not elsewhere classifiable"
                This abbreviation in the **Tabular List** represents "other specified". When a specific code is not available for a condition the **Tabular List** includes an NEC entry under a code to identify the code as the "other specified" code.

        NOS   "Not otherwise specified"
                This abbreviation is the equivalent of unspecified.

7. **Punctuation**

    [ ]   Brackets are used in the **Tabular List** to enclose synonyms, alternative wording or explanatory phrases. Brackets are used in the **Alphabetic Index** to identify manifestation codes.

    ( )   Parentheses are used in both the **Alphabetic Index** and **Tabular List** to enclose supplementary words that may be present or absent in the statement of a disease or procedure without affecting the code number to which it is assigned. The terms within the parentheses are referred to as nonessential modifiers.

    :   Colons are used in the Tabular List after an incomplete term which needs one or more of the modifiers following the colon to make it assignable to a given category.

8. **Use of "and"**

When the term "and" is used in a narrative statement it represents and/or.

9. **Other and Unspecified codes**

a. **"Other" codes**

Codes titled "other" or "other specified" are for use when the information in the medical record provides detail for which a specific code does not exist. **Alphabetic Index** entries with NEC in the line designate "other" codes in the **Tabular List**. These **Alphabetic Index** entries represent specific disease entities for which no specific code exists so the term is included within an "other" code.

b. **"Unspecified" codes**

Codes titled "unspecified" are for use when the information in the medical record is insufficient to assign a more specific code. For those categories for which an unspecified code is not provided, the "other specified" code may represent both other and unspecified.

10. **Includes Notes**

This note appears immediately under a three **character** code title to further define, or give examples of, the content of the category.

11. **Inclusion terms**

List of terms is included under some codes. These terms are the conditions for which that code is to be used. The terms may be synonyms of the code title, or, in the case of "other specified" codes, the terms are a list of the various conditions assigned to that code. The inclusion terms are not necessarily exhaustive. Additional terms found only in the **Alphabetic Index** may also be assigned to a code.

12. **Excludes Notes**

The ICD-10-CM has two types of excludes notes. Each type of note has a different definition for use but they are all similar in that they indicate that codes excluded from each other are independent of each other.

a. **Excludes1**

A type 1 Excludes note is a pure excludes note. It means "NOT CODED HERE!" An Excludes1 note indicates that the code excluded should never be used at the same time as the code above the Excludes1 note. An Excludes1 is used when two conditions cannot occur together, such as a congenital form versus an acquired form of the same condition.

b. Excludes2

A type 2 excludes note represents "Not included here". An excludes2 note indicates that the condition excluded is not part of the condition represented by the code, but a patient may have both conditions at the same time. When an Excludes2 note appears under a code, it is acceptable to use both the code and the excluded code together, when appropriate.

13. Etiology/manifestation convention ("code first", "use additional code" and "in diseases classified elsewhere" notes)

Certain conditions have both an underlying etiology and multiple body system manifestations due to the underlying etiology. For such conditions, the ICD-10-CM has a coding convention that requires the underlying condition be sequenced first followed by the manifestation. Wherever such a combination exists, there is a "use additional code" note at the etiology code, and a "code first" note at the manifestation code. These instructional notes indicate the proper sequencing order of the codes, etiology followed by manifestation.

In most cases the manifestation codes will have in the code title, "in diseases classified elsewhere." Codes with this title are a component of the etiology/ manifestation convention. The code title indicates that it is a manifestation code. "In diseases classified elsewhere" codes are never permitted to be used as **first-listed** or principal diagnosis codes. They must be used in conjunction with an underlying condition code and they must be listed following the underlying condition. See category F02, Dementia in other diseases classified elsewhere, for an example of this convention.

There are manifestation codes that do not have "in diseases classified elsewhere" in the title. For such codes a "use additional code" note will still be present and the rules for sequencing apply.

In addition to the notes in the **Tabular List**, these conditions also have a specific **Alphabetic Index** entry structure. In the **Alphabetic Index** both conditions are listed together with the etiology code first followed by the manifestation codes in brackets. The code in brackets is always to be sequenced second.

An example of the etiology/manifestation convention is dementia in Parkinson's disease. In the **Alphabetic Index**, code G20 is listed first, followed by code F02.80 or F02.81 in brackets. Code G20 represents the underlying etiology, Parkinson's disease, and must be sequenced first, whereas codes F02.80 and F02.81 represent the manifestation of dementia in diseases classified elsewhere, with or without behavioral disturbance.

"Code first" and "Use additional code" notes are also used as sequencing rules in the classification for certain codes that are not part of an etiology/manifestation combination.

See Section I.B.7. Multiple coding for a single condition.

14. "And"

The word "and" should be interpreted to mean either "and" or "or" when it appears in a title.

15. "With"

The word "with" should be interpreted to mean "associated with" or "due to" when it appears in a code title, the Alphabetic Index, or an instructional note in the Tabular List.

The word "with" in the Alphabetic Index is sequenced immediately following the main term, not in alphabetical order.

16. "See" and "See Also"

The "see" instruction following a main term in the **Alphabetic Index** indicates that another term should be referenced. It is necessary to go to the main term referenced with the "see" note to locate the correct code.

A "see also" instruction following a main term in the **Alphabetic Index** instructs that there is another main term that may also be referenced that may provide additional **Alphabetic Index** entries that may be useful. It is not necessary to follow the "see also" note when the original main term provides the necessary code.

17. "Code also note"

A "code also" note instructs that two codes may be required to fully describe a condition, but this note does not provide sequencing direction.

18. Default codes

A code listed next to a main term in the ICD-10-CM **Alphabetic Index** is referred to as a default code. The default code represents that condition that is most commonly associated with the main term, or is the unspecified code for the condition. If a condition is documented in a medical record (for example, appendicitis) without any additional information, such as acute or chronic, the default code should be assigned.

19. Syndromes

Follow the Alphabetic Index guidance when coding syndromes. In the absence of **Alphabetic Index** guidance, assign codes for the documented manifestations of the syndrome.

B. General Coding Guidelines

1. Locating a code in the ICD-10-CM

To select a code in the classification that corresponds to a diagnosis or reason for visit documented in a medical record, first locate the term in the **Alphabetic Index**, and then verify the code in the Tabular List. Read and be guided by instructional notations that appear in both the **Alphabetic Index** and the Tabular List.

It is essential to use both the **Alphabetic Index** and Tabular List when locating and assigning a code. The **Alphabetic Index** does not always provide the full code. Selection of the full code, including laterality and any applicable 7th character can only be done in the **Tabular List**. A dash (-) at the end of an **Alphabetic Index** entry indicates that additional characters are required. Even if a dash is not included at the **Alphabetic Index** entry, it is necessary to refer to the **Tabular List** to verify that no 7th character is required.

2. Level of Detail in Coding

Diagnosis codes are to be used and reported at their highest number of **characters** available.

ICD-10-CM diagnosis codes are composed of codes with 3, 4, 5, 6 or 7 **characters**. Codes with three **characters** are included in ICD-10-CM as the heading of a category of codes that may be further subdivided by the use of fourth and/or fifth **characters and/or sixth characters**, which provide greater detail.

A three-**character** code is to be used only if it is not further subdivided. A code is invalid if it has not been coded to the full number of characters required for that code, including the 7th character, if applicable.

3. Code or codes from A00.0 through T88.9, Z00-Z99.8

The appropriate code or codes from A00.0 through T88.9, Z00-Z99.8 must be used to identify diagnoses, symptoms, conditions, problems, complaints or other reason(s) for the encounter/visit.

4. Signs and symptoms

Codes that describe symptoms and signs, as opposed to diagnoses, are acceptable for reporting purposes when a related definitive diagnosis has not been established (confirmed) by the provider. Chapter 18 of ICD-10-CM, Symptoms, Signs, and Abnormal Clinical and Laboratory Findings, Not Elsewhere Classified (codes R00.0 - R99) contains many, but not all codes for symptoms.

5. Conditions that are an integral part of a disease process

Signs and symptoms that are associated routinely with a disease process should not be assigned as additional codes, unless otherwise instructed by the classification.

6. Conditions that are not an integral part of a disease process

Additional signs and symptoms that may not be associated routinely with a disease process should be coded when present.

7. Multiple coding for a single condition

In addition to the etiology/manifestation convention that requires two codes to fully describe a single condition that affects multiple body systems, there are other single conditions that also require more than one code. "Use additional code" notes are found in the **Tabular List** at codes that are not part of an etiology/manifestation pair where a secondary code is useful to fully describe a condition. The sequencing rule is the same as the etiology/manifestation pair, "use additional code" indicates that a secondary code should be added.

For example, for bacterial infections that are not included in chapter 1, a secondary code from category B95, Streptococcus, Staphylococcus, and Enterococcus, as the cause of diseases classified elsewhere, or B96, Other bacterial agents as the cause of diseases classified elsewhere, may be required to identify the bacterial organism causing the infection. A "use additional code" note will normally be found at the infectious disease code, indicating a need for the organism code to be added as a secondary code.

"Code first" notes are also under certain codes that are not specifically manifestation codes but may be due to an underlying cause. When there is a "code first" note and an underlying condition is present, the underlying condition should be sequenced first.

"Code, if applicable, any causal condition first", notes indicate that this code may be assigned as a principal diagnosis when the causal condition is unknown or not applicable. If a causal condition is known, then the code for that condition should be sequenced as the principal or first-listed diagnosis.

Multiple codes may be needed for late effects, complication codes and obstetric codes to more fully describe a condition. See the specific guidelines for these conditions for further instruction.

8. Acute and Chronic Conditions

If the same condition is described as both acute (subacute) and chronic, and separate subentries exist in the Alphabetic Index at the same indentation level, code both and sequence the acute (subacute) code first.

9. **Combination Code**

A combination code is a single code used to classify:
Two diagnoses, or
A diagnosis with an associated secondary process (manifestation)
A diagnosis with an associated complication

Combination codes are identified by referring to subterm entries in the Alphabetic Index and by reading the inclusion and exclusion notes in the Tabular List.

Assign only the combination code when that code fully identifies the diagnostic conditions involved or when the Alphabetic Index so directs. Multiple coding should not be used when the classification provides a combination code that clearly identifies all of the elements documented in the diagnosis. When the combination code lacks necessary specificity in describing the manifestation or complication, an additional code should be used as a secondary code.

10. **Late Effects (Sequela)**

A late effect is the residual effect (condition produced) after the acute phase of an illness or injury has terminated. There is no time limit on when a late effect code can be used. The residual may be apparent early, such as in cerebral infarction, or it may occur months or years later, such as that due to a previous injury. Coding of late effects generally requires two codes sequenced in the following order: The condition or nature of the late effect is sequenced first. The late effect code is sequenced second.

An exception to the above guidelines are those instances where the code for late effect is followed by a manifestation code identified in the Tabular List and title, or the late effect code has been expanded (at the fourth, fifth or sixth character levels) to include the manifestation(s). The code for the acute phase of an illness or injury that led to the late effect is never used with a code for the late effect.

See Section I.C.9. Sequelae of cerebrovascular disease
See Section I.C.15. Sequelae of complication of pregnancy, childbirth and the puerperium
See Section I.C.19. Code extensions

11. **Impending or Threatened Condition**

Code any condition described at the time of discharge as "impending" or "threatened" as follows:
    If it did occur, code as confirmed diagnosis.
    If it did not occur, reference the Alphabetic Index to determine if the condition has a subentry term for "impending" or "threatened" and also reference main term entries for "Impending" and for "Threatened."

If the subterms are listed, assign the given code.
If the subterms are not listed, code the existing underlying condition(s) and not the condition described as impending or threatened.

12. Reporting Same Diagnosis Code More than Once

Each unique ICD-10-CM diagnosis code may be reported only once for an encounter. This applies to bilateral conditions when there are no distinct codes identifying laterality or two different conditions classified to the same ICD-10-CM diagnosis code.

13. Laterality

For bilateral sites, the final character of the codes in the ICD-10-CM indicates laterality. An unspecified side code is also provided should the side not be identified in the medical record. If no bilateral code is provided and the condition is bilateral, assign separate codes for both the left and right side.

14. Documentation for BMI and Pressure Ulcer Stages

For the Body Mass Index (BMI) and pressure ulcer stage codes, code assignment may be based on medical record documentation from clinicians who are not the patient's provider (i.e., physician or other qualified healthcare practitioner legally accountable for establishing the patient's diagnosis), since this information is typically documented by other clinicians involved in the care of the patient (e.g., a dietitian often documents the BMI and nurses often documents the pressure ulcer stages). However, the associated diagnosis (such as overweight, obesity, or pressure ulcer) must be documented by the patient's provider. If there is conflicting medical record documentation, either from the same clinician or different clinicians, the patient's attending provider should be queried for clarification.

The BMI codes should only be reported as secondary diagnoses. As with all other secondary diagnosis codes, the BMI codes should only be assigned when they meet the definition of a reportable additional diagnosis (see Section III, Reporting Additional Diagnoses).

C. Chapter-Specific Coding Guidelines

In addition to general coding guidelines, there are guidelines for specific diagnoses and/or conditions in the classification. Unless otherwise indicated, these guidelines apply to all health care settings. Please refer to Section II for guidelines on the selection of principal diagnosis.

1. **Chapter 1: Certain Infectious and Parasitic Diseases (A00-B99)**

   a. **Human Immunodeficiency Virus (HIV) Infections**

      1) **Code only confirmed cases**

         Code only confirmed cases of HIV infection/illness. This is an exception to the hospital inpatient guideline Section II, H.

         In this context, "confirmation" does not require documentation of positive serology or culture for HIV; the provider's diagnostic statement that the patient is HIV positive, or has an HIV-related illness is sufficient.

      2) **Selection and sequencing of HIV codes**

         (a) **Patient admitted for HIV-related condition**

             If a patient is admitted for an HIV-related condition, the principal diagnosis should be B20, followed by additional diagnosis codes for all reported HIV-related conditions.

         (b) **Patient with HIV disease admitted for unrelated condition**

             If a patient with HIV disease is admitted for an unrelated condition (such as a traumatic injury), the code for the unrelated condition (e.g., the nature of injury code) should be the principal diagnosis. Other diagnoses would be B20 followed by additional diagnosis codes for all reported HIV-related conditions.

         (c) **Whether the patient is newly diagnosed**

             Whether the patient is newly diagnosed or has had previous admissions/encounters for HIV conditions is irrelevant to the sequencing decision.

         (d) **Asymptomatic human immunodeficiency virus**

             Z21, Asymptomatic human immunodeficiency virus [HIV] infection status, is to be applied when the patient without any documentation of symptoms is listed as being "HIV positive," "known HIV," "HIV test positive," or similar terminology. Do not use this code if the term "AIDS" is used or if the patient is treated for any HIV-related illness or is described as having any condition(s) resulting from his/her HIV positive status; use B20 in these cases.

(e) **Patients with inconclusive HIV serology**

Patients with inconclusive HIV serology, but no definitive diagnosis or manifestations of the illness, may be assigned code R75, Inconclusive laboratory evidence of human immunodeficiency virus [HIV].

(f) **Previously diagnosed HIV-related illness**

Patients with any known prior diagnosis of an HIV-related illness should be coded to B20. Once a patient has developed an HIV-related illness, the patient should always be assigned code B20 on every subsequent admission/encounter. Patients previously diagnosed with any HIV illness (B20) should never be assigned to R75 or Z21, Asymptomatic human immunodeficiency virus [HIV] infection status.

(g) **HIV Infection in Pregnancy, Childbirth and the Puerperium**

During pregnancy, childbirth or the puerperium, a patient admitted (or presenting for a health care encounter) because of an HIV-related illness should receive a principal diagnosis code of O98.7-, Human immunodeficiency [HIV] disease complicating pregnancy, childbirth and the puerperium, followed by B20 and the code(s) for the HIV-related illness(es). Codes from Chapter 15 always take sequencing priority.

Patients with asymptomatic HIV infection status admitted (or presenting for a health care encounter) during pregnancy, childbirth, or the puerperium should receive codes of O98.7- and Z21.

(h) **Encounters for testing for HIV**

If a patient is being seen to determine his/her HIV status, use code Z11.4, Encounter for screening for human immunodeficiency virus [HIV]. Use additional codes for any associated high risk behavior.

If a patient with signs or symptoms is being seen for HIV testing, code the signs and symptoms. An additional counseling code Z71.7, Human **immunodeficiency** virus [HIV] counseling, may be used if counseling is provided during the encounter for the test.

When a patient returns to be informed of his/her HIV test results and the test result is negative, use code Z71.7, Human immunodeficiency virus [HIV] counseling.

If the results are positive, see previous guidelines and assign codes as appropriate.

b. Infectious agents as the cause of diseases classified to other chapters

Certain infections are classified in chapters other than Chapter 1 and no organism is identified as part of the infection code. In these instances, it is necessary to use an additional code from Chapter 1 to identify the organism. A code from category B95, Streptococcus, Staphylococcus, and Enterococcus as the cause of diseases classified to other chapters, B96, Other bacterial agents as the cause of diseases classified to other chapters, or B97, Viral agents as the cause of diseases classified to other chapters, is to be used as an additional code to identify the organism. An instructional note will be found at the infection code advising that an additional organism code is required.

c. Infections resistant to antibiotics

Many bacterial infections are resistant to current antibiotics. It is necessary to identify all infections documented as antibiotic resistant. Assign code Z16, Infection with drug resistant microorganisms, following the infection code for these cases.

d. Sepsis, Severe Sepsis, and Septic Shock

1) Coding of Sepsis and Severe Sepsis

(a) Sepsis

For a diagnosis of sepsis, assign the appropriate code for the underlying systemic infection. If the type of infection or causal organism is not further specified, assign code A41.9, Sepsis, unspecified.

A code from subcategory R65.2, Severe sepsis, should not be assigned unless severe sepsis or an associated acute organ dysfunction is documented.

(i) Negative or inconclusive blood cultures and sepsis

Negative or inconclusive blood cultures do not preclude a diagnosis of sepsis in patients with clinical evidence of the condition, however, the provider should be queried.

(ii)   Urosepsis

The term urosepsis is a nonspecific term. It is not to be considered synonymous with sepsis. It has no default code in the Alphabetic Index. Should a provider use this term, he/she must be queried for clarification.

(iii)   Sepsis with organ dysfunction

If a patient has sepsis and associated acute organ dysfunction or multiple organ dysfunction (MOD), follow the instructions for coding severe sepsis.

(iv)   Acute organ dysfunction that is not clearly associated with the sepsis

If a patient has sepsis and an acute organ dysfunction, but the medical record documentation indicates that the acute organ dysfunction is related to a medical condition other than the sepsis, do not assign a code from subcategory R65.2, Severe sepsis. An acute organ dysfunction must be associated with the sepsis in order to assign the severe sepsis code. If the documentation is not clear as to whether an acute organ dysfunction is related to the sepsis or another medical condition, query the provider.

(b)   **Severe sepsis**

The coding of severe sepsis requires a minimum of 2 codes: first a code for the underlying systemic infection, followed by a code from subcategory R65.2, Severe sepsis. If the causal organism is not documented, assign code A41.9, Sepsis, unspecified, for the infection. Additional code(s) for the associated acute organ dysfunction are also required.

Due to the complex nature of severe sepsis, some cases may require querying the provider prior to assignment of the codes.

2) **Septic shock**

Septic shock is circulatory failure associated with severe sepsis, and therefore, it represents a type of acute organ dysfunction. For all cases of septic shock, the code for the underlying systemic infection should be sequenced first, followed by code R65.21, Severe sepsis with septic shock. Any additional codes for the other acute organ dysfunctions should also be assigned.

Septic shock indicates the presence of severe sepsis. Code R65.21, Severe sepsis with septic shock, must be assigned if septic shock is documented in the medical record, even if the term severe sepsis is not documented.

3) **Sequencing of severe sepsis**

If severe sepsis is present on admission, and meets the definition of principal diagnosis, the underlying systemic infection should be assigned as principal diagnosis followed by the appropriate code from subcategory R65.2 as required by the sequencing rules in the Tabular List. A code from subcategory R65.2 can never be assigned as a principal diagnosis.

When severe sepsis develops during an encounter (it was not present on admission) the underlying systemic infection and the appropriate code from subcategory R65.2 should be assigned as secondary diagnoses.

Severe sepsis may be present on admission but the diagnosis may not be confirmed until sometime after admission. If the documentation is not clear whether severe sepsis was present on admission, the provider should be queried.

4) **Sepsis and severe sepsis with a localized infection**

If the reason for admission is both sepsis or severe sepsis and a localized infection, such as pneumonia or cellulitis, a code(s) for the underlying systemic infection should be assigned first and the code for the localized infection should be assigned as a secondary diagnosis. If the patient has severe sepsis, a code from subcategory R65.2 should also be assigned as a secondary diagnosis. If the patient is admitted with a localized infection, such as pneumonia, and sepsis/severe sepsis doesn't develop until after admission, the localized infection should be assigned first, followed by the appropriate sepsis/severe sepsis codes.

5) **Sepsis due to a postprocedural infection**

Sepsis resulting from a postprocedural infection is a complication of medical care. For such cases, the postprocedural infection code, such as, T80.2, Infections following infusion, transfusion, and therapeutic injection, T81.4, Infection following a procedure, T88.0, Infection following immunization, or O86.0, Infection of obstetric surgical wound, should be coded first, followed by the code for the specific infection. If the patient has severe sepsis the appropriate code from subcategory R65.2 should also be assigned with the additional code(s) for any acute organ dysfunction.

6) **Sepsis and severe sepsis associated with a noninfectious process (condition)**

In some cases a noninfectious process (condition), such as trauma, may lead to an infection which can result in sepsis or severe sepsis. If sepsis or severe sepsis is documented as associated with a noninfectious condition, such as a burn or serious injury, and this condition meets the definition for principal diagnosis, the code for the noninfectious condition should be sequenced first, followed by the code for the resulting infection. If severe sepsis, is present a code from subcategory R65.2 should also be assigned with any associated organ dysfunction(s) codes. It is not necessary to assign a code from subcategory R65.1, Systemic inflammatory response syndrome (SIRS) of non-infectious origin, for these cases.

If the infection meets the definition of principal diagnosis it should be sequenced before the non-infectious condition. When both the associated non-infectious condition and the infection meet the definition of principal diagnosis either may be assigned as principal diagnosis.

Only one code from category R65, Symptoms and signs specifically associated with systemic inflammation and infection, should be assigned. Therefore, when a non-infectious condition leads to an infection resulting in severe sepsis, assign the appropriate code from subcategory R65.2, Severe sepsis. Do not additionally assign a code from subcategory R65.1, Systemic inflammatory response syndrome (SIRS) of non-infectious origin.

See Section I.C.18. SIRS due to non-infectious process

7) **Sepsis and septic shock complicating abortion, pregnancy, childbirth, and the puerperium**

See Section I.C.15. Sepsis and septic shock complicating abortion, pregnancy, childbirth and the puerperium

8) **Newborn sepsis**

See Section I.C.16. Newborn sepsis

2. Chapter 2: Neoplasms (C00-D49)

General guidelines

Chapter 2 of the ICD-10-CM contains the codes for most benign and all malignant neoplasms. Certain benign neoplasms, such as prostatic adenomas, may be found in the specific body system chapters. To properly code a neoplasm it is necessary to determine from the record if the neoplasm is benign, in-situ, malignant, or of uncertain histologic behavior. If malignant, any secondary (metastatic) sites should also be determined.

The neoplasm table in the Alphabetic Index should be referenced first. However, if the histological term is documented, that term should be referenced first, rather than going immediately to the Neoplasm Table, in order to determine which column in the Neoplasm Table is appropriate. For example, if the documentation indicates "adenoma," refer to the term in the Alphabetic Index to review the entries under this term and the instructional note to "see also neoplasm, by site, benign." The table provides the proper code based on the type of neoplasm and the site. It is important to select the proper column in the table that corresponds to the type of neoplasm. The **Tabular List** should then be referenced to verify that the correct code has been selected from the table and that a more specific site code does not exist. *See Section I.C.21. Factors influencing health status and contact with health services, Status, for information regarding Z15.0, codes for genetic susceptibility to cancer.*

a. Treatment directed at the malignancy

If the treatment is directed at the malignancy, designate the malignancy as the principal diagnosis.

The only exception to this guideline is if a patient admission/encounter is solely for the administration of chemotherapy, immunotherapy or radiation therapy, assign the appropriate Z51.-- code as the first-listed or principal diagnosis, and the diagnosis or problem for which the service is being performed as a secondary diagnosis.

b. **Treatment of secondary site**

When a patient is admitted because of a primary neoplasm with metastasis and treatment is directed toward the secondary site only, the secondary neoplasm is designated as the principal diagnosis even though the primary malignancy is still present.

c. **Coding and sequencing of complications**

Coding and sequencing of complications associated with the malignancies or with the therapy thereof are subject to the following guidelines:

1) **Anemia associated with malignancy**

When admission/encounter is for management of an anemia associated with the malignancy, and the treatment is only for anemia, the appropriate code for the malignancy is sequenced as the principal or first-listed diagnosis followed by code D63.0, Anemia in neoplastic disease.

2) **Anemia associated with chemotherapy, immunotherapy and radiation therapy**

When the admission/encounter is for management of an anemia associated with an adverse effect of chemotherapy **or** immunotherapy and the only treatment is for the anemia, the appropriate adverse effect code should be sequenced first, followed by the appropriate codes for the anemia and neoplasm.

When the admission/encounter is for management of an anemia associated with an adverse effect of radiotherapy, the anemia code should be sequenced first, followed by the appropriate neoplasm code and code Y84.2, Radiological procedure and radiotherapy as the cause of abnormal reaction of the patient, or of later complication, without mention of misadventure at the time of the procedure.

3) **Management of dehydration due to the malignancy**

When the admission/encounter is for management of dehydration due to the malignancy and only the dehydration is being treated (intravenous rehydration), the dehydration is sequenced first, followed by the code(s) for the malignancy.

4) **Treatment of a complication resulting from a surgical procedure**

When the admission/encounter is for treatment of a complication resulting from a surgical procedure, designate the complication as the principal or first-listed diagnosis if treatment is directed at resolving the complication.

d. Primary malignancy previously excised

When a primary malignancy has been previously excised or eradicated from its site and there is no further treatment directed to that site and there is no evidence of any existing primary malignancy, a code from category Z85, Personal history of malignant neoplasm, should be used to indicate the former site of the malignancy. Any mention of extension, invasion, or metastasis to another site is coded as a secondary malignant neoplasm to that site. The secondary site may be the principal or first-listed with the Z85 code used as a secondary code.

e. Admissions/Encounters involving chemotherapy, immunotherapy and radiation therapy

1) Episode of care involves surgical removal of neoplasm

When an episode of care involves the surgical removal of a neoplasm, primary or secondary site, followed by adjunct chemotherapy or radiation treatment during the same episode of care, **the code for the neoplasm should be assigned as principal or first-listed diagnosis.**

2) Patient admission/encounter solely for administration of chemotherapy, immunotherapy and radiation therapy

If a patient admission/encounter is solely for the administration of chemotherapy, immunotherapy or radiation therapy assign code Z51.0, Encounter for antineoplastic radiation therapy, or Z51.11, Encounter for antineoplastic chemotherapy, or Z51.12, Encounter for antineoplastic immunotherapy as the first-listed or principal diagnosis. If a patient receives more than one of these therapies during the same admission more than one of these codes may be assigned, in any sequence.

The malignancy for which the therapy is being administered should be assigned as a secondary diagnosis.

3) Patient admitted for radiation therapy, chemotherapy or immunotherapy and develops complications

When a patient is admitted for the purpose of radiotherapy, immunotherapy or chemotherapy and develops complications such as uncontrolled nausea and vomiting or dehydration, the principal or first-listed diagnosis is Z51.0, Encounter for antineoplastic radiation therapy, or Z51.11, Encounter for antineoplastic chemotherapy, or Z51.12, Encounter for antineoplastic immunotherapy followed by any codes for the complications.

f. Admission/encounter to determine extent of malignancy

When the reason for admission/encounter is to determine the extent of the malignancy, or for a procedure such as paracentesis or thoracentesis, the primary malignancy or appropriate metastatic site is designated as the principal or first-listed diagnosis, even though chemotherapy or radiotherapy is administered.

g. Symptoms, signs, and abnormal findings listed in Chapter 18 associated with neoplasms

Symptoms, signs, and ill-defined conditions listed in Chapter 18 characteristic of, or associated with, an existing primary or secondary site malignancy cannot be used to replace the malignancy as principal or first-listed diagnosis, regardless of the number of admissions or encounters for treatment and care of the neoplasm.
See section I.C.21. Factors influencing health status and contact with health services, Encounter for prophylactic organ removal.

h. Admission/encounter for pain control/management

See Section I.C.6. for information on coding admission/encounter for pain control/management.

i. Malignancy in two or more noncontiguous sites

A patient may have more than one malignant tumor in the same organ. These tumors may represent different primaries or metastatic disease, depending on the site. Should the documentation be unclear, the provider should be queried as to the status of each tumor so that the correct codes can be assigned.

j. Disseminated malignant neoplasm, unspecified

Code C80.0, Disseminated malignant neoplasm, unspecified, is for use only in those cases where the patient has advanced metastatic disease and no known primary or secondary sites are specified. It should not be used in place of assigning codes for the primary site and all known secondary sites.

k. Malignant neoplasm without specification of site

Code C80.1, Malignant **(primary)** neoplasm, unspecified, equates to Cancer, unspecified. This code should only be used when no determination can be made as to the primary site of a malignancy. This code should rarely be used in the inpatient setting.

l. **Sequencing of neoplasm codes**

1) **Encounter for treatment of primary malignancy**

If the reason for the encounter is for treatment of a primary malignancy, assign the malignancy as the principal/**first-listed** diagnosis. The primary site is to be sequenced first, followed by any metastatic sites.

2) **Encounter for treatment of secondary malignancy**

When an encounter is for a primary malignancy with metastasis and treatment is directed toward the metastatic (secondary) site(s) only, the metastatic site(s) is designated as the principal/**first-listed** diagnosis. The primary malignancy is coded as an additional code.

3) **Malignant neoplasm in a pregnant patient**

When a pregnant woman has a malignant neoplasm, a code from subcategory **O9A.1-**, Malignant neoplasm complicating pregnancy, childbirth, and the puerperium, should be **sequenced** first, followed by the appropriate code from Chapter 2 to indicate the type of neoplasm.

4) **Encounter for complication associated with a neoplasm**

When an encounter is for management of a complication associated with a neoplasm, such as dehydration, and the treatment is only for the complication, the complication is coded first, followed by the appropriate code(s) for the neoplasm.

The exception to this guideline is anemia. When the admission/encounter is for management of an anemia associated with the malignancy, and the treatment is only for anemia, the appropriate code for the malignancy is sequenced as the principal or first-listed diagnosis followed by code D63.0, Anemia in neoplastic disease.

5) **Complication from surgical procedure for treatment of a neoplasm**

When an encounter is for treatment of a complication resulting from a surgical procedure performed for the treatment of the neoplasm, designate the complication as the principal/**first-listed** diagnosis. See guideline regarding the coding of a current malignancy versus personal history to determine if the code for the neoplasm should also be assigned.

6) **Pathologic fracture due to a neoplasm**

When an encounter is for a pathological fracture due to a neoplasm, if the focus of treatment is the fracture, a code from subcategory M84.5, Pathological fracture in neoplastic disease, should be sequenced first, followed by the code for the neoplasm.

If the focus of treatment is the neoplasm with an associated pathological fracture, the neoplasm code should be sequenced first, followed by a code from M84.5 for the pathological fracture.

m. **Current malignancy versus personal history of malignancy**

When a primary malignancy has been excised but further treatment, such as an additional surgery for the malignancy, radiation therapy or chemotherapy is directed to that site, the primary malignancy code should be used until treatment is completed.

When a primary malignancy has been previously excised or eradicated from its site, there is no further treatment (of the malignancy) directed to that site, and there is no evidence of any existing primary malignancy, a code from category Z85, Personal history of malignant neoplasm, should be used to indicate the former site of the malignancy.

See Section I.C.21. Factors influencing health status and contact with health services, History (of)

n. **Leukemia, *Multiple Myeloma, and Malignant Plasma Cell Neoplasms* in remission versus personal history**

The categories for leukemia, and category C90, Multiple myeloma **and malignant plasma cell neoplasms**, have codes for in remission. There are also codes Z85.6, Personal history of leukemia, and Z85.79, Personal history of other malignant neoplasms of lymphoid, hematopoietic and related tissues. If the documentation is unclear, as to whether the patient is in remission, the provider should be queried.

See Section I.C.21. Factors influencing health status and contact with health services, History (of)

o. **Aftercare following surgery for neoplasm**

See Section I.C.21. Factors influencing health status and contact with health services, Aftercare

p.   Follow-up care for completed treatment of a malignancy

See Section I.C.21. Factors influencing health status and contact with health services, Follow-up

q.   Prophylactic organ removal for prevention of malignancy

See Section I.C. 21, Factors influencing health status and contact with health services, Prophylactic organ removal

r.   Malignant neoplasm associated with transplanted organ

A malignant neoplasm of a transplanted organ should be coded as a transplant complication. Assign first the appropriate code from category T86.-, Complications of transplanted **organs and tissue**, followed by code C80.2, Malignant neoplasm associated with transplanted organ. Use an additional code for the specific malignancy.

3.   Chapter 3: Disease of the blood and blood-forming organs and certain disorders involving the immune mechanism (D50-D89)

Reserved for future guideline expansion

4.   Chapter 4: Endocrine, Nutritional, and Metabolic Diseases (E00-*E89*)

a.   Diabetes mellitus

The diabetes mellitus codes are combination codes that include the type of **diabetes mellitus**, the body system affected, and the complications affecting that body system. As many codes within a particular category as are necessary to describe all of the complications of the disease may be used. They should be sequenced based on the reason for a particular encounter. Assign as many codes from categories E08 – E13 as needed to identify all of the associated conditions that the patient has.

1)   Type of diabetes

The age of a patient is not the sole determining factor, though most type 1 diabetics develop the condition before reaching puberty. For this reason type 1 diabetes mellitus is also referred to as juvenile diabetes.

2) Type of diabetes mellitus not documented

If the type of diabetes mellitus is not documented in the medical record the default is E11.-, Type 2 diabetes mellitus.

3) Diabetes mellitus and the use of insulin

If the documentation in a medical record does not indicate the type of diabetes but does indicate that the patient uses insulin, code E11, Type 2 diabetes mellitus, should be assigned. **Code** Z79.4, Long-term (current) use of insulin, should also be assigned to indicate that the patient uses insulin. Code Z79.4 should not be assigned if insulin is given temporarily to bring a type 2 patient's blood sugar under control during an encounter.

4) Diabetes mellitus in pregnancy and gestational diabetes

See Section I.C.15. Diabetes mellitus in pregnancy.
See Section I.C.15. Gestational (pregnancy induced) diabetes

5) Complications due to insulin pump malfunction

(a) Underdose of insulin due *to* insulin pump failure

An underdose of insulin due to an insulin pump failure should be assigned to a code from subcategory T85.6, Mechanical complication of other specified internal and external prosthetic devices, implants and grafts, that specifies the type of pump malfunction, as the principal or **first-listed** code, followed by code T38.3x6-, Underdosing of insulin and oral hypoglycemic [antidiabetic] drugs. Additional codes for the type of diabetes mellitus and any associated complications due to the underdosing should also be assigned.

(b) Overdose of insulin due to insulin pump failure

The principal or **first-listed** code for an encounter due to an insulin pump malfunction resulting in an overdose of insulin, should also be T85.6-, Mechanical complication of other specified internal and external prosthetic devices, implants and grafts, followed by code T38.3x1-, Poisoning by insulin and oral hypoglycemic [antidiabetic] drugs, accidental (unintentional).

6) **Secondary Diabetes Mellitus**

Codes under **categories** E08, Diabetes mellitus due to underlying condition, and E09, Drug or chemical induced diabetes mellitus, identify complications/manifestations associated with secondary diabetes mellitus. Secondary diabetes is always caused by another condition or event (e.g., cystic fibrosis, malignant neoplasm of pancreas, pancreatectomy, adverse effect of drug, or poisoning).

(a) **Secondary diabetes mellitus and the use of insulin**

For patients who routinely use insulin, code Z79.4, Long-term (current) use of insulin, should also be assigned. Code Z79.4 should not be assigned if insulin is given temporarily to bring a patient's blood sugar under control during an encounter.

(b) **Assigning and sequencing secondary diabetes codes and its causes**

The sequencing of the secondary diabetes codes in relationship to codes for the cause of the diabetes is based on the **Tabular List** instructions for categories E08 and E09. For example, for category E08, Diabetes mellitus due to underlying condition, code first the underlying condition; for category E09, Drug or chemical induced diabetes mellitus, code first the drug or chemical (T36-T65).

(i) **Secondary diabetes mellitus due to pancreatectomy**

For postpancreatectomy diabetes mellitus (lack of insulin due to the surgical removal of all or part of the pancreas), assign code E89.1, **Postprocedural** hypoinsulinemia. Assign a code from category **E13** and **a** code **from subcategory Z90.41-, Acquired absence of pancreas**, as additional codes.

(ii) **Secondary diabetes due to drugs**

Secondary diabetes may be caused by an adverse effect of correctly administered medications, poisoning or late effect of poisoning.

See section I.C.19.e for coding of adverse effects and poisoning, and section I.C.20 for external cause code reporting.

5. Chapter 5: Mental and behavioral disorders (F01 – F99)

a. Pain disorders related to psychological factors

Assign code F45.41, for pain that is exclusively psychological. Code F45.41, Pain disorder **exclusively** related **to** psychological factors, should be used following the appropriate code from category G89, Pain, not elsewhere classified, if there is documentation of a psychological component for a patient with acute or chronic pain.

See Section I.C.6. Pain

b. *Mental and behavioral disorders due to psychoactive substance use*

1) *In Remission*

Selection of codes for "in remission" for categories F10-F19, Mental and behavioral disorders due to psychoactive substance use (categories F10-F19 with -.21) requires the provider's clinical judgment. The appropriate codes for "in remission" are assigned only on the basis of provider documentation (as defined in the Official Guidelines for Coding and Reporting).

2) *Psychoactive Substance Use, Abuse And Dependence*

When the provider documentation refers to use, abuse and dependence of the same substance (e.g. alcohol, opioid, cannabis, etc.), only one code should be assigned to identify the pattern of use based on the following hierarchy:
- If both use and abuse are documented, assign only the code for abuse
- If both abuse and dependence are documented, assign only the code for dependence
- If use, abuse and dependence are all documented, assign only the code for dependence
- If both use and dependence are documented, assign only the code for dependence.

3) *Psychoactive Substance Use*

As with all other diagnoses, the codes for psychoactive substance use (F10.9-, F11.9-, F12.9-, F13.9-, F14.9-, F15.9-, F16.9-) should only be assigned based on provider documentation and when they meet the definition of a reportable diagnosis (see Section III, Reporting Additional Diagnoses). **The codes are to be used only when the psychoactive substance use is associated with a mental or behavioral disorder, and such a relationship is documented by the provider.**

6. Chapter 6: Diseases of Nervous System and Sense Organs (G00-G99)

a. Dominant/nondominant side

Codes from category G81, Hemiplegia and hemiparesis, and subcategories, G83.1, Monoplegia of lower limb, G83.2, Monoplegia of upper limb, and G83.3, Monoplegia, unspecified, identify whether the dominant or nondominant side is affected. Should **the affected side be documented, but not specified as dominant or nondominant**, and the classification system does not indicate a default, **code selection is as follows:**

- For ambidextrous patients, the default should be dominant.
- **If the left side is affected, the default is non-dominant.**
- **If the right side is affected, the default is dominant.**

b. Pain - Category G89

1) General coding information

Codes in category G89, Pain, not elsewhere classified, may be used in conjunction with codes from other categories and chapters to provide more detail about acute or chronic pain and neoplasm-related pain, unless otherwise indicated below.

If the pain is not specified as acute or chronic, post-thoracotomy, postprocedural, or neoplasm-related, do not assign codes from category G89.

A code from category G89 should not be assigned if the underlying (definitive) diagnosis is known, unless the reason for the encounter is pain control/ management and not management of the underlying condition.

When an admission or encounter is for a procedure aimed at treating the underlying condition (e.g., spinal fusion, kyphoplasty), a code for the underlying condition (e.g., vertebral fracture, spinal stenosis) should be assigned as the principal diagnosis. No code from category G89 should be assigned.

(a) **Category G89 Codes as Principal or First-Listed Diagnosis**

Category G89 codes are acceptable as principal diagnosis or the first-listed code:

- When pain control or pain management is the reason for the admission/encounter (e.g., a patient with displaced intervertebral disc, nerve impingement and severe back pain presents for injection of steroid into the spinal canal). The underlying cause of the pain should be reported as an additional diagnosis, if known.

- When a patient is admitted for the insertion of a neurostimulator for pain control, assign the appropriate pain code as the principal or **first-listed** diagnosis. When an admission or encounter is for a procedure aimed at treating the underlying condition and a neurostimulator is inserted for pain control during the same admission/encounter, a code for the underlying condition should be assigned as the principal diagnosis and the appropriate pain code should be assigned as a secondary diagnosis.

(b) **Use of Category G89 Codes in Conjunction with Site Specific Pain Codes**

(i) **Assigning Category G89 and Site-Specific Pain Codes**

Codes from category G89 may be used in conjunction with codes that identify the site of pain (including codes from chapter 18) if the category G89 code provides additional information. For example, if the code describes the site of the pain, but does not fully describe whether the pain is acute or chronic, then both codes should be assigned.

(ii) **Sequencing of Category G89 Codes with Site-Specific Pain Codes**

The sequencing of category G89 codes with site-specific pain codes (including chapter 18 codes), is dependent on the circumstances of the encounter/admission as follows:

- If the encounter is for pain control or pain management, assign the code from category G89 followed by the code identifying the specific site of pain (e.g., encounter for pain management for acute neck pain from trauma is assigned code G89.11, Acute pain due to trauma, followed by code M54.2, Cervicalgia, to identify the site of pain).

- If the encounter is for any other reason except pain control or pain management, and a related definitive diagnosis has not been established (confirmed) by the provider, assign the code for the specific site of pain first, followed by the appropriate code from category G89.

2) **Pain due to devices, implants and grafts**

See Section I.C.19. Pain due to medical devices

3) **Postoperative Pain**

The provider's documentation should be used to guide the coding of postoperative pain, as well as *Section III. Reporting Additional Diagnoses* and *Section IV. Diagnostic Coding and Reporting in the Outpatient Setting.*

The default for post-thoracotomy and other postoperative pain not specified as acute or chronic is the code for the acute form.

Routine or expected postoperative pain immediately after surgery should not be coded.

(a) **Postoperative pain not associated with specific postoperative complication**

Postoperative pain not associated with a specific postoperative complication is assigned to the appropriate postoperative pain code in category G89.

(b) **Postoperative pain associated with specific postoperative complication**

Postoperative pain associated with a specific postoperative complication (such as painful wire sutures) is assigned to the appropriate code(s) found in

Chapter 19, Injury, poisoning, and certain other consequences of external causes. If appropriate, use additional code(s) from category G89 to identify acute or chronic pain (G89.18 or G89.28).

4) Chronic pain

Chronic pain is classified to subcategory G89.2. There is no time frame defining when pain becomes chronic pain. The provider's documentation should be used to guide use of these codes.

5) Neoplasm Related Pain

Code G89.3 is assigned to pain documented as being related, associated or due to cancer, primary or secondary malignancy, or tumor. This code is assigned regardless of whether the pain is acute or chronic.

This code may be assigned as the principal or first-listed code when the stated reason for the admission/encounter is documented as pain control/pain management. The underlying neoplasm should be reported as an additional diagnosis.

When the reason for the admission/encounter is management of the neoplasm and the pain associated with the neoplasm is also documented, code G89.3 may be assigned as an additional diagnosis. It is not necessary to assign an additional code for the site of the pain.

See Section I.C.2 for instructions on the sequencing of neoplasms for all other stated reasons for the admission/encounter (except for pain control/pain management).

6) Chronic pain syndrome

Central pain syndrome (G89.0) and chronic pain syndrome (G89.4) are different than the term "chronic pain," and therefore codes should only be used when the provider has specifically documented this condition.

See Section I.C.5. Pain disorders related to psychological factors

7.   **Chapter 7: Diseases of Eye and Adnexa (H00-H59)**
     Reserved for future guideline expansion

8.   **Chapter 8: Diseases of Ear and Mastoid Process (H60-H95)**
     Reserved for future guideline expansion

9.   **Chapter 9: Diseases of Circulatory System (I00-I99)**

  a.   **Hypertension**

    1)   **Hypertension with Heart Disease**
         Heart conditions classified to I50.- or I51.4-I51.9, are assigned to, a code from category I11, Hypertensive heart disease, when a causal relationship is stated (due to hypertension) or implied (hypertensive). Use an additional code from category I50, Heart failure, to identify the type of heart failure in those patients with heart failure.

         The same heart conditions (I50.-, I51.4-I51.9) with hypertension, but without a stated causal relationship, are coded separately. Sequence according to the circumstances of the admission/encounter.

    2)   **Hypertensive Chronic Kidney Disease**
         Assign codes from category I12, Hypertensive chronic kidney disease, when both hypertension and a condition classifiable to category N18, Chronic kidney disease (CKD), are present. Unlike hypertension with heart disease, ICD-10-CM presumes a cause-and-effect relationship and classifies chronic kidney disease with hypertension as hypertensive chronic kidney disease.
         The appropriate code from category N18 should be used as a secondary code with a code from category I12 to identify the stage of chronic kidney disease.

         See Section I.C.14. Chronic kidney disease.

         If a patient has hypertensive chronic kidney disease and acute renal failure, an additional code for the acute renal failure is required.

    3)   **Hypertensive Heart and Chronic Kidney Disease**
         Assign codes from combination category I13, Hypertensive heart and chronic kidney disease, when both hypertensive

kidney disease and hypertensive heart disease are stated in the diagnosis. Assume a relationship between the hypertension and the chronic kidney disease, whether or not the condition is so designated. If heart failure is present, assign an additional code from category I50 to identify the type of heart failure.

The appropriate code from category N18, Chronic kidney disease, should be used as a secondary code with a code from category I13 to identify the stage of chronic kidney disease.

See Section I.C.14. Chronic kidney disease.

The codes in category I13, Hypertensive heart and chronic kidney disease, are combination codes that include hypertension, heart disease and chronic kidney disease. The Includes note at I13 specifies that the conditions included at I11 and I12 are included together in I13. If a patient has hypertension, heart disease and chronic kidney disease then a code from I13 should be used, not individual codes for hypertension, heart disease and chronic kidney disease, or codes from I11 or I12.

For patients with both acute renal failure and chronic kidney disease an additional code for acute renal failure is required.

4) **Hypertensive Cerebrovascular Disease**
For hypertensive cerebrovascular disease, first assign the appropriate code from categories I60-I69, followed by the appropriate hypertension code.

5) **Hypertensive Retinopathy**
Subcategory H35.0, Background retinopathy and retinal vascular changes, should be used with code I10, Essential (primary) hypertension, to include the systemic hypertension. The sequencing is based on the reason for the encounter.

6) **Hypertension, Secondary**
Secondary hypertension is due to an underlying condition. Two codes are required: one to identify the underlying etiology and one from category I15 to identify the hypertension. Sequencing of codes is determined by the reason for admission/encounter.

7) **Hypertension, Transient**
Assign code R03.0, Elevated blood pressure reading without diagnosis of hypertension, unless patient has an established

diagnosis of hypertension. Assign code O13.-, Gestational [pregnancy-induced] hypertension without significant proteinuria, or O14.-, **Pre-eclampsia**, for transient hypertension of pregnancy.

8)   **Hypertension, Controlled**

This diagnostic statement usually refers to an existing state of hypertension under control by therapy. Assign **the appropriate** code **from categories I10-I15, Hypertensive diseases**.

9)   **Hypertension, Uncontrolled**

Uncontrolled hypertension may refer to untreated hypertension or hypertension not responding to current therapeutic regimen. In either case, assign **the appropriate** code **from categories I10-I15, Hypertensive diseases**.

b.   **Atherosclerotic *Coronary Artery Disease* and *Angina***

ICD-10-CM has combination codes for atherosclerotic heart disease with angina pectoris. The subcategories for these codes are I25.11, Atherosclerotic heart disease of native coronary artery with angina pectoris and I25.7, Atherosclerosis of coronary artery bypass graft(s) and coronary artery of transplanted heart with angina pectoris.

When using one of these combination codes it is not necessary to use an additional code for angina pectoris. A causal relationship can be assumed in a patient with both atherosclerosis and angina pectoris, unless the documentation indicates the angina is due to something other than the atherosclerosis.

If a patient with coronary artery disease is admitted due to an acute myocardial infarction (AMI), the AMI should be sequenced before the coronary artery disease.

See Section I.C.9. Acute myocardial infarction (AMI)

c.   **Intraoperative and Postprocedural *Cerebrovascular Accident***

Medical record documentation should clearly specify the cause- and-effect relationship between the medical intervention and the cerebrovascular accident in order to assign a code for intraoperative or postprocedural cerebrovascular accident.
Proper code assignment depends on whether it was an infarction or hemorrhage and whether it occurred intraoperatively or postoperatively. If it was a cerebral hemorrhage, code assignment depends on the type of procedure performed.

d.   Sequelae of Cerebrovascular Disease

1)   Category I69, Sequelae of Cerebrovascular disease

Category I69 is used to indicate conditions classifiable to categories I60-I67 as the causes of late effects (neurologic deficits), themselves classified elsewhere. These "late effects" include neurologic deficits that persist after initial onset of conditions classifiable to categories I60-I67. The neurologic deficits caused by cerebrovascular disease may be present from the onset or may arise at any time after the onset of the condition classifiable to categories I60-I67.

2)   Codes from category I69 with codes from I60-I67

Codes from category I69 may be assigned on a health care record with codes from I60-I67, if the patient has a current cerebrovascular **disease** and deficits from an old **cerebrovascular disease**.

3)   Code Z86.73

Assign code Z86.73, Personal history of transient ischemic attack (TIA), and cerebral infarction without residual deficits (and not a code from category I69) as an additional code for history of cerebrovascular disease when no neurologic deficits are present.

e.   Acute myocardial infarction (AMI)

1)   ST elevation myocardial infarction (STEMI) and non ST elevation myocardial infarction (NSTEMI)

The ICD-10-CM codes for acute myocardial infarction (AMI) identify the site, such as anterolateral wall or true posterior wall. Subcategories I21.0-I21.2 and code I21.4 are used for ST elevation myocardial infarction (STEMI). Code I21.4, Non-ST elevation (NSTEMI) myocardial infarction, is used for non ST elevation myocardial infarction (NSTEMI) and nontransmural MIs.

If NSTEMI evolves to STEMI, assign the STEMI code. If STEMI converts to NSTEMI due to thrombolytic therapy, it is still coded as STEMI.

When the patient requires continued care for the myocardial infarction, codes from category I21 may continue to be reported for the duration of 4 weeks (28 days) or less from onset, regardless of the healthcare setting, including when a patient is transferred from the acute care setting to the post-acute care setting if the patient is still within the four weeks time frame. For encounters after the 4 weeks time frame and the patient requires continued care related to the myocardial infarction, the appropriate aftercare code should be assigned, rather than a code from category I21. Otherwise, code I25.2, Old myocardial infarction, may be assigned for old or healed myocardial infarction not requiring further care.

2) **Acute myocardial infarction, unspecified**

Code I21.3, ST elevation (STEMI) myocardial infarction of unspecified site, is the default for the unspecified term acute myocardial infarction. If only STEMI or transmural MI without the site is documented, query the provider as to the site, or assign code I21.3.

3) **AMI documented as nontransmural or subendocardial but site provided**

If an AMI is documented as nontransmural or subendocardial, but the site is provided, it is still coded as a subendocardial AMI.

See Section I.C.21.3 for information on coding status post administration of tPA in a different facility within the last 24 hours.

4) **Subsequent acute myocardial infarction**

A code from category I22, Subsequent ST elevation (STEMI) and non ST elevation (NSTEMI) myocardial infarction, is to be used when a patient who has suffered an AMI has a new AMI within the 4 week time frame of the initial AMI. A code from category I22 must be used in conjunction with a code from category I21.

The sequencing of the I22 and I21 codes depends on the circumstances of the encounter. Should a patient who is in the hospital due to an AMI have a subsequent AMI while still in the hospital code I21 would be sequenced first as the reason for admission, with code I22 sequenced as a secondary code. Should a patient have a subsequent AMI after discharge for care of an initial AMI, and the reason for admission is the subsequent AMI, the I22 code should be sequenced first followed by the I21. An I21 code must accompany an I22 code to identify the site of the initial AMI, and to indicate that the patient is still within the 4 week time frame of healing from the initial AMI.

The guidelines for assigning the correct I22 code are the same as for the initial AMI.

10. Chapter 10: Diseases of Respiratory System (J00-J99)

a. Chronic Obstructive Pulmonary Disease [COPD] and Asthma

1) Acute exacerbation of chronic obstructive bronchitis and asthma

The codes in categories J44 and J45 distinguish between uncomplicated cases and those in acute exacerbation. An acute exacerbation is a worsening or a decompensation of a chronic condition. An acute exacerbation is not equivalent to an infection superimposed on a chronic condition, though an exacerbation may be triggered by an infection.

b. Acute Respiratory Failure

1) Acute respiratory failure as principal diagnosis

A code from subcategory J96.0, Acute respiratory failure, or **subcategory** J96.2, Acute and chronic respiratory failure, may be assigned as a principal diagnosis when it is the condition established after study to be chiefly responsible for occasioning the admission to the hospital, and the selection is supported by the Alphabetic Index and Tabular List. However, chapter-specific coding guidelines (such as obstetrics, poisoning, HIV, newborn) that provide sequencing direction take precedence.

2) Acute respiratory failure as secondary diagnosis

Respiratory failure may be listed as a secondary diagnosis if it occurs after admission, or if it is present on admission, but does not meet the definition of principal diagnosis.

3) **Sequencing of acute respiratory failure and another acute condition**

When a patient is admitted with respiratory failure and another acute condition, (e.g., myocardial infarction, cerebrovascular accident, aspiration pneumonia), the principal diagnosis will not be the same in every situation. This applies whether the other acute condition is a respiratory or nonrespiratory condition. Selection of the principal diagnosis will be dependent on the circumstances of admission. If both the respiratory failure and the other acute condition are equally responsible for occasioning the admission to the hospital, and there are no chapter-specific sequencing rules, the guideline regarding two or more diagnoses that equally meet the definition for principal diagnosis *(Section II, C.)* may be applied in these situations.

If the documentation is not clear as to whether acute respiratory failure and another condition are equally responsible for occasioning the admission, query the provider for clarification.

c. **Influenza due to *certain identified influenza* influenza *viruses***

Code only confirmed cases of avian influenza (code J09.0-, Influenza due to identified avian influenza virus) or novel H1N1 or swine flu, code J09.1-. This is an exception to the hospital inpatient guideline Section II, H. (Uncertain Diagnosis).

In this context, "confirmation" does not require documentation of positive laboratory testing specific for avian or novel H1N1 (H1N1 or swine flu) influenza. However, coding should be based on the provider's diagnostic statement that the patient has avian influenza.

If the provider records "suspected or possible or probable avian influenza," the appropriate influenza code from category **J11**, Influenza due to **unspecified** influenza virus, should be assigned. A code from category J09, Influenza due to certain identified influenza viruses, should not be assigned.

d. *Ventilator associated Pneumonia*

1) Documentation of Ventilator associated Pneumonia

As with all procedural or postprocedural complications, code assignment is based on the provider's documentation of the relationship between the condition and the procedure.

Code J95.851, Ventilator associated pneumonia, should be assigned only when the provider has documented ventilator associated pneumonia (VAP). An additional code to identify the organism (e.g., Pseudomonas aeruginosa, code B96.5) should also be assigned. Do not assign an additional code from categories J12-J18 to identify the type of pneumonia.

Code J95.851 should not be assigned for cases where the patient has pneumonia and is on a mechanical ventilator but the provider has not specifically stated that the pneumonia is ventilator-associated pneumonia. If the documentation is unclear as to whether the patient has a pneumonia that is a complication attributable to the mechanical ventilator, query the provider.

2) Ventilator associated Pneumonia Develops after Admission

A patient may be admitted with one type of pneumonia (e.g., code J13, Pneumonia due to Streptococcus pneumonia) and subsequently develop VAP. In this instance, the principal diagnosis would be the appropriate code from categories J12-J18 for the pneumonia diagnosed at the time of admission. Code J95.851, Ventilator associated pneumonia, would be assigned as an additional diagnosis when the provider has also documented the presence of ventilator associated pneumonia.

11. Chapter 11: Diseases of Digestive System (K00-K94)

Reserved for future guideline expansion

12. Chapter 12: Diseases of Skin and Subcutaneous Tissue (L00-L99)

a. Pressure ulcer stage codes

1) Pressure ulcer stages

Codes from category L89, Pressure ulcer, are combination codes that identify the site of the pressure ulcer as well as the stage of the ulcer.

The ICD-10-CM classifies pressure ulcer stages based on severity, which is designated by stages 1-4, unspecified stage and unstageable.

Assign as many codes from category L89 as needed to identify all the pressure ulcers the patient has, if applicable.

2) Unstageable pressure ulcers

Assignment of the code for unstageable pressure ulcer (L89.--0) should be based on the clinical documentation. These codes are used for pressure ulcers whose stage cannot be clinically determined (e.g., the ulcer is covered by eschar or has been treated with a skin or muscle graft) and pressure ulcers that are documented as deep tissue injury but not documented as due to trauma. This code should not be confused with the codes for unspecified stage (L89.--9). When there is no documentation regarding the stage of the pressure ulcer, assign the appropriate code for unspecified stage (L89.--9).

3) Documented pressure ulcer stage

Assignment of the pressure ulcer stage code should be guided by clinical documentation of the stage or documentation of the terms found in the **Alphabetic Index**. For clinical terms describing the stage that are not found in the **Alphabetic Index**, and there is no documentation of the stage, the provider should be queried.

4) Patients admitted with pressure ulcers documented as healed

No code is assigned if the documentation states that the pressure ulcer is completely healed.

5) **Patients admitted with pressure ulcers documented as healing**

Pressure ulcers described as healing should be assigned the appropriate pressure ulcer stage code based on the documentation in the medical record. If the documentation does not provide information about the stage of the healing pressure ulcer, assign the appropriate code for unspecified stage.

If the documentation is unclear as to whether the patient has a current (new) pressure ulcer or if the patient is being treated for a healing pressure ulcer, query the provider.

6) **Patient admitted with pressure ulcer evolving into another stage during the admission**

If a patient is admitted with a pressure ulcer at one stage and it progresses to a higher stage, assign the code for the highest stage reported for that site.

13. Chapter 13: Diseases of the Musculoskeletal System and Connective Tissue (M00-M99)

a. Site and laterality

Most of the codes within Chapter 13 have site and laterality designations. The site represents the bone, joint or the muscle involved. For some conditions where more than one bone, joint or muscle is usually involved, such as osteoarthritis, there is a "multiple sites" code available. For categories where no multiple site code is provided and more than one bone, joint or muscle is involved, multiple codes should be used to indicate the different sites involved.

1) Bone versus joint

For certain conditions, the bone may be affected at the upper or lower end, (e.g., avascular necrosis of bone, M87, Osteoporosis, M80, M81). Though the portion of the bone affected may be at the joint, the site designation will be the bone, not the joint.

b. Acute traumatic versus chronic or recurrent musculoskeletal conditions

Many musculoskeletal conditions are a result of previous injury or trauma to a site, or are recurrent conditions. Bone, joint or muscle conditions that are the result of a healed injury are usually found in chapter 13. Recurrent bone, joint or muscle conditions are also usually found in chapter 13. Any current, acute injury should be coded to the appropriate injury code from chapter 19. Chronic or recurrent conditions should generally be coded with a code from chapter 13. If it is difficult to determine from the documentation in the record which code is best to describe a condition, query the provider.

c. Coding of Pathologic Fractures

7th character A is for use as long as the patient is receiving active treatment for the fracture. Examples of active treatment are: surgical treatment, emergency department encounter, evaluation and treatment by a new physician. 7th character, D is to be used for encounters after the patient has completed active treatment. The other 7th characters, listed under each subcategory in the Tabular List, are to be used for subsequent encounters for treatment of problems associated with the healing, such as malunions, nonunions, and sequelae.
Care for complications of surgical treatment for fracture repairs during the healing or recovery phase should be coded with the appropriate complication codes.

See Section I.C.19. Coding of traumatic fractures.

d. Osteoporosis

Osteoporosis is a systemic condition, meaning that all bones of the musculoskeletal system are affected. Therefore, site is not a component of the codes under category M81, Osteoporosis without current pathological fracture. The site codes under category M80, Osteoporosis with current pathological fracture, identify the site of the fracture, not the osteoporosis.

1) Osteoporosis without pathological fracture

Category M81, Osteoporosis without current pathological fracture, is for use for patients with osteoporosis who do not currently have a pathologic fracture due to the osteoporosis, even if they have had a fracture in the past. For patients with a history of osteoporosis fractures, status code **Z87.310**, Personal history of **(healed)** osteoporosis fracture, should follow the code from M81.

2) Osteoporosis with current pathological fracture

Category M80, Osteoporosis with current pathological fracture, is for patients who have a current pathologic fracture at the time of an encounter. The codes under M80 identify the site of the fracture. A code from category M80, not a traumatic fracture code, should be used for any patient with known osteoporosis who suffers a fracture, even if the patient had a minor fall or trauma, if that fall or trauma would not usually break a normal, healthy bone.

14. Chapter 14: Diseases of Genitourinary System (N00-N99)

a. Chronic kidney disease

1) Stages of chronic kidney disease (CKD)

The ICD-10-CM classifies CKD based on severity. The severity of CKD is designated by stages **1-5**. Stage **2**, code N18.2, equates to mild CKD; stage **3**, code N18.3, equates to moderate CKD; and stage **4**, code N18.4, equates to severe CKD. Code N18.6, End stage renal disease (ESRD), is assigned when the provider has documented end-stage-renal disease (ESRD).

If both a stage of CKD and ESRD are documented, assign code N18.6 only.

2) Chronic kidney disease and kidney transplant status

Patients who have undergone kidney transplant may still have some form of chronic kidney disease (CKD) because the kidney transplant may not fully restore kidney function. Therefore, the presence of CKD alone does not constitute a transplant complication. Assign the appropriate N18 code for the patient's stage of CKD and code Z94.0, Kidney transplant status. If a transplant complication such as failure or rejection or other transplant complication is documented, see section I.C.19.g for information on coding complications of a kidney transplant. If the documentation is unclear as to whether the patient has a complication of the transplant, query the provider.

3) Chronic kidney disease with other conditions

Patients with CKD may also suffer from other serious conditions, most commonly diabetes mellitus and hypertension. The sequencing of the CKD code in relationship to codes for other contributing conditions is based on the conventions in the Tabular List.

See I.C.9. Hypertensive chronic kidney disease.
See I.C.19. Chronic kidney disease and kidney transplant complications.

15.   Chapter 15: Pregnancy, Childbirth, and the Puerperium (O00-*O9A*)

a.   General Rules for Obstetric Cases

1)   Codes from chapter 15 and sequencing priority

Obstetric cases require codes from chapter 15, codes in the range O00-O9A, Pregnancy, Childbirth, and the Puerperium. Chapter 15 codes have sequencing priority over codes from other chapters. Additional codes from other chapters may be used in conjunction with chapter 15 codes to further specify conditions. Should the provider document that the pregnancy is incidental to the encounter, then code Z33.1, Pregnant state, incidental, should be used in place of any chapter 15 codes. It is the provider's responsibility to state that the condition being treated is not affecting the pregnancy.

2)   Chapter 15 codes used only on the maternal record

Chapter 15 codes are to be used only on the maternal record, never on the record of the newborn.

3)   Final character for trimester

The majority of codes in Chapter 15 have a final character indicating the trimester of pregnancy. The timeframes for the trimesters are indicated at the beginning of the chapter. If trimester is not a component of a code it is because the condition always occurs in a specific trimester, or the concept of trimester of pregnancy is not applicable. Certain codes have characters for only certain trimesters because the condition does not occur in all trimesters, but it may occur in more than just one.

Assignment of the final character for trimester should be based on the **provider's documentation of the** trimester **(or number of weeks)** for the current admission/encounter. This applies to the assignment of trimester for pre-existing conditions as well as those that develop during or are due to the pregnancy. **The provider's documentation of the number of weeks may be used to assign the appropriate code identifying the trimester.**

Whenever delivery occurs during the current admission, and there is an "in childbirth" option for the obstetric complication being coded, the "in childbirth" code should be assigned.

4) Selection of trimester for inpatient admissions that encompass more than one trimesters

In instances when a patient is admitted to a hospital for complications of pregnancy during one trimester and remains in the hospital into a subsequent trimester, the trimester character for the antepartum complication code should be assigned on the basis of the trimester when the complication developed, not the trimester of the discharge. If the condition developed prior to the current admission/encounter or represents a pre-existing condition, the trimester character for the trimester at the time of the admission/encounter should be assigned.

5) Unspecified trimester

Each category that includes codes for trimester has a code for "unspecified trimester." The "unspecified trimester" code should rarely be used, such as when the documentation in the record is insufficient to determine the trimester and it is not possible to obtain clarification.

6) *Fetal Extensions*

Where applicable, a 7ᵗʰ character is to be assigned for certain categories (O31, O32, O33.3 - O33.6, O35, O36, O40, O41, O60.1, O60.2, O64, and O69) to identify the fetus for which the complication code applies.

Assign 7ᵗʰ character "0":
- **For single gestations**
- **When the documentation in the record is insufficient to determine the fetus affected and it is not possible to obtain clarification.**
- **When it is not possible to clinically determine which fetus is affected.**

b. Selection of OB Principal or First-listed Diagnosis

1) Routine outpatient prenatal visits

For routine outpatient prenatal visits when no complications are present, a code from category Z34, Encounter for supervision of normal pregnancy, should be used as the first-listed diagnosis. These codes should not be used in conjunction with chapter 15 codes.

2)   **Prenatal outpatient visits for high-risk patients**

For routine prenatal outpatient visits for patients with high-risk pregnancies, a code from category O09, Supervision of high-risk pregnancy, should be used as the first-listed diagnosis. Secondary chapter 15 codes may be used in conjunction with these codes if appropriate.

3)   **Episodes when no delivery occurs**

In episodes when no delivery occurs, the principal diagnosis should correspond to the principal complication of the pregnancy which necessitated the encounter. Should more than one complication exist, all of which are treated or monitored, any of the complications codes may be sequenced first.

4)   **When a delivery occurs**

When a delivery occurs, the principal diagnosis should correspond to the main circumstances or complication of the delivery. In cases of cesarean delivery, the selection of the principal diagnosis should be the condition established after study that was responsible for the patient's admission. If the patient was admitted with a condition that resulted in the performance of a cesarean procedure, that condition should be selected as the principal diagnosis. If the reason for the admission/encounter was unrelated to the condition resulting in the cesarean delivery, the condition related to the reason for the admission/encounter should be selected as the principal diagnosis.

5)   **Outcome of delivery**

A code from category Z37, Outcome of delivery, should be included on every maternal record when a delivery has occurred. These codes are not to be used on subsequent records or on the newborn record.

c.   **Pre-existing conditions versus conditions due to the pregnancy**

Certain categories in Chapter 15 distinguish between conditions of the mother that existed prior to pregnancy (pre-existing) and those that are a direct result of pregnancy. When assigning codes from Chapter 15, it is important to assess if a condition was pre-existing prior to pregnancy or developed during or due to the pregnancy in order to assign the correct code.

Categories that do not distinguish between pre-existing and pregnancy-related conditions may be used for either. It is acceptable to use codes specifically for the puerperium with codes complicating pregnancy and childbirth if a condition arises postpartum during the delivery encounter.

d. Pre-existing hypertension in pregnancy

Category O10, Pre-existing hypertension complicating pregnancy, childbirth and the puerperium, includes codes for hypertensive heart and hypertensive chronic kidney disease. When assigning one of the O10 codes that includes hypertensive heart disease or hypertensive chronic kidney disease, it is necessary to add a secondary code from the appropriate hypertension category to specify the type of heart failure or chronic kidney disease.

See Section I.C.9. Hypertension.

e. Fetal Conditions Affecting the Management of the Mother

1) Codes from categories O35 and O36

Codes from categories O35, Maternal care for known or suspected fetal abnormality and damage, and O36, Maternal care for other fetal problems, are assigned only when the fetal condition is actually responsible for modifying the management of the mother, i.e., by requiring diagnostic studies, additional observation, special care, or termination of pregnancy. The fact that the fetal condition exists does not justify assigning a code from this series to the mother's record.

2) In utero surgery

In cases when surgery is performed on the fetus, a diagnosis code from category O35, Maternal care for known or suspected fetal abnormality and damage, should be assigned identifying the fetal condition. Assign the appropriate procedure code for the procedure performed.

No code from Chapter 16, the perinatal codes, should be used on the mother's record to identify fetal conditions. Surgery performed in utero on a fetus is still to be coded as an obstetric encounter.

f. HIV Infection in Pregnancy, Childbirth and the Puerperium

During pregnancy, childbirth or the puerperium, a patient admitted because of an HIV-related illness should receive a principal diagnosis from subcategory O98.7-, Human immunodeficiency [HIV] disease complicating pregnancy, childbirth and the puerperium, followed by the code(s) for the HIV-related illness(es).

Patients with asymptomatic HIV infection status admitted during pregnancy, childbirth, or the puerperium should receive codes of O98.7- and Z21, Asymptomatic human immunodeficiency virus [HIV] infection status.

g. Diabetes mellitus in pregnancy

Diabetes mellitus is a significant complicating factor in pregnancy. Pregnant women who are diabetic should be assigned a code **from category** O24, Diabetes mellitus in pregnancy, childbirth, and the puerperium, first, followed by the appropriate diabetes code(s) (E08-E13) from Chapter 4.

h. Long term use of insulin

Code Z79.4, Long-term (current) use of insulin, should also be assigned if the diabetes mellitus is being treated with insulin.

i. Gestational (pregnancy induced) diabetes

Gestational (pregnancy induced) diabetes can occur during the second and third trimester of pregnancy in women who were not diabetic prior to pregnancy. Gestational diabetes can cause complications in the pregnancy similar to those of pre-existing diabetes mellitus. It also puts the woman at greater risk of developing diabetes after the pregnancy. Codes for gestational diabetes are in subcategory O24.4, Gestational diabetes mellitus. No other code from category O24, Diabetes mellitus in pregnancy, childbirth, and the puerperium, should be used with a code from O24.4

The codes under subcategory O24.4 include diet controlled and insulin controlled. If a patient with gestational diabetes is treated with both diet and insulin, only the code for insulin-controlled is required. Code Z79.4, Long-term (current) use of insulin, should not be assigned with codes from subcategory O24.4.

An abnormal glucose tolerance in pregnancy is assigned a code from subcategory O99.81, Abnormal glucose complicating pregnancy, childbirth, and the puerperium.

j. Sepsis and septic shock complicating abortion, pregnancy, childbirth and the puerperium

When assigning a chapter 15 code for sepsis complicating abortion, pregnancy, childbirth, and the puerperium, a code for the specific type of infection should be assigned as an additional diagnosis. If severe sepsis is present, a code from subcategory R65.2, Severe sepsis, and code(s) for associated organ dysfunction(s) should also be assigned as additional diagnoses.

k. Puerperal sepsis

Code O85, Puerperal sepsis, should be assigned with a secondary code to identify the causal organism (e.g., for a bacterial infection, assign a code from category B95-B96, Bacterial infections in conditions classified elsewhere). A code from category A40, Streptococcal sepsis, or A41, Other sepsis, should not be used for puerperal sepsis. If applicable, use additional codes to identify severe sepsis (R65.2-) and any associated acute organ dysfunction.

l. Alcohol and tobacco use during pregnancy, childbirth and the puerperium

1) Alcohol use during pregnancy, childbirth and the puerperium

Codes under subcategory O99.31, Alcohol use complicating pregnancy, childbirth, and the puerperium, should be assigned for any pregnancy case when a mother uses alcohol during the pregnancy or postpartum. A secondary code from category F10, Alcohol related disorders, should also be assigned **to identify manifestations of the alcohol use**.

2) Tobacco use during pregnancy, childbirth and the puerperium

Codes under subcategory O99.33, Smoking (tobacco) complicating pregnancy, childbirth, and the puerperium, should be assigned for any pregnancy case when a mother uses any type of tobacco product during the pregnancy or postpartum. A secondary code from category F17, Nicotine dependence, or code Z72.0, Tobacco use, should also be assigned **to identify the type of nicotine dependence**.

m. Poisoning, toxic effects, adverse effects and underdosing in a pregnant patient

A code from subcategory O9A.2, Injury, poisoning and certain other consequences of external causes complicating pregnancy, childbirth, and the puerperium, should be sequenced first, followed by the appropriate poisoning, toxic effect, adverse effect or underdosing code, and then the additional code(s) that specifies the condition caused by the poisoning, toxic effect, adverse effect or underdosing.

See Section I.C.19. Adverse effects, poisoning, underdosing and toxic effects.

n. Normal Delivery, Code O80

1) Encounter for full term uncomplicated delivery
Code O80 should be assigned when a woman is admitted for a full-term normal delivery and delivers a single, healthy infant without any complications antepartum, during the delivery, or postpartum during the delivery episode. Code O80 is always a principal diagnosis. It is not to be used if any other code from chapter 15 is needed to describe a current complication of the antenatal, delivery, or perinatal period. Additional codes from other chapters may be used with code O80 if they are not related to or are in any way complicating the pregnancy.

2) Uncomplicated delivery with resolved antepartum complication
Code O80 may be used if the patient had a complication at some point during the pregnancy, but the complication is not present at the time of the admission for delivery.

3) Outcome of delivery for O80
Z37.0, Single live birth, is the only outcome of delivery code appropriate for use with O80.

o. The Peripartum and Postpartum Periods

1) Peripartum and Postpartum periods
The postpartum period begins immediately after delivery and continues for six weeks following delivery. The peripartum period is defined as the last month of pregnancy to five months postpartum.

2) Peripartum and postpartum complication
A postpartum complication is any complication occurring within the six-week period.

3) Pregnancy-related complications after 6 week period
Chapter 15 codes may also be used to describe pregnancy-related complications after the peripartum or

postpartum period if the provider documents that a condition is pregnancy related.

4) Admission for routine postpartum care following delivery outside hospital

When the mother delivers outside the hospital prior to admission and is admitted for routine postpartum care and no complications are noted, code Z39.0, Encounter for care and examination of mother immediately after delivery, should be assigned as the principal diagnosis.

5) Pregnancy associated cardiomyopathy

Pregnancy associated cardiomyopathy, code O90.3, is unique in that it may be diagnosed in the third trimester of pregnancy but may continue to progress months after delivery. For this reason, it is referred to as peripartum cardiomyopathy. Code O90.3 is only for use when the cardiomyopathy develops as a result of pregnancy in a woman who did not have pre-existing heart disease.

p. Code O94, Sequelae of complication of pregnancy, childbirth, and the puerperium

1) Code O94

Code O94, Sequelae of complication of pregnancy, childbirth, and the puerperium, is for use in those cases when an initial complication of a pregnancy develops a sequelae requiring care or treatment at a future date.

2) After the initial postpartum period

This code may be used at any time after the initial postpartum period.

3) Sequencing of Code O94

This code, like all late effect codes, is to be sequenced following the code describing the sequelae of the complication.

q. Abortions

1) Abortion with Liveborn Fetus

When an attempted termination of pregnancy results in a liveborn fetus, assign a code from subcategory O60.1, Preterm labor with preterm delivery, and a code from category Z37, Outcome of Delivery. The procedure code for the attempted termination of pregnancy should also be assigned.

2) Retained Products of Conception following an abortion

Subsequent encounters for retained products of conception following a spontaneous abortion or elective termination of pregnancy are assigned the appropriate code from category O03, Spontaneous abortion, or **codes O07.4, Failed attempted termination of pregnancy without complication and** Z33.2, Encounter for elective termination of pregnancy. This advice is appropriate even when the patient was discharged previously with a discharge diagnosis of complete abortion.

r. *Abuse in a pregnant patient*

For suspected or confirmed cases of abuse of a pregnant patient, a code(s) from subcategories O9A.3, Physical abuse complicating pregnancy, childbirth, and the puerperium, O9A.4, Sexual abuse complicating pregnancy, childbirth, and the puerperium, and O9A.5, Psychological abuse complicating pregnancy, childbirth, and the puerperium, should be sequenced first, followed by the appropriate codes (if applicable) to identify any associated current injury due to physical abuse, sexual abuse, and the perpetrator of abuse.

See Section I.C.19.f. Adult and child abuse, neglect and other maltreatment.

16. Chapter 16: Newborn (Perinatal) Guidelines (P00-P96)

For coding and reporting purposes the perinatal period is defined as before birth through the 28th day following birth. The following guidelines are provided for reporting purposes

a. General Perinatal Rules

1) Use of Chapter 16 Codes

Codes in this chapter are <u>never</u> for use on the maternal record. Codes from Chapter 15, the obstetric chapter, are never permitted on the newborn record. Chapter 16 **codes** may be used throughout the life of the patient if the condition is still present.

2) Principal Diagnosis for Birth Record

When coding the birth episode in a newborn record, assign a code from category Z38, Liveborn **infants** according to place of birth and type of delivery, as the principal diagnosis. A code from category Z38 is assigned only once, to a newborn at the time of birth. If a newborn is transferred to another institution, a code from category Z38 should not be used at the receiving hospital.

A code from category Z38 is used only on the newborn record, not on the mother's record.

3) Use of Codes from other Chapters with Codes from Chapter 16

Codes from other chapters may be used with codes from chapter 16 if the codes from the other chapters provide more specific detail. Codes for signs and symptoms may be assigned when a definitive diagnosis has not been established. If the reason for the encounter is a perinatal condition, the code from chapter 16 should be sequenced first.

4) Use of Chapter 16 Codes after the Perinatal Period

Should a condition originate in the perinatal period, and continue throughout the life of the patient, the perinatal code should continue to be used regardless of the patient's age.

5) Birth process or community acquired conditions

If a newborn has a condition that may be either due to the birth process or community acquired and the documentation does not indicate which it is, the default is due to the birth process and the code from Chapter 16 should be used.   If the condition is community-acquired, a code from Chapter 16 should not be assigned.

6) Code all clinically significant conditions

All clinically significant conditions noted on routine newborn examination should be coded. A condition is clinically significant if it requires:
- clinical evaluation; or
- therapeutic treatment; or
- diagnostic procedures; or
- extended length of hospital stay; or
- increased nursing care and/or monitoring; or
- has implications for future health care needs

Note: The perinatal guidelines listed above are the same as the general coding guidelines for "additional diagnoses", except for the final point regarding implications for future health care needs. Codes should be assigned for conditions that have been specified by the provider as having implications for future health care needs.

b. **Observation and Evaluation of Newborns for Suspected Conditions not Found**

Assign a code from categories P00-P04 to identify those instances when a healthy newborn is evaluated for a suspected condition that is determined after study not to be present. Do not use a code from categories P00-P04 when the patient has identified signs or symptoms of a suspected problem; in such cases, code the sign or symptom.

c. **Coding Additional Perinatal Diagnoses**

1) **Assigning codes for conditions that require treatment**

Assign codes for conditions that require treatment or further investigation, prolong the length of stay, or require resource utilization.

2) **Codes for conditions specified as having implications for future health care needs**

Assign codes for conditions that have been specified by the provider as having implications for future health care needs.

Note: This guideline should not be used for adult patients.

d. **Prematurity and Fetal Growth Retardation**

Providers utilize different criteria in determining prematurity. A code for prematurity should not be assigned unless it is documented. Assignment of codes in categories P05, Disorders of newborn related to slow fetal growth and fetal malnutrition, and P07, Disorders of newborn related to short gestation and low birth weight, not elsewhere classified, should be based on the recorded birth weight and estimated gestational age. Codes from category P05 should not be assigned with codes from category P07.

When both birth weight and gestational age are available, two codes from category P07 should be assigned, with the code for birth weight sequenced before the code for gestational age.

e. **Low birth weight and immaturity status**

Codes from **category P07, Disorders of newborn related to short gestation and low birth weight, not elsewhere classified, are for use for a child or adult who was premature** or had a low birth weight as a newborn and this is affecting the patient's current health status.

See Section I.C.21. Factors influencing health status and contact with health services, Status.

f. Bacterial Sepsis of Newborn

Category P36, Bacterial sepsis of newborn, includes congenital sepsis. If a perinate is documented as having sepsis without documentation of congenital or community acquired, the default is congenital and a code from category P36 should be assigned. If the P36 code includes the causal organism, an additional code from category B95, Streptococcus, Staphylococcus, and Enterococcus as the cause of diseases classified elsewhere, or B96, Other bacterial agents as the cause of diseases classified elsewhere, should not be assigned. If the P36 code does not include the causal organism, assign an additional code from category B96. If applicable, use additional codes to identify severe sepsis (R65.2-) and any associated acute organ dysfunction.

g. Stillbirth

Code P95, Stillbirth, is only for use in institutions that maintain separate records for stillbirths. No other code should be used with P95. Code P95 should not be used on the mother's record.

17. Chapter 17: Congenital malformations, deformations, and chromosomal abnormalities (Q00-Q99)

Assign an appropriate code(s) from categories Q00-Q99, Congenital malformations, deformations, and chromosomal abnormalities when a malformation/deformation or chromosomal abnormality is documented. A malformation/deformation/or chromosomal abnormality may be the principal/**first-listed** diagnosis on a record or a secondary diagnosis.

When a malformation/deformation/or chromosomal abnormality does not have a unique code assignment, assign additional code(s) for any manifestations that may be present.

When the code assignment specifically identifies the malformation/deformation/or chromosomal abnormality, manifestations that are an inherent component of the anomaly should not be coded separately. Additional codes should be assigned for manifestations that are not an inherent component.

Codes from Chapter 17 may be used throughout the life of the patient. If a congenital malformation or deformity has been corrected, a personal history code should be used to identify the history of the malformation or deformity. Although present at birth, malformation/deformation/or chromosomal abnormality may not be identified until later in life. Whenever the condition is diagnosed by the physician, it is appropriate to assign a code from codes Q00-Q99.

For the birth admission, the appropriate code from category Z38, Liveborn infants, according to place of birth and type of delivery, should be sequenced as the principal diagnosis, followed by any congenital anomaly codes, Q00-**Q99**.

18. Chapter 18: Symptoms, signs, and abnormal clinical and laboratory findings, not elsewhere classified (R00-R99)

Chapter 18 includes symptoms, signs, abnormal results of clinical or other investigative procedures, and ill-defined conditions regarding which no diagnosis classifiable elsewhere is recorded. Signs and symptoms that point to a **specific** diagnosis have been assigned to a category in other chapters of the classification.

a. Use of symptom codes

Codes that describe symptoms and signs are acceptable for reporting purposes when a related definitive diagnosis has not been established (confirmed) by the provider.

b. Use of a symptom code with a definitive diagnosis code

Codes for signs and symptoms may be reported in addition to a related definitive diagnosis when the sign or symptom is not routinely associated with that diagnosis, such as the various signs and symptoms associated with complex syndromes. The definitive diagnosis code should be sequenced before the symptom code.

Signs or symptoms that are associated routinely with a disease process should not be assigned as additional codes, unless otherwise instructed by the classification.

c. Combination codes that include symptoms

ICD-10-CM contains a number of combination codes that identify both the definitive diagnosis and common symptoms of that diagnosis. When using one of these combination codes, an additional code should not be assigned for the symptom.

d. Repeated falls

Code R29.6, Repeated falls, is for use for encounters when a patient has recently fallen and the reason for the fall is being investigated.

Code Z91.81, History of falling, is for use when a patient has fallen in the past and is at risk for future falls. When appropriate, both codes R29.6 and Z91.81 may be assigned together.

e.   *Coma* scale

The coma scale codes (R40.2-) can be used in conjunction with traumatic brain injury codes, **acute cerebrovascular disease** or sequelae of cerebrovascular **disease** codes. These codes are primarily for use by trauma registries, but they may be used in any setting where this information is collected. The coma scale codes should be sequenced after the diagnosis code**(s)**.

These codes, one from each subcategory, are needed to complete the scale. The 7th character indicates when the scale was recorded. The 7th character should match for all three codes.

At a minimum, report the initial score documented on presentation at your facility. This may be a score from the emergency medicine technician (EMT) or in the emergency department. If desired, a facility may choose to capture multiple Glasgow coma scale scores.

f.   **Functional quadriplegia**

Functional quadriplegia (code R53.2) is the lack of ability to use one's limbs or to ambulate due to extreme debility. It is not associated with neurologic deficit or injury, and code R53.2 should not be used for cases of neurologic quadriplegia. It should only be assigned if functional quadriplegia is specifically documented in the medical record.

g.   **SIRS due to Non-Infectious Process**

The systemic inflammatory response syndrome (SIRS) can develop as a result of certain non-infectious disease processes, such as trauma, malignant neoplasm, or pancreatitis. When SIRS is documented with a noninfectious condition, and no subsequent infection is documented, the code for the underlying condition, such as an injury, should be assigned, followed by code R65.10, Systemic inflammatory response syndrome (SIRS) of non-infectious origin without acute organ dysfunction, or code R65.11, Systemic inflammatory response syndrome (SIRS) of non-infectious origin with acute organ dysfunction. If an associated acute organ dysfunction is documented, the appropriate code(s) for the specific type of organ dysfunction(s) should be assigned in addition to code R65.11. If acute organ dysfunction is documented, but it cannot be determined if the acute organ dysfunction is associated with SIRS or due to another condition (e.g., directly due to the trauma), the provider should be queried.

g.   **Death NOS**

Code R99, Ill-defined and unknown cause of mortality, is only for use in the very limited circumstance when a patient who has already died is brought into an emergency department or other healthcare facility and is pronounced dead upon arrival. It does not represent the discharge disposition of death.

19. Chapter 19: Injury, poisoning, and certain other consequences of external causes (S00-T88)

a. Code Extensions

Most categories in chapter 19 have 7th character extensions that are required for each applicable code. Most categories in this chapter have three extensions (with the exception of fractures): A, initial encounter, D, subsequent encounter and S, sequela.

Extension "A", initial encounter is used while the patient is receiving active treatment for the injury. Examples of active treatment are: surgical treatment, emergency department encounter, and evaluation and treatment by a new physician.

Extension "D" subsequent encounter is used for encounters after the patient has received active treatment of the injury and is receiving routine care for the injury during the healing or recovery phase. Examples of subsequent care are: cast change or removal, removal of external **or** internal fixation device, medication adjustment, other aftercare and follow up visits following injury treatment.

The aftercare Z codes should not be used for aftercare for injuries. For aftercare of an injury, assign the acute injury code with the 7th character "D" (subsequent encounter).

Extension "S", sequela, is for use for complications or conditions that arise as a direct result of an injury, such as scar formation after a burn. The scars are sequelae of the burn. When using extension "S", it is necessary to use both the injury code that precipitated the sequela and the code for the sequela itself. The "S" is added only to the injury code, not the sequela code. The "S" extension identifies the injury responsible for the sequela. The specific type of sequela (e.g. scar) is sequenced first, followed by the injury code.

b. Coding of Injuries

When coding injuries, assign separate codes for each injury unless a combination code is provided, in which case the combination code is assigned. **Code T07, Unspecified multiple injuries** should not be assigned unless information for a more specific code is not available. **Traumatic** injury codes (S00-T14.9) are not to be used for normal, healing surgical wounds or to identify complications of surgical wounds.

The code for the most serious injury, as determined by the provider and the focus of treatment, is sequenced first.

1) Superficial injuries

Superficial injuries such as abrasions or contusions are not coded when associated with more severe injuries of the same site.

2) Primary injury with damage to nerves/blood vessels

When a primary injury results in minor damage to peripheral nerves or blood vessels, the primary injury is sequenced first with additional code(s) for injuries to nerves and spinal cord (such as category S04), and/or injury to blood vessels (such as category S15). When the primary injury is to the blood vessels or nerves, that injury should be sequenced first.

c. Coding of Traumatic Fractures

The principles of multiple coding of injuries should be followed in coding fractures. Fractures of specified sites are coded individually by site in accordance with both the provisions within categories S02, S12, S22, S32, S42, S49, S52, S59, S62, S72, S79, S82, S89, S92 and the level of detail furnished by medical record content.

A fracture not indicated as open or closed should be coded to closed. A fracture not indicated whether displaced or not displaced should be coded to displaced.

More specific guidelines are as follows:

1) Initial vs. Subsequent Encounter for Fractures

Traumatic fractures are coded using the appropriate 7th character extension for initial encounter (A, B, C) while the patient is receiving active treatment for the fracture. Examples of active treatment are: surgical treatment, emergency department encounter, and evaluation and treatment by a new physician. **The appropriate 7th character for initial encounter should also be assigned for a patient who delayed seeking treatment for the fracture or nonunion.**

Fractures are coded using the appropriate 7th character extension for subsequent care for encounters after the patient has completed active treatment of the fracture and is receiving routine care for the fracture during the healing or recovery phase. Examples of fracture aftercare are: cast change or removal, removal of external or internal fixation device, medication adjustment, and follow-up visits following fracture treatment.

Care for complications of surgical treatment for fracture repairs during the healing or recovery phase should be coded with the appropriate complication codes.

Care of complications of fractures, such as malunion and nonunion, should be reported with the appropriate 7th character extensions for subsequent care with nonunion (K, M, N,) or subsequent care with malunion (P, Q, R).

A code from category M80, not a traumatic fracture code, should be used for any patient with known osteoporosis who suffers a fracture, even if the patient had a minor fall or trauma, if that fall or trauma would not usually break a normal, healthy bone.
See Section I.C.13. Osteoporosis.

The aftercare Z codes should not be used for aftercare for **traumatic fractures**. For aftercare of **a traumatic fracture**, assign the acute **fracture** code with the **appropriate** 7th character.

2) Multiple fractures sequencing

Multiple fractures are sequenced in accordance with the severity of the fracture.

d. Coding of Burns and Corrosions

The ICD-10-CM **makes a distinction** between burns and corrosions. The burn codes are for thermal burns, except sunburns, that come from a heat source, such as a fire or hot appliance. The burn codes are also for burns resulting from electricity and radiation. Corrosions are burns due to chemicals. The guidelines are the same for burns and corrosions.

Current burns (T20-T25) are classified by depth, extent and by agent (X code). Burns are classified by depth as first degree (erythema), second degree (blistering), and third degree (full-thickness involvement). Burns of the eye and internal organs (T26-T28) are classified by site, but not by degree.

1) Sequencing of burn and related condition codes

Sequence first the code that reflects the highest degree of burn when more than one burn is present.

a. When the reason for the admission or encounter is for treatment of external multiple burns, sequence first the code that reflects the burn of the highest degree.

b. When a patient has both internal and external burns, the circumstances of admission govern the selection of the principal diagnosis or first-listed diagnosis.

c. When a patient is admitted for burn injuries and other related conditions such as smoke inhalation and/or respiratory failure, the circumstances of admission govern the selection of the principal or first-listed diagnosis.

2) **Burns of the same local site**

Classify burns of the same local site (three-**character** category level, T20-T28) but of different degrees to the subcategory identifying the highest degree recorded in the diagnosis.

3) **Non-healing burns**

Non-healing burns are coded as acute burns.
Necrosis of burned skin should be coded as a non-healed burn.

4) **Infected Burn**

For any documented infected burn site, use an additional code for the infection.

5) **Assign separate codes for each burn site**

When coding burns, assign separate codes for each burn site. Category T30, Burn and corrosion, body region unspecified is extremely vague and should rarely be used.

6) **Burns and Corrosions Classified According to Extent of Body Surface Involved**

Assign codes from category T31, Burns classified according to extent of body surface involved, or T32, Corrosions classified according to extent of body surface involved, when the site of the burn is not specified or when there is a need for additional data. It is advisable to use category T31 as additional coding when needed to provide data for evaluating burn mortality, such as that needed by burn units. It is also advisable to use category T31 as an additional code for reporting purposes when there is mention of a third-degree burn involving 20 percent or more of the body surface.

Categories T31 and T32 are based on the classic "rule of nines" in estimating body surface involved: head and neck are assigned nine percent, each arm nine percent, each leg 18 percent, the anterior trunk 18 percent, posterior trunk 18 percent, and genitalia one percent. Providers may change these percentage assignments where necessary to accommodate infants and children who have proportionately larger heads than adults, and patients who have large buttocks, thighs, or abdomen that involve burns.

7) **Encounters for treatment of late effects of burns**

Encounters for the treatment of the late effects of burns or corrosions (i.e., scars or joint contractures) should be coded with a burn or corrosion code with the 7th character "S" **for** sequela.

8) **Sequelae with a late effect code and current burn**

When appropriate, both a code for a current burn or corrosion with 7th character extension "A" or "D" and a burn or corrosion code with extension "S" may be assigned on the same record (when both a current burn and sequelae of an old burn exist). Burns and corrosions do not heal at the same rate and a current healing wound may still exist with sequela of a healed burn or corrosion.

9) **Use of an external cause code with burns and corrosions**

An external cause code should be used with burns and corrosions to identify the source and intent of the burn, as well as the place where it occurred.

e. **Adverse Effects, Poisoning , Underdosing and Toxic Effects**

Codes in categories T36-T65 are combination codes that include the substances related to adverse effects, poisonings, toxic effects and underdosing, as well as the external cause. No additional external cause code is required for poisonings, toxic effects, adverse effects and underdosing codes.

A code from categories T36-T65 is sequenced first, followed by the code(s) that specify the nature of the adverse effect, poisoning, or toxic effect. Note: This sequencing instruction does not apply to underdosing codes (fifth or sixth character "6", for example T36.0x6-).

1) **Do not code directly from the Table of Drugs**

Do not code directly from the Table of Drugs and Chemicals. Always refer back to the Tabular List.

2) Use as many codes as necessary to describe

Use as many codes as necessary to describe completely all drugs, medicinal or biological substances.

3) If the same code would describe the causative agent

If the same code would describe the causative agent for more than one adverse reaction, poisoning, toxic effect or underdosing, assign the code only once.

4) If two or more drugs, medicinal or biological substances

If two or more drugs, medicinal or biological substances are reported, code each individually unless **a** combination code is listed in the Table of Drugs and Chemicals.

5) The occurrence of drug toxicity is classified in ICD-10-CM as follows:

(a) **Adverse Effect**

Assign the appropriate code for adverse effect (for example, T36.0x5-) when the drug was correctly prescribed and properly administered. Use additional code(s) for all manifestations of adverse effects. Examples of manifestations are tachycardia, delirium, gastrointestinal hemorrhaging, vomiting, hypokalemia, hepatitis, renal failure, or respiratory failure.

(b) **Poisoning**

When coding a poisoning or reaction to the improper use of a medication (e.g., overdose, wrong substance given or taken in error, wrong route of administration), assign the appropriate code from categories T36-T50. Poisoning codes have an associated intent: accidental, intentional self-harm, assault and undetermined. Use additional code(s) for all manifestations of poisonings.

If there is also a diagnosis of abuse or dependence on the substance, the abuse or dependence is coded as an additional code.

Examples of poisoning include:

(i)   Error was made in drug prescription

Errors made in drug prescription or in the administration of the drug by provider, nurse, patient, or other person.

(ii)   Overdose of a drug intentionally taken

If an overdose of a drug was intentionally taken or administered and resulted in drug toxicity, it would be coded as a poisoning.

(iii)   Nonprescribed drug taken with correctly prescribed and properly administered drug

If a nonprescribed drug or medicinal agent was taken in combination with a correctly prescribed and properly administered drug, any drug toxicity or other reaction resulting from the interaction of the two drugs would be classified as a poisoning.

(iv)   Interaction of drug(s) and alcohol

When a reaction results from the interaction of a drug(s) and alcohol, this would be classified as poisoning.

See Section I.C.4. if poisoning is the result of insulin pump malfunctions.

(c)   **Underdosing**

Underdosing refers to taking less of a medication than is prescribed by a provider or a manufacturer's instruction. For underdosing, assign the code from categories T36-T50 (fifth or sixth character "6").

Codes for underdosing should never be assigned as principal or first-listed codes. If a patient has a relapse or exacerbation of the medical condition for which the drug is prescribed because of the reduction in dose, then the medical condition itself should be coded.

Noncompliance (Z91.12-, Z91.13-) or complication of care (Y63.61, Y63.8-Y63.9) codes are to be used with an underdosing code to indicate intent, if known.

(d) **Toxic Effects**

When a harmful substance is ingested or comes in contact with a person, this is classified as a toxic effect. The toxic effect codes are in categories T51-T65.

Toxic effect codes have an associated intent: accidental, intentional self-harm, assault and undetermined.

f. Adult and child abuse, neglect and other maltreatment

Sequence first the appropriate code from categories T74.- **(Adult and child abuse, neglect and other maltreatment, confirmed)** or T76.- **(Adult and child abuse, neglect and other maltreatment, suspected)** for abuse, neglect and other maltreatment, followed by any accompanying mental health or injury code(s).

If the documentation in the medical record states abuse or neglect it is coded as confirmed **(T74.-)**. It is coded as suspected if it is documented as suspected **(T76.-)**.

For cases of confirmed abuse or neglect an external cause code from the assault section (X92-Y08) should be added to identify the cause of any physical injuries. A perpetrator code (Y07) should be added when the perpetrator of the abuse is known. For suspected cases of abuse or neglect, do not report external cause or perpetrator code.

If a suspected case of abuse, neglect or mistreatment is ruled out during an encounter code Z04.71, Suspected adult physical and sexual abuse, ruled out, or code Z04.72, Suspected child physical and sexual abuse, ruled out, should be used, not a code from T76.

See Section I.C.15.r Abuse in a pregnant patient.

g. Complications of care

1) Complications of care

(a) **Documentation of complications of care**

As with all procedural or postprocedural complications, code assignment is based on the provider's documentation of the relationship between the condition and the procedure.

2) Pain due to medical devices

Pain associated with devices, implants or grafts left in a surgical site (for example painful hip prosthesis) is assigned to the appropriate code(s) found in Chapter 19, Injury, poisoning, and certain other consequences of external causes. Specific codes for pain due to medical devices are found in the T code section of the ICD-10-CM. Use additional code(s) from category G89 to identify acute or chronic pain due to presence of the device, implant or graft (G89.18 or G89.28).

3) Transplant complications

(a) Transplant complications other than kidney

Codes under category T86, Complications of transplanted organs and tissues, are for use for both complications and rejection of transplanted organs. A transplant complication code is only assigned if the complication affects the function of the transplanted organ. Two codes are required to fully describe a transplant complication: the appropriate code from category T86 and a secondary code that identifies the complication.

Pre-existing conditions or conditions that develop after the transplant are not coded as complications unless they affect the function of the transplanted organs.

See I.C.21.c.3 for transplant organ removal status
See I.C.2.r for malignant neoplasm associated with transplanted organ.

(b) Chronic kidney disease and kidney transplant complications

Patients who have undergone kidney transplant may still have some form of chronic kidney disease (CKD) because the kidney transplant may not fully restore kidney function. Code T86.1- should be assigned for documented complications of a kidney transplant, such as transplant failure or rejection or other transplant complication. Code T86.1- should not be assigned for post kidney transplant patients who have chronic kidney (CKD) unless a transplant complication such as transplant failure or rejection is documented. If the documentation is unclear as to whether the patient has a complication of the transplant, query the provider.

For patients with CKD following a kidney transplant, but who do not have a complication such as failure or rejection, *see section I.C.14. Chronic kidney disease and kidney transplant status*.

4) Complication codes that include the external cause

As with certain other T codes, some of the complications of care codes have the external cause included in the code. The code includes the nature of the complication as well as the type of procedure that caused the complication. No external cause code indicating the type of procedure is necessary for these codes.

5) Complications of care codes within the body system chapters

Intraoperative and postprocedural complication codes are found within the body system chapters with codes specific to the organs and structures of that body system. These codes should be sequenced first, followed by a code(s) for the specific complication, if applicable.

20. Chapter 20: External Causes of Morbidity (V01-Y99)

Introduction: These guidelines are provided for the reporting of external causes of morbidity codes in order that there will be standardization in the process. These codes are secondary codes for use in any health care setting.

External cause codes are intended to provide data for injury research and evaluation of injury prevention strategies. These codes capture how the injury or health condition happened (cause), the intent (unintentional or accidental; or intentional, such as suicide or assault), the place where the event occurred the activity of the patient at the time of the event, and the person's status (e.g., civilian, military).

a. General External Cause Coding Guidelines

1) Used with any code in the range of A00.0-T88.9, Z00-Z99

An external cause code may be used with any code in the range of A00.0-T88.9, Z00-Z99, classification that is a health condition due to an external cause. Though they are most applicable to injuries, they are also valid for use with such things as infections or diseases due to an external source, and other health conditions, such as a heart attack that occurs during strenuous physical activity.

2) **External cause code used for length of treatment**

Assign the external cause code, with the appropriate 7th character (initial encounter, subsequent encounter or sequela) for each encounter for which the injury or condition is being treated.

3) **Use the full range of external cause codes**

Use the full range of external cause codes to completely describe the cause, the intent, the place of occurrence, and if applicable, the activity of the patient at the time of the event, and the patient's status, for all injuries, and other health conditions due to an external cause.

4) **Assign as many external cause codes as necessary**

Assign as many external cause codes as necessary to fully explain each cause. If only one external code can be recorded, assign the code most related to the principal diagnosis.

5) **The selection of the appropriate external cause code**

The selection of the appropriate external cause code is guided by the **Alphabetic Index of** External Causes and by Inclusion and Exclusion notes in the Tabular List.

6) **External cause code can never be a principal diagnosis**

An external cause code can never be a principal (**first-listed**) diagnosis.

7) **Combination external cause codes**

Certain of the external cause codes are combination codes that identify sequential events that result in an injury, such as a fall which results in striking against an object. The injury may be due to either event or both. The combination external cause code used should correspond to the sequence of events regardless of which caused the most serious injury.

8) **No external cause code needed in certain circumstances**

No external cause code from Chapter 20 is needed if the external cause and intent are included in a code from another chapter (e.g. **T36.0x1**- Poisoning by penicillins, accidental (unintentional)).

b. **Place of Occurrence Guideline**

Codes from category Y92, Place of occurrence of the external cause, are secondary codes for use after other external cause codes to identify the location of the patient at the time of injury or other condition.

A place of occurrence code is used only once, at the initial encounter for treatment. No 7th characters are used for Y92. Only one code from Y92 should be recorded on a medical record. A place of occurrence code should be used in conjunction with an activity code, Y93.

Do not use place of occurrence code Y92.9 if the place is not stated or is not applicable.

c. **Activity Code**

Assign a code from category Y93, Activity code, to describe the activity of the patient at the time the injury or other health condition occurred.

An activity code is used only once, at the initial encounter for treatment. Only one code from Y93 should be recorded on a medical record. An activity code should be used in conjunction with a place of occurrence code, Y92.

The activity codes are not applicable to poisonings, adverse effects, misadventures or late effects.

Do not assign Y93.9, Unspecified activity, if the activity is not stated.

A code from category Y93 is appropriate for use with external cause and intent codes if identifying the activity provides additional information about the event.

d. **Place of Occurrence, Activity, *and Status* Codes Used with other External Cause Code**

When applicable, place of occurrence, activity, and external cause status codes are sequenced after the main external cause code(s). Regardless of the number of external cause codes assigned, there should be only one place of occurrence code, one activity code, and one external cause status code assigned to an encounter.

e. **If the Reporting Format Limits the Number of External Cause Codes**

If the reporting format limits the number of external cause codes that can be used in reporting clinical data, report the code for the cause/intent most related to the principal diagnosis. If the format permits capture of additional external cause codes, the cause/intent, including medical misadventures, of the additional events should be reported rather than the codes for place, activity, or external status.

f.   Multiple External Cause Coding Guidelines

More than one external cause code is required to fully describe the external cause of an illness **or** injury. The assignment of external cause codes should be sequenced in the following priority:

If two or more events cause separate injuries, an external cause code should be assigned for each cause. The **first-listed** external cause code will be selected in the following order:

External codes for child and adult abuse take priority over all other external cause codes.

See Section I.C.19., Child and Adult abuse guidelines.

External cause codes for terrorism events take priority over all other external cause codes except child and adult abuse.

External cause codes for cataclysmic events take priority over all other external cause codes except child and adult abuse and terrorism.

External cause codes for transport accidents take priority over all other external cause codes except cataclysmic events, child and adult abuse and terrorism.

Activity and external cause status codes are assigned following all causal (intent) external cause codes.

The first-listed external cause code should correspond to the cause of the most serious diagnosis due to an assault, accident, or self-harm, following the order of hierarchy listed above.

g.   Child and Adult Abuse Guideline

Adult and child abuse, neglect and maltreatment are classified as assault. Any of the assault codes may be used to indicate the external cause of any injury resulting from the confirmed abuse.

For confirmed cases of abuse, neglect and maltreatment, when the perpetrator is known, a code from Y07, Perpetrator of maltreatment and neglect, should accompany any other assault codes.

See Section I.C.19. Adult and child abuse, neglect and other maltreatment

h. Unknown or Undetermined Intent Guideline

If the intent (accident, self-harm, assault) of the cause of an injury or other condition is unknown or unspecified, code the intent as accidental intent. All transport accident categories assume accidental intent.

1) Use of undetermined intent

External cause codes for events of undetermined intent are only for use if the documentation in the record specifies that the intent cannot be **determined.**

i. Late Effects of External Cause Guidelines

1) Late effect external cause codes

Late effects are reported using the external cause code with the 7th character extension "S" for sequela. These codes should be used with any report of a late effect or sequela resulting from a previous injury.

2) Late effect external cause code with a related current injury

A late effect external cause code should never be used with a related current nature of injury code.

3) Use of late effect external cause codes for subsequent visits

Use a late effect external cause code for subsequent visits when a late effect of the initial injury is being treated. Do not use a late effect external cause code for subsequent visits for follow-up care (e.g., to assess healing, to receive rehabilitative therapy) of the injury when no late effect of the injury has been documented.

j. Terrorism Guidelines

1) Cause of injury identified by the Federal Government (FBI) as terrorism

When the cause of an injury is identified by the Federal Government (FBI) as terrorism, the first-listed external cause code should be a code from category Y38, Terrorism. The definition of terrorism employed by the FBI is found at the inclusion note at the beginning of category Y38. Use additional code for place of occurrence (Y92.-). More than one Y38 code may be assigned if the injury is the result of more than one mechanism of terrorism.

2) **Cause of an injury is suspected to be the result of terrorism**

When the cause of an injury is suspected to be the result of terrorism a code from category Y38 should not be assigned. Suspected cases should be classified as assault.

3) **Code Y38.9, Terrorism, secondary effects**

Assign code Y38.9, Terrorism, secondary effects, for conditions occurring subsequent to the terrorist event. This code should not be assigned for conditions that are due to the initial terrorist act.

It is acceptable to assign code Y38.9 with another code from Y38 if there is an injury due to the initial terrorist event and an injury that is a subsequent result of the terrorist event.

k. **External cause status**

A code from category Y99, External cause status, should be assigned whenever any other external cause code is assigned for an encounter, including an Activity code, except for the events noted below. Assign a code from category Y99, External cause status, to indicate the work status of the person at the time the event occurred. The status code indicates whether the event occurred during military activity, whether a non-military person was at work, whether an individual including a student or volunteer was involved in a non-work activity at the time of the causal event.

A code from Y99, External cause status, should be assigned, when applicable, with other external cause codes, such as transport accidents and falls. The external cause status codes are not applicable to poisonings, adverse effects, misadventures or late effects.
Do not assign a code from category Y99 if no other external cause codes (cause, activity) are applicable for the encounter.

An external cause status code is used only once, at the initial encounter for treatment. Only one code from Y99 should be recorded on a medical record.

Do not assign code Y99.9, Unspecified external cause status, if the status is not stated.

21. **Chapter 21: Factors influencing health status and contact with health services (Z00-Z99)**

Note: The chapter specific guidelines provide additional information about the use of Z codes for specified encounters.

a. **Use of Z codes in any healthcare setting**

Z codes are for use in any healthcare setting. Z codes may be used as either a **first-listed** (principal diagnosis code in the inpatient setting) or secondary code, depending on the circumstances of the encounter. Certain Z codes may only be used as **first-listed** or principal diagnosis.

b. **Z Codes indicate a reason for an encounter**

Z codes are not procedure codes. A corresponding procedure code must accompany a Z code to describe **any** procedure performed.

c. **Categories of Z Codes**

1) **Contact/Exposure**

Category Z20 indicates contact with, and suspected exposure to, communicable diseases. These codes are for patients who do not show any sign or symptom of a disease but are suspected to have been exposed to it by close personal contact with an infected individual or are in an area where a disease is epidemic.

Category Z77, indicates contact with and suspected exposures hazardous to health.

Contact/exposure codes may be used as a **first-listed** code to explain an encounter for testing, or, more commonly, as a secondary code to identify a potential risk.

2) **Inoculations and vaccinations**

Code Z23 is for encounters for inoculations and vaccinations. It indicates that a patient is being seen to receive a prophylactic inoculation against a disease. Procedure codes are required to identify the actual administration of the injection and the type(s) of immunizations given. Code Z23 may be used as a secondary code if the inoculation is given as a routine part of preventive health care, such as a well-baby visit.

3) **Status**

Status codes indicate that a patient is either a carrier of a disease or has the sequelae or residual of a past disease or condition. This includes such things as the presence of prosthetic or mechanical devices resulting from past treatment. A status code is informative, because the status may affect the course of treatment and its outcome. A status code is distinct from a history code. The history code indicates that the patient no longer has the condition.

A status code should not be used with a diagnosis code from one of the body system chapters, if the diagnosis code includes the information provided by the status code. For example, code Z94.1, Heart transplant status, should not be used with a code from subcategory T86.2, Complications of heart transplant. The status code does not provide additional information. The complication code indicates that the patient is a heart transplant patient.

For encounters for weaning from a mechanical ventilator, assign **a** code **from subcategory** J96.1, Chronic respiratory failure, followed by code Z99.11, Dependence on respirator [ventilator] status.

The status Z codes/categories are:

Z14   Genetic carrier
        Genetic carrier status indicates that a person carries a gene, associated with a particular disease, which may be passed to offspring who may develop that disease. The person does not have the disease and is not at risk of developing the disease.

Z15   Genetic susceptibility to disease
        Genetic susceptibility indicates that a person has a gene that increases the risk of that person developing the disease.

        Codes from category Z15 should not be used as principal or first-listed codes. If the patient has the condition to which he/she is susceptible, and that condition is the reason for the encounter, the code for the current condition should be sequenced first. If the patient is being seen for follow-up after completed treatment for this condition, and the condition no longer exists, a follow-up code should be sequenced first, followed by the appropriate personal history and genetic susceptibility codes. If the purpose of the encounter is genetic counseling associated with procreative management, code Z31.5, Encounter for genetic counseling, should be assigned as the first-listed code, followed by a code from category Z15. Additional codes should be assigned for any applicable family or personal history.

Z16   Infection with drug-resistant microorganisms
This code indicates that a patient has an infection that is resistant to drug treatment. Sequence the infection code first.

Z17   Estrogen receptor status

Z18   **Retained foreign body fragments**

Z21   Asymptomatic HIV infection status
This code indicates that a patient has tested positive for HIV but has manifested no signs or symptoms of the disease.

Z22   Carrier of infectious disease
Carrier status indicates that a person harbors the specific organisms of a disease without manifest symptoms and is capable of transmitting the infection.

Z28.3   Underimmunization status

Z33.1   Pregnant state, incidental
This code is a secondary code only for use when the pregnancy is in no way complicating the reason for visit. Otherwise, a code from the obstetric chapter is required.

Z66   Do not resuscitate
This code may be used when it is documented by the provider that a patient is on do not resuscitate status at any time during the stay.

Z67   Blood type

Z68   Body mass index (BMI)

Z74.01   Bed confinement status

Z76.82   Awaiting organ transplant status

Z78   Other specified health status
Code Z78.1, Physical restraint status, may be used when it is documented by the provider that a patient has been put in restraints during the current encounter. Please note that this code should not be reported when it is documented by the provider that a patient is temporarily restrained during a procedure.

Z79   Long-term (current) drug therapy
Codes from this category indicate a patient's continuous use of a prescribed drug (including such things as aspirin therapy) for the long-term treatment of a condition or for prophylactic use. It is not for use for patients who have addictions to drugs. This subcategory is not for use of medications for detoxification or maintenance programs to prevent withdrawal symptoms in patients with drug dependence (e.g., methadone maintenance for opiate dependence). Assign the appropriate code for the drug dependence instead.

Assign a code from Z79 if the patient is receiving a medication for an extended period as a prophylactic measure (such as for the prevention of deep vein thrombosis) or as treatment of a chronic condition (such as arthritis) or a disease requiring a lengthy course of treatment (such as cancer). Do not assign a code from category Z79 for medication being administered for a brief period of time to treat an acute illness or injury (such as a course of antibiotics to treat acute bronchitis).

Z88   Allergy status to drugs, medicaments and biological substances
Except: Z88.9, Allergy status to unspecified drugs, medicaments and biological substances status

Z89   Acquired absence of limb

Z90   Acquired absence of organs, not elsewhere classified

Z91.0-   Allergy status, other than to drugs and biological substances

Z92.82   Status post administration of tPA (rtPA) in a different facility within the last 24 hours prior to admission to a current facility

Assign code Z92.82, Status post administration of tPA (rtPA) in a different facility within the last 24 hours prior to admission to current facility, as a secondary diagnosis when a patient is received by transfer into a facility and documentation indicates they were administered tissue plasminogen activator (tPA) within the last 24 hours prior to admission to the current facility.

This guideline applies even if the patient is still receiving the tPA at the time they are received into the current facility.

The appropriate code for the condition for which the tPA was administered (such as cerebrovascular disease or myocardial infarction) should be assigned first.

Code Z92.82 is only applicable to the receiving facility record and not to the transferring facility record.

Z93	Artificial opening status
Z94	Transplanted organ and tissue status
Z95	Presence of cardiac and vascular implants and grafts
Z96	Presence of other functional implants
Z97	Presence of other devices
Z98	Other postprocedural states

Assign code Z98.85, Transplanted organ removal status, to indicate that a transplanted organ has been previously removed. This code should not be assigned for the encounter in which the transplanted organ is removed. The complication necessitating removal of the transplant organ should be assigned for that encounter.

See section I.C19.g.3. for information on the coding of organ transplant complications.

Z99	Dependence on enabling machines and devices, not elsewhere classified

Note: Categories Z89-Z90 and Z93-Z99 are for use only if there are no complications or malfunctions of the organ or tissue replaced, the amputation site or the equipment on which the patient is dependent.

4) **History (of)**

There are two types of history Z codes, personal and family. Personal history codes explain a patient's past medical condition that no longer exists and is not receiving any treatment, but that has the potential for recurrence, and therefore may require continued monitoring.

Family history codes are for use when a patient has a family member(s) who has had a particular disease that causes the patient to be at higher risk of also contracting the disease.

Personal history codes may be used in conjunction with follow-up codes and family history codes may be used in conjunction with screening codes to explain the need for a test or procedure. History codes are also acceptable on any medical record regardless of the reason for visit. A history of an illness, even if no longer present, is important information that may alter the type of treatment ordered.

The history Z code categories are:
Z80	Family history of primary malignant neoplasm
Z81	Family history of mental and behavioral disorders
Z82	Family history of certain disabilities and chronic diseases (leading to disablement)
Z83	Family history of other specific disorders
Z84	Family history of other conditions
Z85	Personal history of malignant neoplasm
Z86	Personal history of certain other diseases
Z87	Personal history of other diseases and conditions
Z91.4-	Personal history of psychological trauma, not elsewhere classified
Z91.5	Personal history of self-harm
Z91.8-	Other specified personal risk factors, not elsewhere classified
Z92	Personal history of medical treatment Except: Z92.0, Personal history of contraception Except: Z92.82, Status post administration of tPA (rtPA) in a different facility within the last 24 hours prior to admission to a current facility

5) **Screening**

Screening is the testing for disease or disease precursors in seemingly well individuals so that early detection and treatment can be provided for those who test positive for the disease (e.g., screening mammogram).

The testing of a person to rule out or confirm a suspected diagnosis because the patient has some sign or symptom is a diagnostic examination, not a screening. In these cases, the sign or symptom is used to explain the reason for the test.

A screening code may be a **first-listed** code if the reason for the visit is specifically the screening exam. It may also be used as an additional code if the screening is done during an office visit for other health problems. A screening code is not necessary if the screening is inherent to a routine examination, such as a pap smear done during a routine pelvic examination.

Should a condition be discovered during the screening then the code for the condition may be assigned as an additional diagnosis.

The Z code indicates that a screening exam is planned. A procedure code is required to confirm that the screening was performed.

The screening Z codes/categories:

Z11   Encounter for screening for infectious and parasitic diseases
Z12   Encounter for screening for malignant neoplasms
Z13   Encounter for screening for other diseases and disorders
        Except: Z13.9, Encounter for screening, unspecified
Z36   Encounter for antenatal screening for mother

6)   Observation

There are two observation Z code categories. They are for use in very limited circumstances when a person is being observed for a suspected condition that is ruled out. The observation codes are not for use if an injury or illness or any signs or symptoms related to the suspected condition are present. In such cases the diagnosis/symptom code is used with the corresponding external cause code.

The observation codes are to be used as principal diagnosis only. Additional codes may be used in addition to the observation code but only if they are unrelated to the suspected condition being observed.

Codes from subcategory Z03.7, Encounter for suspected maternal and fetal conditions ruled out, may either be used as a **first-listed** or as an additional code assignment depending on the case. They are for use in very limited circumstances on a maternal record when an encounter is for a suspected maternal or fetal condition that is ruled out during that encounter (for example, a maternal or fetal condition may be suspected due to an abnormal test result). These codes should not be used when the condition is confirmed. In those cases, the confirmed condition should be coded. In addition, these codes are not for use if an illness or any signs or symptoms related to the suspected condition or problem are present. In such cases the diagnosis/symptom code is used.

Additional codes may be used in addition to the code from subcategory Z03.7, but only if they are unrelated to the suspected condition being evaluated.

Codes from subcategory Z03.7 may not be used for encounters for antenatal screening of mother. *See Section I.C.21.c.5, Screening.*

For encounters for suspected fetal condition that are inconclusive following testing and evaluation, assign the appropriate code from category O35, O36, O40 or O41. The observation Z code categories:

Z03   Encounter for medical observation for suspected diseases and conditions ruled out

Z04   Encounter for examination and observation for other reasons
Except: Z04.9, Encounter for examination and observation for unspecified reason

7)   **Aftercare**

Aftercare visit codes cover situations when the initial treatment of a disease has been performed and the patient requires continued care during the healing or recovery phase, or for the long-term consequences of the disease. The aftercare Z code should not be used if treatment is directed at a current, acute disease. The diagnosis code is to be used in these cases. Exceptions to this rule are codes Z51.0, Encounter for antineoplastic radiation therapy, and codes from subcategory Z51.1, Encounter for antineoplastic chemotherapy and immunotherapy. These codes are to be **first-listed**, followed by the diagnosis code when a patient's encounter is solely to receive radiation therapy, chemotherapy, or immunotherapy for the treatment of a neoplasm. If the reason for the encounter is more than one type of antineoplastic therapy, code Z51.0 and a code from subcategory Z51.1 may be assigned together, in which case one of these codes would be reported as a secondary diagnosis.

The aftercare Z codes should also not be used for aftercare for injuries. For aftercare of an injury, assign the acute injury code with the **appropriate** 7th character (**for** subsequent encounter).

The aftercare codes are generally **first-listed** to explain the specific reason for the encounter. An aftercare code may be used as an additional code when some type of aftercare is provided in addition to the reason for admission and no diagnosis code is applicable. An example of this would be the closure of a colostomy during an encounter for treatment of another condition.

Aftercare codes should be used in conjunction with other aftercare codes or diagnosis codes to provide better detail on the specifics of an aftercare encounter visit, unless otherwise directed by the classification. Should a patient receive multiple types of antineoplastic therapy during the same encounter, code Z51.0, Encounter for antineoplastic radiation therapy, and codes from subcategory Z51.1, Encounter for antineoplastic chemotherapy and immunotherapy, may be used together on a record. The sequencing of multiple aftercare codes depends on the circumstances of the encounter.

Certain aftercare Z code categories need a secondary diagnosis code to describe the resolving condition or sequelae. For others, the condition is included in the code title.

Additional Z code aftercare category terms include fitting and adjustment, and attention to artificial openings.

Status Z codes may be used with aftercare Z codes to indicate the nature of the aftercare. For example code Z95.1, Presence of aortocoronary bypass graft, may be used with code Z48.812, Encounter for surgical aftercare following surgery on the circulatory system, to indicate the surgery for which the aftercare is being performed. A status code should not be used when the aftercare code indicates the type of status, such as using Z43.0, Encounter for attention to tracheostomy, with Z93.0, Tracheostomy status.

The aftercare Z category/codes:
Z42 Encounter for plastic and reconstructive surgery following medical procedure or healed injury
Z43 Encounter for attention to artificial openings
Z44 Encounter for fitting and adjustment of external prosthetic device
Z45 Encounter for adjustment and management of implanted device
Z46 Encounter for fitting and adjustment of other devices
Z47 Orthopedic aftercare
Z48 Encounter for other postprocedural aftercare
Z49 Encounter for care involving renal dialysis
Z51 Encounter for other aftercare

8) **Follow-up**

The follow-up codes are used to explain continuing surveillance following completed treatment of a disease, condition, or injury. They imply that the condition has been fully treated and no longer exists. They should not be confused with aftercare codes, or injury codes with **a** 7th character **for subsequent encounter,** that explain ongoing care of a healing condition or its sequelae. Follow-up codes may be used in conjunction with history codes to provide the full picture of the healed condition and its treatment. The follow-up code is sequenced first, followed by the history code.

A follow-up code may be used to explain multiple visits. Should a condition be found to have recurred on the follow-up visit, then the **diagnosis** code for the condition should be assigned **in place of the follow-up code**.

The follow-up Z code categories:

Z08   Encounter for follow-up examination after completed treatment for malignant neoplasm

Z09   Encounter for follow-up examination after completed treatment for conditions other than malignant neoplasm

Z39   Encounter for maternal postpartum care and examination

9) **Donor**

Codes in category Z52, Donors of organs and tissues, are used for living individuals who are donating blood or other body tissue. These codes are only for individuals donating for others, not for self-donations. They are not used to identify cadaveric donations.

10) **Counseling**

Counseling Z codes are used when a patient or family member receives assistance in the aftermath of an illness or injury, or when support is required in coping with family or social problems. They are not used in conjunction with a diagnosis code when the counseling component of care is considered integral to standard treatment.

The counseling Z codes/categories:

Z30.0-   Encounter for general counseling and advice on contraception

Z31.5	Encounter for genetic counseling
Z31.6-	Encounter for general counseling and advice on procreation
Z32.2	Encounter for childbirth instruction
Z32.3	Encounter for childcare instruction
Z69	Encounter for mental health services for victim and perpetrator of abuse
Z70	Counseling related to sexual attitude, behavior and orientation
Z71	Persons encountering health services for other counseling and medical advice, not elsewhere classified
Z76.81	Expectant mother prebirth pediatrician visit

11) Encounters for Obstetrical and Reproductive Services

See Section I.C.15. Pregnancy, Childbirth, and the Puerperium, for further instruction on the use of these codes.

Z codes for pregnancy are for use in those circumstances when none of the problems or complications included in the codes from the Obstetrics chapter exist (a routine prenatal visit or postpartum care). Codes in category Z34, Encounter for supervision of normal pregnancy, are always **first-listed** and are not to be used with any other code from the OB chapter.

The outcome of delivery, category Z37, should be included on all maternal delivery records. It is always a secondary code. Codes in category Z37 should not be used on the newborn record.

Z codes for family planning (contraceptive) or procreative management and counseling should be included on an obstetric record either during the pregnancy or the postpartum stage, if applicable.

Z codes/categories for obstetrical and reproductive services:

Z30	Encounter for contraceptive management
Z31	Encounter for procreative management
Z32.2	Encounter for childbirth instruction
Z32.3	Encounter for childcare instruction
Z33	Pregnant state
Z34	Encounter for supervision of normal pregnancy
Z36	Encounter for antenatal screening of mother
Z37	Outcome of delivery
Z39	Encounter for maternal postpartum care and examination
Z76.81	Expectant mother prebirth pediatrician visit

12) Newborns and Infants

See Section I.C.16. Newborn (Perinatal) Guidelines, for further instruction on the use of these codes.

Newborn Z codes/categories:

Z76.1   Encounter for health supervision and care of foundling

Z00.1-   Encounter for routine child health examination

Z38   Liveborn infants according to place of birth and type of delivery

13) Routine and administrative examinations

The Z codes allow for the description of encounters for routine examinations, such as, a general check-up, or, examinations for administrative purposes, such as, a pre-employment physical. The codes are not to be used if the examination is for diagnosis of a suspected condition or for treatment purposes. In such cases the diagnosis code is used. During a routine exam, should a diagnosis or condition be discovered, it should be coded as an additional code. Pre-existing and chronic conditions and history codes may also be included as additional codes as long as the examination is for administrative purposes and not focused on any particular condition.

Some of the codes for routine health examinations distinguish between "with" and "without" abnormal findings. Code assignment depends on the information that is known at the time the encounter is being coded. For example, if no abnormal findings were found during the examination, but the encounter is being coded before test results are back, it is acceptable to assign the code for "without abnormal findings." When assigning a code for "with abnormal findings," additional code(s) should be assigned to identify the specific abnormal finding(s).

Pre-operative examination and pre-procedural laboratory examination Z codes are for use only in those situations when a patient is being cleared for a procedure or surgery and no treatment is given.

The Z codes/categories for routine and administrative examinations:

Z00   Encounter for general examination without complaint, suspected or reported diagnosis

Z01	Encounter for other special examination without complaint, suspected or reported diagnosis
Z02	Encounter for administrative examination Except: Z02.9, Encounter for administrative examinations, unspecified
Z32.0-	Encounter for pregnancy test

14) Miscellaneous Z codes

The miscellaneous Z codes capture a number of other health care encounters that do not fall into one of the other categories. Certain of these codes identify the reason for the encounter; others are for use as additional codes that provide useful information on circumstances that may affect a patient's care and treatment.

Prophylactic Organ Removal

For encounters specifically for prophylactic removal of an organ (such as prophylactic removal of breasts due to a genetic susceptibility to cancer or a family history of cancer), the principal or **first-listed** code should be a code from category Z40, Encounter for prophylactic surgery, followed by the appropriate codes to identify the associated risk factor (such as genetic susceptibility or family history).

If the patient has a malignancy of one site and is having prophylactic removal at another site to prevent either a new primary malignancy or metastatic disease, a code for the malignancy should also be assigned in addition to a code from subcategory Z40.0, Encounter for prophylactic surgery for risk factors related to malignant neoplasms. A Z40.0 code should not be assigned if the patient is having organ removal for treatment of a malignancy, such as the removal of the testes for the treatment of prostate cancer.

Miscellaneous Z codes/categories:

Z28	Immunization not carried out Except: Z28.3, Underimmunization status
Z40	Encounter for prophylactic surgery
Z41	Encounter for procedures for purposes other than remedying health state Except: Z41.9, Encounter for procedure for purposes other than remedying health state, unspecified
Z53	Persons encountering health services for specific procedures and treatment, not carried out
Z55	Problems related to education and literacy
Z56	Problems related to employment and unemployment

Z57	Occupational exposure to risk factors
Z58	Problems related to physical environment
Z59	Problems related to housing and economic circumstances
Z60	Problems related to social environment
Z62	Problems related to upbringing
Z63	Other problems related to primary support group, including family circumstances
Z64	Problems related to certain psychosocial circumstances
Z65	Problems related to other psychosocial circumstances
Z72	Problems related to lifestyle
Z73	Problems related to life management difficulty
Z74	Problems related to care provider dependency Except: Z74.01, Bed confinement status
Z75	Problems related to medical facilities and other health care
Z76.0	Encounter for issue of repeat prescription
Z76.3	Healthy person accompanying sick person
Z76.4	Other boarder to healthcare facility
Z76.5	Malingerer [conscious simulation]
Z91.1-	Patient's noncompliance with medical treatment and regimen
Z91.89	Other specified personal risk factors, not elsewhere classified

15) **Nonspecific Z codes**

Certain Z codes are so non-specific, or potentially redundant with other codes in the classification, that there can be little justification for their use in the inpatient setting. Their use in the outpatient setting should be limited to those instances when there is no further documentation to permit more precise coding. Otherwise, any sign or symptom or any other reason for visit that is captured in another code should be used.

Nonspecific Z codes/categories:

Z02.9	Encounter for administrative examinations, unspecified
Z04.9	Encounter for examination and observation for unspecified reason
Z13.9	Encounter for screening, unspecified
Z41.9	Encounter for procedure for purposes other than remedying health state, unspecified
Z52.9	Donor of unspecified organ or tissue
Z86.59	**Personal history of other mental and behavioral disorders**

| Z88.9 | Allergy status to unspecified drugs, medicaments and biological substances status |
| Z92.0 | Personal history of contraception |

16) **Z Codes That May Only be Principal/First-Listed Diagnosis**

The following Z codes/categories may only be reported as the principal/first-listed diagnosis, except when there are multiple encounters on the same day and the medical records for the encounters are combined:

Z00	Encounter for general examination without complaint, suspected or reported diagnosis
Z01	Encounter for other special examination without complaint, suspected or reported diagnosis
Z02	Encounter for administrative examination
Z03	Encounter for medical observation for suspected diseases and conditions ruled out
Z04	**Encounter for examination and observation for other reasons**
Z33.2	Encounter for elective termination of pregnancy
Z31.81	Encounter for male factor infertility in female patient
Z31.82	Encounter for Rh incompatibility status
Z31.83	Encounter for assisted reproductive fertility procedure cycle
Z31.84	Encounter for fertility preservation procedure
Z34	Encounter for supervision of normal pregnancy
Z39	Encounter for maternal postpartum care and examination
Z38	Liveborn infants according to place of birth and type of delivery
Z42	Encounter for plastic and reconstructive surgery following medical procedure or healed injury
Z51.0	Encounter for antineoplastic radiation therapy
Z51.1-	Encounter for antineoplastic chemotherapy and immunotherapy
Z52	Donors of organs and tissues
	Except: Z52.9, Donor of unspecified organ or tissue
Z76.1	Encounter for health supervision and care of foundling
Z76.2	Encounter for health supervision and care of other healthy infant and child
Z99.12	Encounter for respirator [ventilator] dependence during power failure

Section II. Selection of Principal Diagnosis

The circumstances of inpatient admission always govern the selection of principal diagnosis. The principal diagnosis is defined in the Uniform Hospital Discharge Data Set (UHDDS) as "that condition established after study to be chiefly responsible for occasioning the admission of the patient to the hospital for care."

The UHDDS definitions are used by hospitals to report inpatient data elements in a standardized manner. These data elements and their definitions can be found in the July 31, 1985, Federal Register (Vol. 50, No, 147), pp. 31038-40.

Since that time the application of the UHDDS definitions has been expanded to include all non-outpatient settings (acute care, short term, long term care and psychiatric hospitals; home health agencies; rehab facilities; nursing homes, etc).

In determining principal diagnosis the coding conventions in the ICD-10-CM, **the Tabular List and Alphabetic Index** take precedence over these official coding guidelines. *(See Section I.A., Conventions for the ICD-10-CM)*

The importance of consistent, complete documentation in the medical record cannot be overemphasized. Without such documentation the application of all coding guidelines is a difficult, if not impossible, task.

A. Codes for symptoms, signs, and ill-defined conditions

Codes for symptoms, signs, and ill-defined conditions from Chapter 18 are not to be used as principal diagnosis when a related definitive diagnosis has been established.

B. Two or more interrelated conditions, each potentially meeting the definition for principal diagnosis.

When there are two or more interrelated conditions (such as diseases in the same ICD-10-CM chapter or manifestations characteristically associated with a certain disease) potentially meeting the definition of principal diagnosis, either condition may be sequenced first, unless the circumstances of the admission, the therapy provided, the Tabular List, or the Alphabetic Index indicate otherwise.

C. Two or more diagnoses that equally meet the definition for principal diagnosis

In the unusual instance when two or more diagnoses equally meet the criteria for principal diagnosis as determined by the circumstances of admission, diagnostic workup and/or therapy provided, and the Alphabetic Index, Tabular List, or another coding guidelines does not provide sequencing direction, any one of the diagnoses may be sequenced first.

D. Two or more comparative or contrasting conditions.

In those rare instances when two or more contrasting or comparative diagnoses are documented as "either/or" (or similar terminology), they are coded as if the diagnoses were confirmed and the diagnoses are sequenced according to the circumstances of the admission. If no further determination can be made as to which diagnosis should be principal, either diagnosis may be sequenced first.

E. A symptom(s) followed by contrasting/comparative diagnoses

When a symptom(s) is followed by contrasting/comparative diagnoses, the symptom code is sequenced first. All the contrasting/comparative diagnoses should be coded as additional diagnoses.

F. Original treatment plan not carried out

Sequence as the principal diagnosis the condition, which after study occasioned the admission to the hospital, even though treatment may not have been carried out due to unforeseen circumstances.

G. Complications of surgery and other medical care

When the admission is for treatment of a complication resulting from surgery or other medical care, the complication code is sequenced as the principal diagnosis. If the complication is classified to the T80-T88 series and the code lacks the necessary specificity in describing the complication, an additional code for the specific complication should be assigned.

H. Uncertain Diagnosis

If the diagnosis documented at the time of discharge is qualified as "probable", "suspected", "likely", "questionable", "possible", or "still to be ruled out", or other similar terms indicating uncertainty, code the condition as if it existed or was established. The bases for these guidelines are the diagnostic workup, arrangements for further workup or observation, and initial therapeutic approach that correspond most closely with the established diagnosis.

Note: This guideline is applicable only to inpatient admissions to short-term, acute, long-term care and psychiatric hospitals.

I. Admission from Observation Unit

1. Admission Following Medical Observation

When a patient is admitted to an observation unit for a medical condition, which either worsens or does not improve, and is subsequently admitted as an inpatient of the same hospital for this same medical condition, the principal diagnosis would be the medical condition which led to the hospital admission.

2. **Admission Following Post-Operative Observation**

When a patient is admitted to an observation unit to monitor a condition (or complication) that develops following outpatient surgery, and then is subsequently admitted as an inpatient of the same hospital, hospitals should apply the Uniform Hospital Discharge Data Set (UHDDS) definition of principal diagnosis as "that condition established after study to be chiefly responsible for occasioning the admission of the patient to the hospital for care."

J. Admission from Outpatient Surgery

When a patient receives surgery in the hospital's outpatient surgery department and is subsequently admitted for continuing inpatient care at the same hospital, the following guidelines should be followed in selecting the principal diagnosis for the inpatient admission:

- If the reason for the inpatient admission is a complication, assign the complication as the principal diagnosis.
- If no complication, or other condition, is documented as the reason for the inpatient admission, assign the reason for the outpatient surgery as the principal diagnosis.
- If the reason for the inpatient admission is another condition unrelated to the surgery, assign the unrelated condition as the principal diagnosis.

Section III. Reporting Additional Diagnoses

GENERAL RULES FOR OTHER (ADDITIONAL) DIAGNOSES

For reporting purposes the definition for "other diagnoses" is interpreted as additional conditions that affect patient care in terms of requiring:

clinical evaluation; or
therapeutic treatment; or
diagnostic procedures; or
extended length of hospital stay; or
increased nursing care and/or monitoring.

The UHDDS item #11-b defines Other Diagnoses as "all conditions that coexist at the time of admission, that develop subsequently, or that affect the treatment received and/or the length of stay. Diagnoses that relate to an earlier episode which have no bearing on the current hospital stay are to be excluded." UHDDS definitions apply to inpatients in acute care, short-term, long term care and psychiatric hospital setting. The UHDDS definitions are used by acute care short-term hospitals to report inpatient data elements in a standardized manner. These data elements and their definitions can be found in the July 31, 1985, Federal Register (Vol. 50, No, 147), pp. 31038-40.

Since that time the application of the UHDDS definitions has been expanded to include all non-outpatient settings (acute care, short term, long term care and psychiatric hospitals; home health agencies; rehab facilities; nursing homes, etc).

The following guidelines are to be applied in designating "other diagnoses" when neither the Alphabetic Index nor the Tabular List in ICD-10-CM provide direction. The listing of the diagnoses in the patient record is the responsibility of the attending provider.

A. Previous conditions

If the provider has included a diagnosis in the final diagnostic statement, such as the discharge summary or the face sheet, it should ordinarily be coded. Some providers include in the diagnostic statement resolved conditions or diagnoses and status-post procedures from previous admission that have no bearing on the current stay. Such conditions are not to be reported and are coded only if required by hospital policy.

However, history codes (categories Z80-Z87) may be used as secondary codes if the historical condition or family history has an impact on current care or influences treatment.

B. Abnormal findings

Abnormal findings (laboratory, x-ray, pathologic, and other diagnostic results) are not coded and reported unless the provider indicates their clinical significance. If the findings are outside the normal range and the attending provider has ordered other tests to evaluate the condition or prescribed treatment, it is appropriate to ask the provider whether the abnormal finding should be added.

Please note: This differs from the coding practices in the outpatient setting for coding encounters for diagnostic tests that have been interpreted by a provider.

C. Uncertain Diagnosis

If the diagnosis documented at the time of discharge is qualified as "probable", "suspected", "likely", "questionable", "possible", or "still to be ruled out" or other similar terms indicating uncertainty, code the condition as if it existed or was established. The bases for these guidelines are the diagnostic workup, arrangements for further workup or observation, and initial therapeutic approach that correspond most closely with the established diagnosis.

Note: This guideline is applicable only to inpatient admissions to short-term, acute, long-term care and psychiatric hospitals.

Section IV. Diagnostic Coding and Reporting Guidelines for Outpatient Services

These coding guidelines for outpatient diagnoses have been approved for use by hospitals/providers in coding and reporting hospital-based outpatient services and provider-based office visits.

Information about the use of certain abbreviations, punctuation, symbols, and other conventions used in the ICD-10-CM Tabular List (code numbers and titles), can be found in Section IA of these guidelines, under "Conventions Used in the Tabular List." Information about the correct sequence to use in finding a code is also described in Section I.

The terms encounter and visit are often used interchangeably in describing outpatient service contacts and, therefore, appear together in these guidelines without distinguishing one from the other.

Though the conventions and general guidelines apply to all settings, coding guidelines for outpatient and provider reporting of diagnoses will vary in a number of instances from those for inpatient diagnoses, recognizing that:

> The Uniform Hospital Discharge Data Set (UHDDS) definition of principal diagnosis applies only to inpatients in acute, short-term, long-term care and psychiatric hospitals.

> Coding guidelines for inconclusive diagnoses (probable, suspected, rule out, etc.) were developed for inpatient reporting and do not apply to outpatients.

A. Selection of first-listed condition

> In the outpatient setting, the term first-listed diagnosis is used in lieu of principal diagnosis.

> In determining the first-listed diagnosis the coding conventions of ICD-10-CM, as well as the general and disease specific guidelines take precedence over the outpatient guidelines.

> Diagnoses often are not established at the time of the initial encounter/visit. It may take two or more visits before the diagnosis is confirmed.

> The most critical rule involves beginning the search for the correct code assignment through the Alphabetic Index. Never begin searching initially in the Tabular List as this will lead to coding errors.

1. **Outpatient Surgery**

    When a patient presents for outpatient surgery (same day surgery), code the reason for the surgery as the first-listed diagnosis (reason for the encounter), even if the surgery is not performed due to a contraindication.

2. **Observation Stay**

    When a patient is admitted for observation for a medical condition, assign a code for the medical condition as the first-listed diagnosis.

    When a patient presents for outpatient surgery and develops complications requiring admission to observation, code the reason for the surgery as the first reported diagnosis (reason for the encounter), followed by codes for the complications as secondary diagnoses.

B. Codes from A00.0 through T88.9, Z00-Z99

The appropriate code(s) from A00.0 through T88.9, Z00-Z99 must be used to identify diagnoses, symptoms, conditions, problems, complaints, or other reason(s) for the encounter/visit.

C. Accurate reporting of ICD-10-CM diagnosis codes

For accurate reporting of ICD-10-CM diagnosis codes, the documentation should describe the patient's condition, using terminology which includes specific diagnoses as well as symptoms, problems, or reasons for the encounter. There are ICD-10-CM codes to describe all of these.

D. Codes that describe symptoms and signs

Codes that describe symptoms and signs, as opposed to diagnoses, are acceptable for reporting purposes when a diagnosis has not been established (confirmed) by the provider. Chapter 18 of ICD-10-CM, Symptoms, Signs, and Abnormal Clinical and Laboratory Findings Not Elsewhere Classified (codes R00-R99) contain many, but not all codes for symptoms.

E. Encounters for circumstances other than a disease or injury

ICD-10-CM provides codes to deal with encounters for circumstances other than a disease or injury. The Factors Influencing Health Status and Contact with Health Services codes (Z00-**Z99) are** provided to deal with occasions when circumstances other than a disease or injury are recorded as diagnosis or problems.
See Section I.C.21. Factors influencing health status and contact with health services.

F. Level of Detail in Coding

1. ICD-10-CM codes with *3, 4, 5, 6 or 7 characters*

ICD-10-CM is composed of codes with 3, 4, 5, 6 or 7 **characters**. Codes with three **characters** are included in ICD-10-CM as the heading of a category of codes that may be further subdivided by the use of **fourth,** fifth, sixth or seventh **characters to** provide greater specificity.

2. Use of full number of *characters* required for a code

A three-**character** code is to be used only if it is not further subdivided. A code is invalid if it has not been coded to the full number of characters required for that code, including the 7th character extension, if applicable.

G. ICD-10-CM code for the diagnosis, condition, problem, or other reason for encounter/visit

List first the ICD-10-CM code for the diagnosis, condition, problem, or other reason for encounter/visit shown in the medical record to be chiefly responsible for the services provided. List additional codes that describe any coexisting conditions. In some cases the first-listed diagnosis may be a symptom when a diagnosis has not been established (confirmed) by the physician.

H. Uncertain diagnosis

Do not code diagnoses documented as "probable", "suspected," "questionable," "rule out," or "working diagnosis" or other similar terms indicating uncertainty. Rather, code the condition(s) to the highest degree of certainty for that encounter/visit, such as symptoms, signs, abnormal test results, or other reason for the visit.

Please note: This differs from the coding practices used by short-term, acute care, long-term care and psychiatric hospitals.

I. Chronic diseases

Chronic diseases treated on an ongoing basis may be coded and reported as many times as the patient receives treatment and care for the condition(s)

J. Code all documented conditions that coexist

Code all documented conditions that coexist at the time of the encounter/visit, and require or affect patient care treatment or management. Do not code conditions that were previously treated and no longer exist. However, history codes (categories Z80-Z87) may be used as secondary codes if the historical condition or family history has an impact on current care or influences treatment.

K. Patients receiving diagnostic services only

For patients receiving diagnostic services only during an encounter/visit, sequence first the diagnosis, condition, problem, or other reason for encounter/visit shown in the medical record to be chiefly responsible for the outpatient services provided during the encounter/visit. Codes for other diagnoses (e.g., chronic conditions) may be sequenced as additional diagnoses.

For encounters for routine laboratory/radiology testing in the absence of any signs, symptoms, or associated diagnosis, assign Z01.89, Encounter for other specified special examinations. If routine testing is performed during the same encounter as a test to evaluate a sign, symptom, or diagnosis, it is appropriate to assign both the V code and the code describing the reason for the non-routine test.

For outpatient encounters for diagnostic tests that have been interpreted by a physician, and the final report is available at the time of coding, code any confirmed or definitive diagnosis(es) documented in the interpretation. Do not code related signs and symptoms as additional diagnoses.

Please note: This differs from the coding practice in the hospital inpatient setting regarding abnormal findings on test results.

L. Patients receiving therapeutic services only

For patients receiving therapeutic services only during an encounter/visit, sequence first the diagnosis, condition, problem, or other reason for encounter/visit shown in the medical record to be chiefly responsible for the outpatient services provided during the encounter/visit. Codes for other diagnoses (e.g., chronic conditions) may be sequenced as additional diagnoses.

The only exception to this rule is that when the primary reason for the admission/encounter is chemotherapy or radiation therapy, the appropriate Z code for the service is listed first, and the diagnosis or problem for which the service is being performed listed second.

M. Patients receiving preoperative evaluations only

For patients receiving preoperative evaluations only, sequence first a code from subcategory Z01.81, Encounter for pre-procedural examinations, to describe the pre-op consultations. Assign a code for the condition to describe the reason for the surgery as an additional diagnosis. Code also any findings related to the pre-op evaluation.

N. Ambulatory surgery

For ambulatory surgery, code the diagnosis for which the surgery was performed. If the postoperative diagnosis is known to be different from the preoperative diagnosis at the time the diagnosis is confirmed, select the postoperative diagnosis for coding, since it is the most definitive.

O. Routine outpatient prenatal visits

See Section I.C.15. Routine outpatient prenatal visits.

P. Encounters for general medical examinations with abnormal findings

The subcategories for encounters for general medical examinations, Z00.0-, provide codes for with and without abnormal findings. Should a general medical examination result in an abnormal finding, the code for general medical examination with abnormal finding should be assigned as the **first-listed** diagnosis. A secondary code for the abnormal finding should also be coded.

Q. Encounters for routine health screenings

See Section I.C.21. Factors influencing health status and contact with health services, Screening

Appendix I
Present on Admission Reporting Guidelines
(Effective with 2011 update)

Introduction

These guidelines are to be used as a supplement to the *ICD-10-CM Official Guidelines for Coding and Reporting* to facilitate the assignment of the Present on Admission (POA) indicator for each diagnosis and external cause of injury code reported on claim forms (UB-04 and 837 Institutional).

These guidelines are not intended to replace any guidelines in the main body of the *ICD-10-CM Official Guidelines for Coding and Reporting*. The POA guidelines are not intended to provide guidance on when a condition should be coded, but rather, how to apply the POA indicator to the final set of diagnosis codes that have been assigned in accordance with Sections I, II, and III of the official coding guidelines. Subsequent to the assignment of the ICD-10-CM codes, the POA indicator should then be assigned to those conditions that have been coded.

As stated in the Introduction to the ICD-10-CM Official Guidelines for Coding and Reporting, a joint effort between the healthcare provider and the coder is essential to achieve complete and accurate documentation, code assignment, and reporting of diagnoses and procedures. The importance of consistent, complete documentation in the medical record cannot be overemphasized. Medical record documentation from any provider involved in the care and treatment of the patient may be used to support the determination of whether a condition was present on admission or not. In the context of the official coding guidelines, the term "provider" means a physician or any qualified healthcare practitioner who is legally accountable for establishing the patient's diagnosis.

These guidelines are not a substitute for the provider's clinical judgment as to the determination of whether a condition was/was not present on admission. The provider should be queried regarding issues related to the linking of signs/symptoms, timing of test results, and the timing of findings.

General Reporting Requirements

All claims involving inpatient admissions to general acute care hospitals or other facilities that are subject to a law or regulation mandating collection of present on admission information.

Present on admission is defined as present at the time the order for inpatient admission occurs -- conditions that develop during an outpatient encounter, including emergency department, observation, or outpatient surgery, are considered as present on admission.

POA indicator is assigned to principal and secondary diagnoses (as defined in Section II of the Official Guidelines for Coding and Reporting) and the external cause of injury codes.

Issues related to inconsistent, missing, conflicting or unclear documentation must still be resolved by the provider.

If a condition would not be coded and reported based on UHDDS definitions and current official coding guidelines, then the POA indicator would not be reported.

Reporting Options
> Y - Yes
> N - No
> U - Unknown
> W – Clinically undetermined
> Unreported/Not used (or "1" for Medicare usage) – (Exempt from POA reporting)

Reporting Definitions
> Y = present at the time of inpatient admission
> N = not present at the time of inpatient admission
> U = documentation is insufficient to determine if condition is present on admission
> W = provider is unable to clinically determine whether condition was present on admission or not

Timeframe for POA Identification and Documentation

There is no required timeframe as to when a provider (per the definition of "provider" used in these guidelines) must identify or document a condition to be present on admission. In some clinical situations, it may not be possible for a provider to make a definitive diagnosis (or a condition may not be recognized or reported by the patient) for a period of time after admission. In some cases it may be several days before the provider arrives at a definitive diagnosis. This does not mean that the condition was not present on admission. Determination of whether the condition was present on admission or not will be based on the applicable POA guideline as identified in this document, or on the provider's best clinical judgment.

If at the time of code assignment the documentation is unclear as to whether a condition was present on admission or not, it is appropriate to query the provider for clarification.

Assigning the POA Indicator

Condition is on the "Exempt from Reporting" list
> Leave the "present on admission" field blank if the condition is on the list

of ICD-10-CM codes for which this field is not applicable. This is the only circumstance in which the field may be left blank.

POA Explicitly Documented
Assign Y for any condition the provider explicitly documents as being present on admission.

Assign N for any condition the provider explicitly documents as not present at the time of admission.

Conditions diagnosed prior to inpatient admission
Assign "Y" for conditions that were diagnosed prior to admission (example: hypertension, diabetes mellitus, asthma)

Conditions diagnosed during the admission but clearly present before admission
Assign "Y" for conditions diagnosed during the admission that were clearly present but not diagnosed until after admission occurred.

Diagnoses subsequently confirmed after admission are considered present on admission if at the time of admission they are documented as suspected, possible, rule out, differential diagnosis, or constitute an underlying cause of a symptom that is present at the time of admission.

Condition develops during outpatient encounter prior to inpatient admission
Assign Y for any condition that develops during an outpatient encounter prior to a written order for inpatient admission.

Documentation does not indicate whether condition was present on admission
Assign "U" when the medical record documentation is unclear as to whether the condition was present on admission. "U" should not be routinely assigned and used only in very limited circumstances. Coders are encouraged to query the providers when the documentation is unclear.

Documentation states that it cannot be determined whether the condition was or was not present on admission
Assign "W" when the medical record documentation indicates that it cannot be clinically determined whether or not the condition was present on admission.

Chronic condition with acute exacerbation during the admission
If a single code identifies both the chronic condition and the acute exacerbation, see POA guidelines pertaining to combination codes.

If a single code only identifies the chronic condition and not the acute exacerbation (e.g., acute exacerbation of chronic leukemia), assign "Y."

Conditions documented as possible, probable, suspected, or rule out at the time of discharge

> If the final diagnosis contains a possible, probable, suspected, or rule out diagnosis, and this diagnosis was based on signs, symptoms or clinical findings suspected at the time of inpatient admission, assign "Y."

> If the final diagnosis contains a possible, probable, suspected, or rule out diagnosis, and this diagnosis was based on signs, symptoms or clinical findings that were not present on admission, assign "N".

Conditions documented as impending or threatened at the time of discharge

> If the final diagnosis contains an impending or threatened diagnosis, and this diagnosis is based on symptoms or clinical findings that were present on admission, assign "Y".

> If the final diagnosis contains an impending or threatened diagnosis, and this diagnosis is based on symptoms or clinical findings that were not present on admission, assign "N".

Acute and Chronic Conditions

> Assign "Y" for acute conditions that are present at time of admission and N for acute conditions that are not present at time of admission.

> Assign "Y" for chronic conditions, even though the condition may not be diagnosed until after admission.

> If a single code identifies both an acute and chronic condition, see the POA guidelines for combination codes.

Combination Codes

> Assign "N" if any part of the combination code was not present on admission (e.g., COPD with acute exacerbation and the exacerbation was not present on admission; gastric ulcer that does not start bleeding until after admission; asthma patient develops status asthmaticus after admission)

> Assign "Y" if all parts of the combination code were present on admission (e.g., patient with acute prostatitis admitted with hematuria)

> If the final diagnosis includes comparative or contrasting diagnoses, and both were present, or suspected, at the time of admission, assign "Y".

> For infection codes that include the causal organism, assign "Y" if the infection (or signs of the infection) was present on admission, even though the culture results may not be known until after admission (e.g., patient is admitted with pneumonia and the provider documents pseudomonas as the causal organism a few days later).

Same Diagnosis Code for Two or More Conditions

When the same ICD-10-CM diagnosis code applies to two or more conditions during the same encounter (e.g. two separate conditions classified to the same ICD-10-CM diagnosis code):

Assign "Y" if all conditions represented by the single ICD-10-CM code were present on admission (e.g. bilateral unspecified age-related cataracts).

Assign "N" if any of the conditions represented by the single ICD-10-CM code was not present on admission (e.g. traumatic secondary and recurrent hemorrhage and seroma is assigned to a single code T79.2, but only one of the conditions was present on admission).

Obstetrical conditions

Whether or not the patient delivers during the current hospitalization does not affect assignment of the POA indicator. The determining factor for POA assignment is whether the pregnancy complication or obstetrical condition described by the code was present at the time of admission or not.

If the pregnancy complication or obstetrical condition was present on admission (e.g., patient admitted in preterm labor), assign "Y".

If the pregnancy complication or obstetrical condition was not present on admission (e.g., 2nd degree laceration during delivery, postpartum hemorrhage that occurred during current hospitalization, fetal distress develops after admission), assign "N".

If the obstetrical code includes more than one diagnosis and any of the diagnoses identified by the code were not present on admission assign "N".
(e.g., Category O11, Pre-existing hypertension with pre-eclampsia)

Perinatal conditions

Newborns are not considered to be admitted until after birth. Therefore, any condition present at birth or that developed in utero is considered present at admission and should be assigned "Y". This includes conditions that occur during delivery (e.g., injury during delivery, meconium aspiration, exposure to streptococcus B in the vaginal canal).

Congenital conditions and anomalies

Assign "Y" for congenital conditions and anomalies (except for codes Q00-Q99 which are exempt). Congenital conditions are always considered present on admission.

External cause of injury codes

Assign "Y" for any external cause code representing an external cause of morbidity that occurred prior to inpatient admission (e.g., patient fell out of bed at home, patient fell out of bed in emergency room prior to admission)

Assign "N" for any external cause code representing an external cause of morbidity that occurred during inpatient hospitalization (e.g., patient fell out of hospital bed during hospital stay, patient experienced an adverse reaction to a medication administered after inpatient admission)

Categories and Codes
Exempt from
Diagnosis Present on Admission Requirement

Note: "Diagnosis present on admission" for these code categories are exempt because they represent circumstances regarding the healthcare encounter or factors influencing health status that do not represent a current disease or injury or are always present on admission

B90–B94, Sequelae of infectious and parasitic diseases

E64, Sequelae of malnutrition and other nutritional deficiences

I25.2, Old myocardial infarction

I69, Sequelae of cerebrovascular disease

O09, Supervision of high risk pregnancy

O66.5, Attempted application of vacuum extractor and forceps

O80, Encounter for full-term uncomplicated delivery

O94, Sequelae of complication of pregnancy, childbirth, and the puerperium

P00, Newborn (suspected to be) affected by maternal conditions that may be unrelated to present pregnancy

Q00 – Q99, Congenital malformations, deformations and chromosomal abnormalities

S00-T88.9, Injury, poisoning and certain other consequences of external causes with 7th character representing subsequent encounter or sequela

V00.121, Fall from non-in-line roller-skates

V00.131, Fall from skateboard

V00.141, Fall from scooter (nonmotorized)

V00.311, Fall from snowboard

V00.321, Fall from snow-skis

V40-V49, Car occupant injured in transport accident

V80-V89, Other land transport accidents

V90-V94, Water transport accidents

V95-V97, Air and space transport accidents

W03, Other fall on same level due to collision with another person

 W09, Fall on and from playground equipment

W15, Fall from cliff

W17.0, Fall into well

W17.1, Fall into storm drain or manhole

W18.01 Striking against sports equipment with subsequent fall

W20.8, Other cause of strike by thrown, projected or falling object

W21, Striking against or struck by sports equipment

W30, Contact with agricultural machinery

W31, Contact with other and unspecified machinery

W32-W34, Accidental handgun discharge and malfunction

W35- W40, Exposure to inanimate mechanical forces

W52, Crushed, pushed or stepped on by crowd or human stampede

W89, Exposure to man-made visible and ultraviolet light

X02, Exposure to controlled fire in building or structure

X03, Exposure to controlled fire, not in building or structure

X04, Exposure to ignition of highly flammable material

X52, Prolonged stay in weightless environment

X71-X83, Intentional self-harm

Y21, Drowning and submersion, undetermined intent

Y22, Handgun discharge, undetermined intent

Y23, Rifle, shotgun and larger firearm discharge, undetermined intent

Y24, Other and unspecified firearm discharge, undetermined intent

Y30, Falling, jumping or pushed from a high place, undetermined intent

Y35, Legal intervention

Y37, Military operations

Y36, Operations of war

Y38, Terrorism

Y92, Place of occurrence of the external cause

Y93, Activity code

Y99, External cause status

Z00, Encounter for general examination without complaint, suspected or reported diagnosis

Z01, Encounter for other special examination without complaint, suspected or reported diagnosis

Z02, Encounter for administrative examination

Z03, Encounter for medical observation for suspected diseases and conditions ruled out

Z08, Encounter for follow-up examination following completed treatment for malignant neoplasm

Z09, Encounter for follow-up examination after completed treatment for conditions other than malignant neoplasm

Z11, Encounter for screening for infectious and parasitic diseases

Z11.8, Encounter for screening for other infectious and parasitic diseases

Z12, Encounter for screening for malignant neoplasms

Z13, Encounter for screening for other diseases and disorders

Z13.4, Encounter for screening for certain developmental disorders in childhood

Z13.5, Encounter for screening for eye and ear disorders

Z13.6, Encounter for screening for cardiovascular disorders

Z13.83, Encounter for screening for respiratory disorder NEC

Z13.89, Encounter for screening for other disorder (inclusion term) Encounter for screening for genitourinary disorders)

Z13.89, Encounter for screening for other disorder

Z14, Genetic carrier

Z15, Genetic susceptibility to disease

Z17, Estrogen receptor status

Z18, Retained foreign body fragments

Z22, Carrier of infectious disease

Z23, Encounter for immunization

Z28, Immunization not carried out and underimmunization status

Z28.3, Underimmunization status

Z30, Encounter for contraceptive management

Z31, Encounter for procreative management

Z34, Encounter for supervision of normal pregnancy

Z36, Encounter for antenatal screening of mother

Z37, Outcome of delivery

Z38, Liveborn infants according to place of birth and type of delivery

Z39, Encounter for maternal postpartum care and examination

Z41, Encounter for procedures for purposes other than remedying health state

Z42, Encounter for plastic and reconstructive surgery following medical procedure or healed injury

Z43, Encounter for attention to artificial openings

Z44, Encounter for fitting and adjustment of external prosthetic device

Z45, Encounter for adjustment and management of implanted device

Z46, Encounter for fitting and adjustment of other devices

Z47.8, Encounter for other orthopedic aftercare

Z49, Encounter for care involving renal dialysis

 Z51, Encounter for other aftercare

Z51.5, Encounter for palliative care

Z51.8, Encounter for other specified aftercare

Z52, Donors of organs and tissues

Z59, Problems related to housing and economic circumstances

Z63, Other problems related to primary support group, including family circumstances

Z65, Problems related to other psychosocial circumstances

Z65.8 Other specified problems related to psychosocial circumstances

Z67.1 – Z67.9 Blood type

Z68, Body mass index (BMI)

Z72, Problems related to lifestyle

Z74.01, Bed confinement status

Z76, Persons encountering health services in other circumstances

Z77.110- Z77.128, Environmental pollution and hazards in the physical environment

Z78, Other specified health status

Z79, Long term (current) drug therapy

Z80, Family history of primary malignant neoplasm

Z81, Family history of mental and behavioral disorders

Z82, Family history of certain disabilities and chronic diseases (leading to disablement)

Z83, Family history of other specific disorders

Z84, Family history of other conditions

Z85, Personal history of primary malignant neoplasm

Z86, Personal history of certain other diseases

Z87, Personal history of other diseases and conditions

Z87.828, Personal history of other (healed) physical injury and trauma

Z87.891, Personal history of nicotine dependence

Z88, Allergy status to drugs, medicaments and biological substances

Z89, Acquired absence of limb

Z90.710, Acquired absence of both cervix and uterus

Z91.0, Allergy status, other than to drugs and biological substances
Z91.4, Personal history of psychological trauma, not elsewhere classified

Z91.5, Personal history of self-harm

Z91.8, Other specified risk factors, not elsewhere classified

Z92, Personal history of medical treatment

Z93, Artificial opening status

Z94, Transplanted organ and tissue status

Z95, Presence of cardiac and vascular implants and grafts

Z97, Presence of other devices

Z98, Other postprocedural states

Z99, Dependence on enabling machines and devices, not elsewhere classified

Subject Index

malunion of, 182, 232
nonunions of, 182
open, 230, 231, 233, 234
osteoporosis pathological, 179–180, 236
pathological, 181–182, 232
pathological, due to neoplasm, 76–77
in patient having AIDS, 59–60
sequencing, 231, 232
spontaneous, 182
stress, 182–183, 223
subsequent care for, 231
traumatic, 59, 181, 231, 233, 235, 236
types of, 230
unspecified, 59
wedge compression, 233
Fractures, multiple, 236
Functional, definition of, 265
Functional quadriplegia, 217

G

Gait, definition of, 275
Gallbladder
calculus in, 47, 169
in digestive system, 156
as part of biliary system, 168
word root of, 279
Gastritis, 161–162, 245
Gastroesophageal reflux disease, 158, 159
General health examinations, 252
Genetic carrier, 255
Genetic counseling, 255
Genetic susceptibility to disease, 255
Genital prolapse, 188–189
Glasgow coma scale, 217, 219
Glaucoma, 120–121
Glomerulonephritis, 183
Glomerular diseases, 183–184
Growth and development terms, definitions of, 264
Gums, word root of, 279

H

Health and Human Services (HHS), U.S. Department of, committee study of code sets by, 6

Healthcare Common Procedure Coding System (HCPCS) as an official code set, 7
Health Insurance Portability and Accountability Act of 1996 (HIPAA)
administrative simplification provisions of, 6
conversion to ICD-10-CM/PCS required by, 6
Hearing
anatomy of organs for, 283
word roots associated with, 282
Hearing loss, 124–125
psychogenic, 102
Heart
anatomy of, 269
diagram of, 270
Heart attack. *See* Myocardial infarction
Heart failure, 132, 133, 138–139
Helminthiases section, 52
Hematemesis, definition of, 279
Hemiplegia and hemiparesis, 114, 140, 141
Hemoglobin, definition of, 270
Hemolytic uremic syndrome, 184–185
Hemophilia, genetic carrier, 255
Hernia
bladder, 188
diaphragmatic, 164
epigastric, 163–164
femoral, 163, 164
hiatal, 165
incisional, 163
inguinal, 163, 164
laterality of, 164
other abdominal, 164
recurrent, 164
spigelian, 164
umbilical, 163, 164, 165
unspecified, 164
ventral, 164
Herpes viruses, 157
High blood pressure, 133. *See also* Hypertension
History codes
distinguished from sequelae codes, 255
family, 259
personal, 259

History of previous conditions, 45
History, personal (of), as main term, 77
Human immunodeficiency virus confirmation of, 60
contact with and exposure to, 60
diagnosis of, 56–57
encounter screening for, 61
ICD-10-CM Official guidelines for diseases of, 58–62
inconclusive laboratory evidence of, 61
sequencing, 59–60
symptoms of, 57
transmission of, 56
Human immunodeficiency virus (HIV) disease section, 52, 56–67
Human immunodeficiency virus (HIV) infection
asymptomatic, 60, 61–62, 255
chronic, 56
from mother to infant, 56
patients symptomatic of, 58
in pregnancy, childbirth and the puerperium, 61–62, 196, 204–205
Hydrocephalus, 110, 275
Hydronephrosis, 186
Hyperglycemia, definition of, 275
Hyperplasia, definition of, 264
Hypertension, 128–133
benign, 129, 131, 138
cardiorenal, 132
with cardiovascular disease, 131
with chronic kidney disease, 131
controlled, 130
essential (primary), 129, 130–131
essential unspecified, 129
ICD-10-CM Official Guidelines for, 129–130, 133, 134
malignant, 129
in pregnancy, preexisting, 195
renovascular, 133
secondary, 129, 130, 133
transient, 130
uncontrolled, 130
Hypertensive cerebrovascular disease, 130
Hypertensive chronic kidney disease, 129, 185

Index of ICD-10-CM Codes

4–Character Subcategories of Anatomic Site, Etiology, or Severity

5-Character Subcategories of Anatomic Site, Etiology, or Severity

6-Character Subclassifications of Anatomic Site, Etiology, or Severity

7-Character Extension Codes

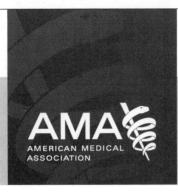
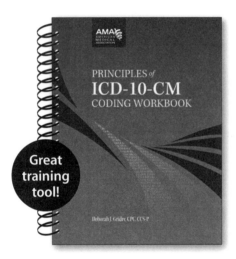